ONE MEAL
AT A TIME

BOOKS BY MARTIN KATAHN, PH.D.

The 200 Calorie Solution

Beyond Diet

The Rotation Diet

The Rotation Diet Cookbook
(with Terry Katahn)

The T-Factor Diet

ONE MEAL AT A TIME

THE INCREDIBLY SIMPLE LOW-FAT DIET FOR A HAPPIER, HEALTHIER, LONGER LIFE

Martin Katahn, Ph.D.

W·W·NORTON & COMPANY

NEW YORK   LONDON

Individual needs for physical fitness and diet can vary from person to person. You should ask your doctor about your own personal needs before changing your diet and starting a fitness program. Consulting with your doctor is especially important if you are under medical care or taking any medication. A change in your diet and level of activity may require that adjustments be made in the kind of treatment or the nature of the medications that you are receiving.

The text of this book is composed in 10/12 Garamond, with the display set in
Gill Sans Bold and Technica Heavy and Medium.
Composition and manufacturing by the Haddon Craftsmen, Inc.
Book design by Margaret M. Wagner.

First Edition.

Library of Congress Cataloging-in-Publication Data
Katahn, Martin.
One meal at a time : a low-fat diet for a happier, healthier,
longer life / by Martin Katahn.
p.   cm.
Includes index.
1. Low-fat diet.   I. Title.
RM237.7.K37   1991
613.2'8—dc20   90-27263

ISBN 0-393-03002-4

W. W. Norton & Company, Inc., 500 Fifth Avenue, New York, N.Y. 10110
W. W. Norton & Company, Ltd., 10 Coptic Street, London WC1A 1PU

1 2 3 4 5 6 7 8 9 10

CONTENTS

Acknowledgments

I would like to express my appreciation, first and foremost, to Ms. Jamie Pope-Cordle, M.S., R.D., for supplying much of the material for the chapter on adolescent and childhood nutrition, developing and testing many of the recipes, putting together menus for nutrient analyses and doing those analyses, gathering the material for the expanded Nutrient Counter contained in this book, and for her comments and suggestions on the manuscript. This book could not have been done without her help.

Many others also have made invaluable contributions, and I would like to thank:

James O. Hill, Ph.D., for his comments, criticism, and suggestions on the scientific background sections of this book.

Harriet Simpkins for coordinating groups in the Vanderbilt Weight Management Program and for being a source of information and encouragement to the thousands of persons who have called for help from all over the country during these past seven years.

Cea Pannell for the bread recipes that I have included and for testing scores of others before we settled on these special choices.

All the members of my family—my wife Enid, and Terri and

David—for creating and testing recipes, and reading and criticizing the manuscript.

Mary Bomar, who has been Enid's personal representative for many years. Mary tends our home office and does literally everything that's necessary to keep us both going, from booking concerts to moving in and taking care of T'ai, our much loved shepherd-malamute, when we are both on the road.

ESHA Research for the Food Processor II Nutrient and Diet Analysis System, which we use to analyze our recipes and menus, and especially Elizabeth Geltz-Hands for always being available for help and advice whenever we need her.

Starling Lawrence, my editor at W. W. Norton, with whom I've worked for ten years and produced seven books, together with Artie and Richard Pine, my literary agents for the same period of time. What a stroke of luck it was that I chanced across Artie's and Richard's names in *Writer's Digest,* after six publishers had turned down my first book in 1981. (I chose to write to the Pines because they had represented Wayne Dyer and Billy Jean King, and I'm a psychologist and tennis player.) The Pines had faith and went straight to Star, knowing he had worked with other respected scientists writing in the nutrition field. I wish every author were as fortunate as I am and had such a team in his corner.

All my other friends at W. W. Norton, most of whom have assisted in the production of my books for the entire ten years of our relationship: Fran Rosencrantz, director of publicity, for continuing to watch over me like a mother while working me to death on what always prove to be the very best possible book tours; Debra Makay, my manuscript editor, whose job was especially difficult this time around due to the greatly expanded Nutrient Counter included in this book; Erik Burns, Jeannie Luciano, and Iva Ashner for their editorial assistance; Hugh O'Neill for his design and production of the attractive book jacket; Margaret Wagner for the design of the text; and production manager Andrew Marasia, for once again producing the books on an almost impossible time schedule.

Dona Tapp, again for the seventh time, for keeping herself ready to jump in for the final proofreading at a moment's notice, so that Andy could meet his production schedule.

Thank you all very much.

ONE MEAL
AT A TIME

CHAPTER 1

INTRODUCTION

We have a problem—a very serious problem.

Mother Nature has turned the tables on us. When it comes to selecting a healthful diet in a world of plenty, she has planted within us the seeds of our own destruction. Let me begin my explanation by asking you to do a little experiment.

Think about the foods you like the most—the entrees, snacks, desserts—the foods that stimulate your appetite and really turn you on. Let's focus on a dessert tray at a favorite restaurant. Imagine that this tray holds a hot fudge sundae, an apple strudel, a piece of cake, an assortment of cheeses with sliced apple and grapes, and apple pie à la mode.

What will be your preference: The strudel? The pie à la mode? The hot fudge sundae?

Or will you ask for a plate of fresh fruit, skip the cheese?

As any restaurant manager will tell you, almost everyone will choose either the pie, the strudel, the sundae, or the piece of cake. My hat is off to you if you would *prefer* the fresh fruit without any trimmings—you probably don't need to read this book. But then, perhaps you're just better at resisting temptation!

My point is this: With very rare exceptions, human beings like fat in their food. A tray of desserts is brought to the table because the management knows it will sell twice as much from a tableside tray compared with a simple recitation of what's available. The sight will stimulate your appetite even when your stomach is full. Although some people do choose the healthier alternatives, fresh fruit and sweet but fat-free desserts such as sherbet always play second fiddle to the sweet, *fat-laden* pies, cakes, and ice cream sundaes.

The same is true for foods that contain fat naturally, such as meat and poultry. Almost all of us prefer the fattier, juicier cuts of meat to the lean. The preference is so strong that when one major fast-food chain tried to take the lead in reducing the fat in its hamburgers a few years ago, and experimented with meat that was only 2 percent less fat than its regular grind, it was noticed in the test population and rejected.

Yes, human beings, like just about all omnivorous animals, will not only choose but *overeat* on fatty foods when they are freely available. The fatty-food preference has been built into our systems through millions of years of evolution. When life is threatened by famine and disease, a love of fatty foods helps us lay down some extra body fat to provide the energy to keep us alive long enough to reproduce. But when safe passage through these early years of life is largely assured by advances in public health and medical science, and we are blessed with a constant food supply, there comes a terrifying downside. From the Surgeon General's Report to the report of the Committee on Diet and Health of the National Research Council to the proclamations of major professional health organizations, there is unanimity:

Too much fat in the diet is the greatest nutritional hazard in America.
IT'S DEADLY!
Eating too much fat is going to KILL or make MILLIONS of us ill with heart disease, certain forms of cancer, and other diseases related to diabetes, hypertension, and obesity—five, ten, even twenty years before our time.

It would take about ten atomic bombs scattered across America (perish the thought) to equal the death and illness caused each year by too much fat in our diets! Yet we blindly do it to ourselves.

Fortunately, it doesn't have to be this way. You, certainly, can do a great deal to help make sure you are not one of these millions on the high-fat road to self-destruction, if you choose to. I think I can show you how to make that choice an easy one with the One Meal at a

Time program. But first, let me summarize the bad news—the statistics that have been compiled by epidemiologists, who study the incidence of diseases in the American population.

THE GLOOMY NUMBERS

Between 1.25 and 1.5 million people will have a heart attack this year. About 500,000 people will die of ischemic heart disease, where a blood vessel supplying oxygen and nutrients to the heart becomes blocked and part of the muscle that does the heart's work dies. Almost half of the people who have a heart attack are suffering or dying five or sometimes even twenty years before they needed to, and a major ingredient in the early onset of their disease or premature death is too much fat in their diets.

It's primarily the saturated fat in the diet that can increase your cholesterol level. A high cholesterol level in turn contributes to the development of fatty lumps in your arteries (atherosclerosis) and ultimately to heart disease. The deadly process starts early in life, leading many health professionals to encourage the lowering of fat consumption among children as early as two years of age, if they are eating a high-fat diet.

Diet may be almost as important in the promotion of cancer as it is in heart disease: Of the approximately 500,000 deaths due to cancer this year, from 10 to as high as 70 percent can be linked to what we eat. (Scientists argue the exact percentage because it has proven harder to show the link between the various forms of cancer and different features of our diets than it has been to demonstrate the link between heart disease and diet.) But whatever the actual percentage of cancers related to diet, there is little dispute over the following conclusion:

Contrary to what you might expect from the media coverage given to herbicides, pesticides, preservatives, and other unnatural toxins in foods, *it's fat in the diet once again that is by far the single greatest nutritional hazard.* Almost 99 percent of all cancer-related deaths linked to nutritional factors are due either to too much fat in the diet or to carcinogens naturally present in food.

In fact, when you consider all of the diet-related illnesses, you can take all the herbicides, pesticides, preservatives, and other unnatural chemicals that find their way into our food supply, put them in a bucket, and they don't do a tiny fraction of the damage that's done by eating too much fat!

Finally, if you're one of the 50 million Americans who are more than 20 percent above desirable weight, you're carrying a significant extra risk for heart disease, hypertension, gallbladder disease, and diabetes. Once again, *it's primarily the overconsumption of fat that leads to the surplus calories that are making you fat.*

It all adds up to this:

Heart disease and cancer cause 70 percent of all deaths in the United States. In actual numbers, over 1 million Americans die each year from a form of heart disease or cancer that has some relationship to diet. Each year, somewhere near twice this number become afflicted with one of these diseases and *then proceed to live and suffer with their illness for the rest of their lives at untold costs in pain and medical bills.*

Many millions more will be affected by an obesity-related illness, such as non-insulin-dependent diabetes, gallbladder disease, or hypertension. *Depending on the disease, up to half of the illnesses and deaths occur before the age of 65.*

All ills considered, in round numbers, there is at least a 50-50 chance that you will encounter some preventable or postponable illness *related to too much fat in your diet* before you reach the age of 65.

However, as I said before, it doesn't *have* to be this way.

Even the more conservative among health professionals estimate that at least half of this early suffering and death, or about one-quarter of the total, could be prevented if we got rid of the risky behaviors that contribute to these degenerative diseases. Some authorities feel that the percentage of preventable early disease and mortality may be as high as 80 percent.

Let me use an analogy: In some sense we all face a loaded gun! We all die someday. When it comes to figuring the odds, in a rough and general way, on coming down with some diet-related degenerative disease before age 65, the gun has four chambers and one of them is loaded no matter what you do. There are both genetic and environmental factors that are indeed out of our control. But *you, yourself,* can put another bullet in one of the chambers with an unhealthy life-style; cigarette smoking, eating a high-fat diet, and a lack of physical activity are chief among the unhealthy life-style factors. So, think about it. Would you want the loaded four-chambered gun in the hand of fate to hold one or two bullets? That second bullet is in your hands and I want to help you throw it away.

But how could Mother Nature play such a mean trick on us, to instill in us a love of the very foods—things high in fat, blended with sugar or a bit of salt and other flavorings—tempting us to load that second bullet and end up "shooting ourselves in the foot" or even killing ourselves before our time?

THE EVOLUTIONARY BACKGROUND FOR OUR LOVE OF FATTY FOODS

For thousands of years, the inheritance of a tendency to be fat, or to like fatty foods that would contribute to the easy storage of body fat, was very important for our survival as a species. It worked like this:

Until just a few generations ago, the major threats to human existence were famine and infectious disease. The average life span ranged between 35 and 40 years. There have been places and times in our history when, because of famine or infectious disease, less than half of all children born lived to reproduce themselves. The diet-related impact of famine is obvious, of course, but infectious disease as a diet-related factor in the first years of life may have been even more important. When you have a fever, your metabolic rate (and thus your need for more fuel) goes up by about 7 percent with each degree rise in body temperature. Instead of being able to eat more to supply the needed energy, however, there is often loss of appetite or an inability to retain food, plus diarrhea. Under such circumstances, being born fat or inheriting a good appetite and a taste for things that would put down fat fast when a child was healthy gave that child a survival advantage in case of illness.

People living in the Western world find it hard to appreciate the pressure that frequent famine and disease can place on our existence, so I'd like to explain the situation in a bit more detail. We are fortunate to have had a fairly constant food supply for the past few hundred years. We also have conquered the threat of infectious disease that still decimates the population in many parts of the world. But even today, two-thirds of the people on earth, outside the Western world, still face a famine every two years and perhaps 25 percent face serious food shortages every year. As a result, at least 15 million die. (Perhaps it's worth noting that without a supply of Western grain there would be a widespread food shortage in Russia and most of

Eastern Europe. Without making the headlines, millions have actually died in China and South America because of food shortages in recent years. As I write, a more serious famine than has been seen in many years is beginning to sweep across several African countries, along with politically controlled food shortages.) When food is limited, people born with a tendency to store fat and those who have gained a bit of extra weight because of their appetite for fatty foods will be better equipped to survive and reproduce themselves, *and they will pass along the fat trait and quite possibly a genetically based love of fatty foods to their offspring.*

Infectious disease exerted (and continues to exert in many places of the world) an influence similar to that of famine in the development of a species that loves fatty foods and that stores fat easily. Before the development of good sanitation, immunization procedures, and antibiotics, diseases such as diptheria, scarlet fever, whooping cough, measles, smallpox, tetanus, polio, typhoid, and cholera were commonplace and often struck during the first few years of life. The problem still exists in parts of Asia and Africa, where 10 to 20 percent of the newborn die within the first year of life. The rate is 1 percent or less in the developed countries.

As I mentioned earlier, in the presence of infection we get a fever. With a temperature of 103 to 104 degrees, a child will burn up 35 to 40 percent more calories than normal. Extra fat gives the body more of a fighting chance by supplying a larger store of energy to help live through the fever and survive the illness. As in the case of famine, inheriting either a tendency to be fat or a liking for fatty foods provides a survival advantage, and these tendencies are passed to the offspring of the survivors.

I hope you can see how these evolutionary pressures have provided most of us with our inherited tendencies toward the love of fatty foods and, as a consequence, our awesome ability to gain weight when these foods are easily available. I hope you also can see that, from a biological standpoint, we are still "primitives." Our food preferences reflect important survival tendencies and inclinations *given primitive conditions.* However, without famine and disease, as time passes beyond our reproductive years, these former assets become liabilities.

Life expectancy in the United States today has increased about 40 years over that of a century ago. However, the same food preferences that for centuries helped us battle starvation and infectious disease and reach the age of 35 or 40 have now become a key element in the onset of a whole new set of life-shortening *degenerative* diseases. These degenerative diseases, primarily heart disease and cancer, have become the major causes of illness and death after the age of 35 or 40. The primary dietary factor is simply *too much fat.*

I have so far focused on the overconsumption of fat because it is our greatest nutritional hazard. However, the *underconsumption* of other nutrients is associated with the onset of the same set of degenerative diseases, especially heart disease and cancer. I'm speaking of the underconsumption of dietary fiber, certain vitamins and minerals, and other substances found in complex carbohydrates. Each of these aspects bears on the other, because, at any given caloric intake, *the more fat we consume, the less we eat of other foods that have protective health benefits.*

I will give you more details on the relationship between your diet and your health and present the scientific rationale for my recommendations in Chapter 2 and in Appendix A. Now, given all this basic information on the paradoxical preference for fatty foods and its deadly impact on our health, I want to point out some additional aspects of our present-day food environment that have made developing a healthful diet so much of a problem. This knowledge can be of vital importance. Once you are fully aware of how your eating environment affects your appetite and eating behavior, you will be in a much better position to do something about it.

THE PROBLEM IN TODAY'S WORLD

Food processors, bakers, and restaurant chefs take advantage of our preference for fatty foods, cleverly flavored, and present us with a very difficult task when it comes to making any changes in our diets. They create "supernormal" stimuli to entice us beyond the limits of a normal, healthy appetite. By "supernormal" I mean that they create foods that don't exist in nature, but which constitute a scientific blending of the flavors the human animal, because of our evolutionary history, tends to like best. Given a plate of chocolate-chip or buttery oatmeal-raisin cookies and a plate of fresh fruit, most people will opt first for the cookies even though they would happily have eaten the fruit if only fruit were available.

Stop right here and continue with another aspect to the little experiment I asked you to do at the beginning of this chapter and you will undoubtedly see what I'm getting at. Just think of an apple or a carrot, envisioning it as clearly as you can in your mind's eye for five seconds. Now, erase that picture and think of a chocolate-chip cookie, a piece of cheesecake, or some other favorite fatty food, visualizing that as clearly as you can for five seconds.

Did you notice a change in the sensation in your mouth as you thought about these different foods? If you are like most people, you will have noticed a much greater "readiness to eat" when you thought about the cookie or cake than when you thought about the carrot or apple. Just the thought alone or the thought plus a mental picture of a preferred fatty snack or dessert can lead to salivation and an increase in gastric secretion and insulin levels. If this little experiment in fantasy did not convince you, try it in reality—compare your *physical* reactions in the actual presence of these different foods. Put them right in front of your nose and watch what happens.

The point I am trying to make is that our preference for these foods, and what is often an abnormal appetite for them, is in reality a biological, not a moral, issue. They turn you on!

And we are surrounded by them. No matter where you go, there they are.

So what's the solution? If you wish to stay healthy as long as possible, how can you deal with this strong inborn preference for the fatty foods that surround us, enticing us to eat a deadly high-fat diet?[1]

[1] I viewed an interesting illustration of this preference and of the environmental controls over this preference a few years ago when I was leading a section of a health-promotion workshop for Tennessee state government employees. Every morning, Monday through Thursday, about 5 or 10 minutes before our scheduled coffee break, the innkeeper at the state park where the workshop was being held put large bowls of fruit on the table at the end of the conference room. Every morning, all the fruit was eaten during the break.

On Friday, however, the innkeeper also brought in large platters of her homemade chocolate-chip and oatmeal-raisin cookies and placed them alongside the bowls of fruit. Participants started murmuring and squirming in their chairs even as she entered and the aroma spread around the room. When the break began a few minutes later, a majority of the group rose quickly and surged toward the table of food. I intended to do a count and compare the amounts of the two types of food that were selected, but my job was easier than I expected: ALL the cookies disappeared immediately and only ONE piece of fruit was eaten during the break.

The main point that I want to make I think is obvious in the light of the main text which reminded me of this event. But there is another, not-so-obvious point. The innkeeper had provided us with exactly the kind of environment and balance in our

ONE MEAL AT A TIME SOLUTION

I hope I have convinced you with my previous recital of disease statistics that the problem of too much fat in our diets really exists, and that there is a critical need to cut that consumption if we wish to maximize our potential for a healthier, happier, longer life. The *practical* question is: How do we get from where we are to where we need to go?

Let's start with where we are.

According to government surveys, the average American diet contains about 38 percent of its calories from fat. Recent research indicates that this figure most certainly underestimates that consumption by 100 to 200 calories, or up to 20 grams of fat per day. About half of the population is obtaining even more than 40 percent of calories from fat (often, in terms of weight, over 100 grams of fat per day). This is the diet that's killing millions of us before our time. The American Heart Association, along with the National Research Council, recommends that we cut our consumption to 30 percent or less. All agree that less is better, since the latest research shows that, once the atherosclerotic process has started, a diet of 30 percent fat will not arrest or reverse it in most people.

Although it's not necessary for beginning the One Meal at a Time program, I will, if you like, show you in Chapter 3 how to calculate the percentage of fat and the number of fat grams in your present diet.

Where do we need to go?

Research in laboratories all over the world shows that significant reductions in cholesterol levels and other risk factors for disease are obtained when people eating diets containing about 40 percent of calories from fat reduce that consumption to about 25 percent fat. In addition, research in natural settings shows that premature heart disease is almost nonexistent in cultures where people eat less than 10 percent of their calories in saturated fat.

---

diet that meets my recommendations. *Four out of five days she provided us with no-fat snacks; on the fifth we had a treat. The innkeeper made it easy for us by making sure no-fat snacks were the only things available 80 percent of the time—she was actually controlling our eating environment in a healthy way!*

The One Meal at a Time program targets an average of 25 percent fat overall, with less than 10 percent of total calories from saturated fat.

Once again, I will show you how to calculate all of this if you wish to. The Nutrient Counter in Appendix B will give you the information you need to implement a diet at any level of fat content you please. One of the most attractive features of the program is that once you learn where the fat is in your food with the simple One Meal at a Time fat-gram approach, you will be done with counting anything. You will not need to turn into a human adding machine.

How do we get there?

This is the most important question.

It's relatively easy to state where we are and set targets for a healthful diet. It's quite another matter to devise a program that you can easily put into practice. If the program does not suit the demands of our modern life-style and the choices that we have available in our supermarkets and restaurants for eating and cooking at home and dining out, it's absolutely doomed to failure. If you don't enjoy it, you won't stick with it. Most of all, if you find that there are too many changes to make all at once and that it's too difficult to learn in the first place, you won't get by square one.

The One Meal at a Time program takes all of these issues into account. It's a simple, step-by-step plan that's based on how people actually learn new skills or succeed in changing undesirable old habits.

It's different from any other plan available to you at this time. Let me illustrate and explain.

If you have ever read a book on changing your diet—for example, on how to lower your cholesterol level or lose weight—what do you usually see? You see many days, even weeks, of menus that require a complete and immediate change in the way you eat—from what you buy in the supermarket, to the way you prepare foods at home, to what you order in restaurants—all to be done in one fell swoop. I'll never forget what one man said to me when I suggested he read what I think, from a preventive medicine standpoint, is a very good book. (There is a list of supplemental readings in Appendix A.) He said, "I know that book, I tried reading and doing it, and I just gave up. It's too complicated. I had to measure and count everything I ate, down to the teaspoonful, all day long."

I went back and looked at the book. He was right. I realized that I was appreciating the book from a professional standpoint. It presents a tremendous amount of excellent information. It was a professional's "dream," but from a practical, layperson's standpoint, it was a "nightmare."

Think about it for a moment: Isn't it unreasonable to expect you to learn a complete set of dietary directions, perhaps involving record keeping and many calculations, and then implement an entirely new eating pattern overnight? People just don't learn that way.

We eat different meals,
made up of many different foods,
prepared in different ways,
at different times of the day,
with different people,
in different places.

We can't always predict what we are going to encounter in each of these situations, but we need to learn to cope with all of them.

Changes will require different methods of food selection and preparation, and different choices in our different eating environments. That's a lot of differences, and it's no wonder people have a difficult time making changes. Information alone won't work and there is no way in the world you can learn to do it all at once.

To learn a new pattern of eating, and to implement it successfully, we need to start at the beginning and build that pattern in the way people actually learn—in an understandable, workable, step-by-step fashion. You may not remember the details, but that's the way you learned reading, writing, and arithmetic. It's the way good teachers and coaches help you to become skilled with a musical instrument or in a sport. None of these is done overnight.

The more you make your learning process conscious, the easier it will be. To help, I'll discuss some important features of the way people learn in Chapter 3. Fortunately, in contrast with learning to read and write, or to play tennis or a musical instrument, it's not going to take you years to develop the expertise to implement a low-fat diet.

The One Meal at a Time program is divided into four easy steps. Each step takes one week, although some people prefer to stay with one or another step for two weeks before concentrating on the next step. In general, plan on taking from four to seven weeks.

The One Meal at a Time program takes each meal by itself as a task to be learned and mastered. There's the breakfast meal, then lunches, and then dinners. Snacks are also an integral part of a healthful diet. Although you will be learning where the fat is in all of your foods as you progress through the program, you won't have to try to do everything at once. You can deal with each meal, and snacks, one at a time. In addition, you don't have to be *perfect!*

There's room for anything you like, from cheeseburgers to ice cream sundaes, as long as, *over time,* you eat a diet that meets the guidelines you set for it. You must appreciate that the nutritional quality of your diet is *not* determined by any single food or meal, but by what you eat averaged out over weeks and months. As I will illustrate in Chapter 3, as long as you eat a low-fat diet about 80 percent of the time, there's room for the special occasions on which higher-fat foods are served.

Your first job is to learn how to design a set of breakfasts that you can live with and enjoy. Since so many people skip this meal—probably the most important for the day—I hope I can convince you to experiment with starting the day with a good breakfast. Working with your preferences, I'll show you how to make sure you're getting all the many benefits of a good healthful breakfast in your total diet. For people unable to eat on waking, I will have some special words of advice. As with all meals, you need to learn how to design a healthful breakfast eating out in your favorite restaurants, as well as at home. Thus there are two parts to each step of the One Meal at a Time program—dining out and eating at home.

I will give you suggestions for some standard breakfasts that are simple and quick to make at home, or to obtain when you are eating out. But I will also give you some delicious recipes for those special occasions when you want to do a little celebrating, as for a weekend brunch.

Most people find that they can master the breakfast issue in one week. In the end you will probably rotate three or four breakfasts, with slight variations, most of the time. Each will be a low-fat breakfast, with hearty breads or cereals, that gives you a good start on the day and helps keep you satisfied throughout.

Your second job is to deal with lunch—at home and away from home. You will need a set of lunches among which you rotate, *most of the time,* at home and away from home if you eat out frequently. I'll give you suggestions and recipes for the quick and easy "standard" lunches, and then for special occasions, which take more care and time. Most people take a week to master the lunch situation.

Your third job is the evening meal. Since most people rotate among 10 to 12 different basic dishes (with slight variations, of course), it takes about two weeks to cover the evening meal thoroughly, sampling most of my basic suggestions, together with some of the dishes for special occasions. I will show you how to prepare all of the traditional dishes—meats, fish, pasta, casseroles, and so on—in the styles most people tend to prefer. I will give you loads of suggestions for a very flexible eating plan that includes a variety of satisfying desserts. I'll show you simple principles for modifying your present recipes, but I hope you will try all of mine. I love to cook and I enjoy eating! As for eating out, you will discover how to get what you want, prepared the way you want it, in your favorite restaurants.

Your fourth job is discovering the wide array of low-fat snacks that are available to you, in place of the high-fat ones you may now be including in your diet. There are some real surprises here. You will see that there is never any reason to deny yourself when you have an urge to nibble. Indeed, people who adopt a nibbling pattern of eating (many small meals and snacks a day) tend to weigh less and have lower cholesterol levels than people who eat three or fewer large meals a day.

The One Meal at a Time plan will prove to you that a healthy diet is not tasteless, boring, or difficult to achieve.

Over the first few days and weeks that you use the One Meal at a Time program, you will be learning how to maximize the nutritional value of your diet in other health-related ways, in addition to learning the fat content of all the foods you like to eat. You can, if you like, begin from the start to make whatever changes come easily throughout the day. *But your main job will be to do one thing at a time.* That's the easiest way to learn to incorporate permanent changes in your diet.

I want to close this section with a word to people who want to lose weight but have a taste for high-fat foods. High-fat foods are usually the primary cause of a person's weight problems, along with a sedentary life-style. If you are overweight and have been eating a high-fat diet, *permanent weight loss is almost guaranteed when you switch to a low-fat diet and increase physical activity.* There is no need to cut or even try to count calories. But you must stop dieting! If you have a problem managing your weight, whether it's 5 or 75 pounds you want to lose, I think I can offer you the only real solution in Chapter 10.

LOOKING FORWARD

In the next chapter I'm going to summarize the recent research on the relationship between your diet and your health. You will see that you can do a great deal to change the odds and increase the likelihood of obtaining many extra years of good health, if not extra years of life itself.

I very much hope you will follow my recommendations, not only for yourself but for those around you. Your behavior influences others; every person who makes a change for the better makes it easier for someone else. This is especially true if you have anything to do with food selection and preparation for family and friends. You do a great deal to ensure the good health of everyone close to you, easily and enjoyably, with the One Meal at a Time program.

Here's a partial list of the things that go along with good health, just in case you haven't thought about them lately:

- No serious aches, pains, nausea, or fatigue caused by what was an avoidable illness.
- No medical bills to worry about.
- A clear mind that can be dedicated to your life's purposes instead of the concerns that go along with an avoidable illness.
- Good spirits to go along with continued enjoyment of your family and friends.
- No limitations on your physical activity.
- No burden placed on others for your care or financial support.
- No side effects—for example, weight gain, nausea, impotence, bloating, constipation—from the drugs you might have to take to help control an illness.

You probably can think of some others.

Good health is itself a great payoff, but the One Meal at a Time program makes good health taste good, too.

CHAPTER 2

THE SCIENTIFIC
BACKGROUND

I really need to hammer this point home:

Too much fat is the greatest hazard in the American diet.

Too much saturated fat is the primary dietary culprit in heart disease. Too much fat of any kind is associated with certain cancers, including colon, prostate, ovarian, breast, and endometrial cancer. Obesity, obviously caused by taking in more energy than we expend, is almost always caused by too much fat in the diet and almost never by too much carbohydrate or protein. Obesity in turn is related to hypertension, gallbladder disease, and non-insulin-dependent diabetes.

Look at the health-related figures[1] on the next page for people in the United States:

[1]These rounded figures are based on information obtained from a number of different sources, including the National Center for Health Statistics, the American Cancer Society, the National Research Council report "Diet and Health," and published research articles on the different illnesses. They include an estimate of cases undiagnosed in diabetes and gallbladder disease. Estimates of the overweight include children and adolescents, as well as adults, and are based on recently relaxed, and controversial, guidelines. Many experts believe that the number of people in this country who are overweight to the point where it presents a potential health hazard may be closer to 60 million rather than 50 million.

20 MILLION PEOPLE HAVE HEART DISEASE.

12 MILLION PEOPLE HAVE CANCER.

30 MILLION PEOPLE HAVE HIGH BLOOD PRESSURE.

20 MILLION PEOPLE HAVE GALLBLADDER DISEASE.

11 MILLION PEOPLE HAVE DIABETES.

50 MILLION PEOPLE ARE MORE THAN 20 PERCENT OVER DESIRABLE WEIGHT.

Although there is overlap in categories (for example, some overweight people have hypertension), we are talking about well over *100 million* people who are predisposed to or already have a degenerative disease because of their weight.

Overall, about half of the 80 million or so people who already are ill (not simply overweight) are under 65 years of age.

Conservatively speaking, at least half of these sick people under age 65 could have prevented their illness entirely, or at least postponed it for some untold number of years.

So much for the disease statistics. I list them to emphasize that about 20 million people are sick in this country and don't need to be! The hundreds of billions of dollars in costs and the untold pain associated with these diseases *can be eliminated.* [2] If you are a sedentary person eating a high-fat diet, reducing the fat and becoming active can give you the likelihood of many extra years of a happier, healthier life. And if you are a cigarette smoker and quit, you will be doing what is probably the single greatest thing you can do in your favor.

In the rest of this chapter I'll present some of the facts about the dietary causes of the diseases I have mentioned. I also will tell you what you can expect when you make the changes I recommend in the One Meal at a Time program. [3] But, frankly, I'm tempted to say that you really don't have to read all this "heavy stuff" to get started with the One Meal at a Time program. If you've been lectured at till it's coming out your ears instead of going in, and if you already feel well informed about the relationship of a high-fat diet to each of the diseases I've just listed, you probably don't need convincing. If that's the case, go ahead and skip this chapter. On the other hand, I do

---

[2] At the present time we spend about $600 billion a year in health care in this country.
[3] Technical details, an expanded discussion, and references will be found in Appendix A.

discuss some interesting findings, including the most recent research. So if you're a bit curious about how I'm going to present the evidence, you might want to skim this material to see if anything attracts your attention.

THE ROLE OF DIETARY FAT IN HEART DISEASE, CANCER, AND OTHER DEGENERATIVE DISEASES

SATURATED, MONOUNSATURATED, AND POLYUNSATURATED FATS

Before I explain the disastrous impact of too much fat in the American diet, I want to clarify some misunderstandings about the kinds of fat that are found in our foods. The fats and oils that are contained in our foods are composed of *combinations* of various fatty acids. These fatty acids are called *saturated, monounsaturated, and polyunsaturated* depending upon certain chemical characteristics that prove to have different effects on our health.[4]

Figure 2–1 shows the percentage of saturated, monounsaturated, and polyunsaturated fatty acids found in different fats and oils, such as olive oil, chicken fat, butter, and so on. You will see that no fat or oil is composed entirely of one or the other kind of fatty acid, but certain ones predominate. Thus, we label butter a saturated fat because a little over 60 percent of the fatty acids contained in butter are saturated (actually about 62 percent). The vegetable oils contain much less saturated fat, and are predominately either monounsaturated (olive and canola oils) or polyunsaturated (safflower and soybean oils).

---

[4]Fatty acids are, in part, composed of carbon and hydrogen atoms stretched out in a chain. When each of the carbon atoms in the chain is attached to two hydrogen atoms, one on each side, the fat is *saturated*. The carbon atoms work in pairs. If two adjacent carbon atoms are each missing one of their hydrogen atoms, they attach to each other in what is called a double bond and the fatty acid is called *monounsaturated*. In *polyunsaturated* fatty acids, four or more carbon atoms lack hydrogen connections, and two or more double bonds are formed.

Hydrogenation of fats (such as corn, soybean, and cottonseed oils, which contain primarily polyunsaturated fatty acids) to make margarine and shortening for baked goods adds hydrogen atoms to the chain, breaking some of the double bonds and increasing the saturation of the fat. Hydrogenated fats appear to have unhealthy effects on your serum cholesterol level. I'll discuss this elsewhere in the chapter.

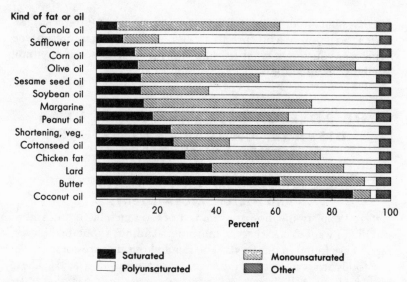

FIGURE 2–1. FATTY ACID CONTENT OF FATS AND OILS.

As you can see from Figure 2–1, the vegetable oils tend to contain only 15 percent or less saturated fatty acids. Olive oil and canola oil are 74 and 55 percent *monounsaturated,* respectively. Safflower and soybean oils contain 75 and 58 percent *polyunsaturated* fatty acids, respectively.[5]

In general, saturated fats tend to be hard at room temperature, and mono- and polyunsaturated fats liquid. Coconut oil as well as palm and palm kernel oils are exceptions to this rule: They are among the most highly saturated fats of all.

Fats that are hard at room temperature, like animal fat, butter, and margarine, can clog your pipes. So can coconut and palm oils.

[5]Fats and oils contain a small amount of other fatty substances that differ in chemical structure from saturated, monounsaturated, and polyunsaturated fatty acids. These are simply classified as "other" for discussion of the health concerns in this chapter since they are of minor importance.

Figure 2–2 shows the percentage of saturated, monounsaturated, and polyunsaturated fatty acids contained in the fats found in foods such as beef, pork, tuna fish, eggs, and so on. The fat in milk is butterfat, and is therefore just as saturated as butter itself. The fats found in fish, poultry, pork, and beef contain, in that order, increasing amounts of saturated fatty acids.

When oils such as soybean, cottonseed, and corn are hydrogenated, hydrogen atoms are attached to carbon atoms found in the chains of fatty acids, and the oils become more saturated. Oils are hydrogenated in order to stiffen products such as margarine, improve the texture of certain foods such as baked goods, and increase shelf life. However, the process produces a kind of fatty acid that may be especially dangerous if you are eating more than a small amount. I'll discuss this matter later in this chapter.

For now, here is a point to remember:

Because the fats and oils in our foods are combinations of the various fatty acids, you may actually be eating more saturated fat when you eat a food "made with pure vegetable shortening" than when you eat something containing butter, lard, or coconut oil. It depends, of course, on *the total amount of fat in the food.* For example,

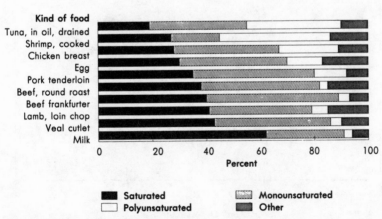

FIGURE 2–2. FATTY ACID CONTENT OF FATS AS FOUND IN SELECTED FOODS.

chocolate-chip cookies and granola bars "made with pure vegetable shortening" can contain more saturated fat than a ginger snap (sometimes containing lard or coconut oil), *because the chocolate-chip cookies and granola bars can contain 5 to 10 times more fat per serving.*

However, both total fat and saturated fat, together with cholesterol in the diet, have important health consequences.

DIETARY FAT, CHOLESTEROL, AND HEART DISEASE

Too much *saturated* fat in the diet is strongly related to atherosclerosis and heart disease. Saturated fat, much more than dietary cholesterol itself, is responsible for raising serum cholesterol, or the amount of cholesterol circulating in your blood. The cholesterol level in your blood is measured in milligrams per deciliter (mg/dl).

As you can see in Figure 2–3, as total serum cholesterol goes up, there is a direct relationship to death from heart disease, with the death rate in men aged 35 to 57 doubling between serum cholesterol levels of 153 and 226 mg/dl, and doubling again between 226 and 290 mg/dl.

Studies of different cultures confirm the relationship between serum cholesterol and heart disease. For example, Japanese males

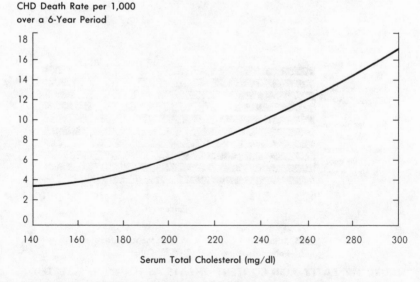

CHD Death Rate per 1,000
over a 6-Year Period

Serum Total Cholesterol (mg/dl)

FIGURE 2–3. SERUM CHOLESTEROL AND CORONARY HEART DISEASE (CHD) MORTALITY.

living in California have about three times the rate of heart disease as Japanese males living in Japan, and they average almost 50 mg/dl higher cholesterol levels. Experts agree that the increase for Japanese living in the United States is due primarily to the adoption of a Western diet. Unfortunately, the increase is now being seen in Japan itself as a Western diet becomes more popular. Although most studies in the past have been done with men, similar trends are now being found in women after menopause.[6]

There are many studies that show it is saturated fat in the diet that accounts for both the elevation in serum cholesterol and the increase in death from heart disease. Among them is one that showed when people who normally use olive oil and other foods containing primarily monounsaturated and polyunsaturated fats switch to butterfat and other saturated fats for research purposes, their cholesterol levels quickly increased an average of 20 to 30 mg/dl. Another study compared different populations, each eating high-fat diets. When the fat was primarily monounsaturated (olive oil), as it is in Crete, the study found very little heart disease even though 40 percent of calories came from fat. That percentage is similar to total fat consumption in the United States, where there is a high rate of heart disease. However, in Crete, only about 8 percent of the total calories comes from saturated fat, while in the United States we eat an average of 16 to 18 percent saturated fat. Many people in this country actually eat as much as 32 percent of total calories in saturated fat.

THE GOOD AND THE BAD ABOUT CHOLESTEROL

First of all, cholesterol is not a fat like butter, oil, and margarine, and it supplies no energy (calories) to the human body, as does fat. Cholesterol is sometimes called "fat-like," however, because it is a waxy substance with a resemblance to fat. Cholesterol performs many essential functions in our bodies. It's used in the formation of the membranes in all cells and in the myelin sheath that coats our nerves. It's also used in the production of bile acids, which aid in fat digestion, and in making hormones like estrogen and other steroids.

All the cholesterol our bodies need can be synthesized in our

---

[6]Prior to menopause, women tend to have lower total-cholesterol and low-density lipoprotein (LDL) levels and relatively higher high-density lipoprotein (HDL) levels than men. Estrogen production may be responsible for this protective state of affairs prior to menopause. The important difference between LDL and HDL will be discussed later in this chapter.

livers—we don't need to obtain any from food to satisfy our requirements. In fact, under normal circumstances, our livers produce much
more cholesterol than is contained in our diets. The average American consumes between 400 and 500 milligrams of cholesterol per
day and produces another 1,500 milligrams or so of cholesterol in
the liver. Although certain genetic predispositions exist which lead
to high serum cholesterol levels, for the great majority of us a high
cholesterol level is produced primarily by too much saturated fat in
the diet, and secondarily by too much dietary cholesterol. And, as is
true of dietary fat, most of us also eat too much cholesterol.

Cholesterol is found only in foods of animal origin. *Both the fat and
the lean part of meat contain cholesterol.* Thus, while you can eliminate a
great deal of saturated fat by purchasing lean cuts and trimming well,
you cannot completely avoid cholesterol by trimming the fat. In dairy products, however, *only the fat contains cholesterol, which is why skim milk and
nonfat yogurt are virtually cholesterol free.*

Cholesterol is bundled with fat and protein as it is carried in the
bloodstream. One particular kind of bundle, called low-density lipoprotein, or LDL, is the dangerous kind. Following some damage to
the wall of a coronary artery, it's primarily cholesterol from LDL that
combines with other articles in the bloodstream and accumulates on
and with the tissue that forms over the damaged area, gradually
closing off the opening through which the blood flows. The process
is called atherosclerotic cardiovascular disease. No one is exactly
sure what causes the initial injuries to the arterial walls, or who is
susceptible to them. It could be wear and tear from surges in blood
pressure or adrenaline, some other substance in the blood produced
by too much saturated fat in the diet, possibly the result of a certain
virus infection or immune system reaction, or simply an inherent
weakness in the nature of the walls themselves. But there is no question that atherosclerotic cardiovascular disease runs in families and is
aggravated by diet and lack of exercise.

Another form of lipoprotein, called high-density lipoprotein
(HDL) because it has relatively more protein and less fat in the
molecule compared with LDL, tends to protect against heart disease.
HDL may carry cholesterol back to the liver for disposal or reuse,
and help keep the arteries clean.[7]

---

[7]From a clinical, or health, standpoint, it's your total cholesterol level, LDL, and HDL
that relate to the risk of heart disease. However, recent research suggests that it may

What are the comparative effects of dietary fat and cholesterol on heart disease?

Although we have been barraged with warnings about too much cholesterol by professional organizations and the media, saturated fat is now recognized by all experts to be considerably more important as a causal factor in heart disease. There are several reasons for this shift in emphasis.

First, your serum cholesterol level is likely to be far more sensitive to a shift in saturated-fat intake than to a change in the amount of cholesterol you eat. Between 85 and 90 percent of people who reduce their intake of saturated fat will see a reduction in their serum cholesterol levels, while only about 30 to 35 percent of those who change their cholesterol intake will see any appreciable change.

Second, the amount of change you will experience in your serum cholesterol level as a result of reducing fat in your diet is likely to be greater than that you can obtain from reducing dietary cholesterol, for what tends to feel like a similar amount of attention and effort. For example, most people who cut saturated-fat intake in half (which would get them under 10 percent of calories from saturated fat) will achieve *twice* the serum cholesterol reduction they could achieve by cutting dietary cholesterol in half (which would get them down to between 200 and 300 milligrams of cholesterol in their daily diets).

Third, saturated fat and cholesterol in the diet may work together, one potentiating the effect of the other. In fact, a high-cholesterol diet may have a limited impact on many people unless they also eat a diet that's high in saturated fat. This is clearly shown in animal studies where serum cholesterol levels increase to a far greater extent when the animals' diets are high in both saturated fat and cholesterol than when their diets are low in fat and high only in cholesterol.

These three findings lead us to an important practical consideration: To maximize the healthful impact you can make with changes in your diet, it's good to work at reducing both saturated fat and cholesterol together. It turns out to be relatively easy with a focus on fat,

---

be certain characteristics of the protein part of the LDL and HDL molecules that determine whether the cholesterol gets deposited on your artery walls or gets carried back to the liver and removed from your bloodstream. Other recent research implicates an abnormal form of LDL that is attacked by the immune system and deposited on arterial walls. Since these findings do not have a direct bearing on the treatment of heart disease at the present time, I'll relegate further discussion to Appendix A.

because when you take aim at your major sources of saturated fat, which are animal and dairy products, you also score big on reducing dietary cholesterol as a by-product, without much extra effort.

Finally, here is an important point that is often overlooked because of the emphasis that's been placed on the impact of saturated fat and dietary cholesterol on serum cholesterol levels. *The consumption of both saturated fat and dietary cholesterol increases the likelihood of heart disease, even among people who have cholesterol levels in the normal range.*

Forty percent of the people who have heart disease actually have *normal* cholesterol levels. Of course, in the absence of a high cholesterol level, much of the predisposition to heart disease may still be accounted for by other hereditary factors, age, sex, diabetes, smoking, and lack of exercise. But even after the effects of these other factors plus a high serum cholesterol level are taken into account, there is still an unexplained, independent contribution to disease that's made by a high-fat or high-cholesterol diet. To put it another way, people who eat a high-fat diet or a high-cholesterol diet may be more likely to get heart disease even if their cholesterol levels remain normal.

What are the dangerous levels for total serum cholesterol, LDL, and HDL?

Scientists have tried very hard to determine the effects of each component of the lipoproteins that carry cholesterol in the body. As a result, research has shown that

- total cholesterol level
- the LDL component by itself
- and the *ratio* of total cholesterol to the HDL component

all have the ability to *predict* heart disease in large groups of people.

When it comes to treating you as an individual, however, if you have a high cholesterol level, most medical authorities feel that the LDL component is the one to use as the primary guide for effective treatment. That's because it's the cholesterol in the LDL component that is most likely to be deposited on the walls of your arteries.

Medical authorities agree that you should cut the fat and cholesterol in your diet if any one of the following measures is over the suggested limits:

- A total cholesterol of over 200 mg/dl.
- An LDL fraction of over 130 mg/dl.[8]
- A total cholesterol/HDL ratio of 4.5 or over.[9]

Let me explain the rationale for each of these boundaries.

1. As total cholesterol levels increase from 200 to 240 mg/dl, people become about twice as likely to die of heart disease.
2. Even stronger relationships are found between the LDL component and heart disease. In fact, the clearest direct evidence for a reduction in individual risk is related to a reduction in the LDL component. You may know about this already since much publicity has been given to the finding that for every 1 percent reduction in LDL level, there is approximately a 2 percent reduction in the risk of heart disease.
3. The ratio of total cholesterol to HDL attempts to take into consideration the protective effects of HDL. A *low ratio* results when HDL is high relative to LDL; this is the *desirable* state of affairs. A high ratio indicates relatively more LDL and less HDL, which is an undesirable state of affairs.

Here are some examples to help explain these points.

If total cholesterol is 200 mg/dl and HDL is 40 mg/dl, the total/HDL ratio is 200/40 = 5.0. That would be considered slightly high. However, if total cholesterol is 200 mg/dl and HDL is 50 mg/dl, the total/HDL ratio is 4.0, and that would be considered in the "good" range.

Although evidence linking the protective effects of HDL is not as strong as the evidence linking high LDL levels to heart disease, many physicians feel that the protective effects of HDL may be most important for people who have total cholesterol levels in the 200 to 240 mg/dl range. This is actually the range in which most heart attacks occur simply because there are many more people with cho-

[8]Some authorities suggest 160 mg/dl of LDL as the threshold for dietary action as long as an individual has fewer than two other risk factors for heart disease (for example, family history of cardiovascular disease, cigarette smoking, diabetes, hypertension, obesity, low HDL cholesterol, and being a man, which in itself bears a greater risk for cardiovascular disease). However, in my opinion, LDL as high as 160 mg/dl is associated with moderate risk of heart disease even if no other risk factor is present.
[9]Because there are differences in risk between men and women, and changes with aging, many physicians prefer to see slightly lower figures than the ones I have suggested for women under 50, compared with men, and allow for slightly higher figures than these in everyone from about 50 years of age on up.

lesterol levels in this range than there are people with levels greater than 240 mg/dl. A *low* total/HDL ratio might have its protective effect in the 200 to 240 mg/dl range in the following way:

Should you find, to begin with, that your cholesterol is as high as 240 mg/dl, and that the HDL fraction is 45 mg/dl, you would have a relatively high risk for heart disease as a function of the total count and very little evidence for a protective effect from HDL because of the relatively high total/HDL ratio of 5.3 (240/45).[10]

Should you do something to obtain a reduction in your total cholesterol of 40 points with no change in HDL, which is probably an overly modest expectation for most people as a result of proper diet, exercise, and weight loss (if called for), your new ratio would be 4.4 (200/45). While total cholesterol at 200 mg/dl is borderline, the ratio reflects considerable improvement.

Many people can obtain a small but potentially important elevation in HDL as a function of weight loss, increasing physical activity (see Chapter 13), and quitting smoking or stopping the use of birth control pills, should these factors apply. Even a 5 mg/dl increase in HDL, combined with that decrease of 40 mg/dl from an initial level of 240 mg/dl, would lead to a rather large change in the total/HDL ratio: 200/50 = 4.0. Thus although total serum cholesterol remains the same as in the preceding example, the increase in HDL reduces the ratio and suggests a possibly greater protective effect.

You may have heard that moderate alcohol consumption can promote an increase in HDL. For a short time after the discovery of the protective effects of HDL we thought this was true. It turns out, however, that alcohol consumption at any level may have *no* desirable impact. Recent research shows that there are several different components in the HDL fraction and that alcohol consumption does not increase the component within HDL that has the beneficial effect.

If you don't already know your cholesterol level, I think it's a good idea to have it evaluated before you start the One Meal at a

[10]The calculation of LDL requires that your triglyceride level be taken into account and cannot be computed directly by subtracting only HDL from total serum cholesterol. The formula calls for taking 20 percent of your triglyceride level, provided triglycerides are below 400 mg/dl, adding it to your HDL level, and subtracting that combined figure from total serum cholesterol. Thus, if your triglyceride level is 100 mg/dl, you would add 20 to your HDL, and subtract that figure from your total serum cholesterol to get your LDL level.

Time program. You need to know it because of its importance to your health to begin with, but you can use changes in your cholesterol level to measure the impact of changes in your diet and level of physical activity.

It's best to go to your own physician for the required blood sample for a cholesterol test so that it can be sent to a laboratory that can be trusted to give reliable measurements. This is important because not all laboratories are well regulated. Results with the same blood sample can vary by as much as 50 mg/dl from one laboratory to another. In addition, having your own physician's technician draw the blood will assure standard conditions in case of repeated testing, since differences in your body position,[11] stress, or your diet over the previous three or four days can affect the outcome. Your physician is much more likely than some independent laboratory or clinic to have on file, or to obtain from you during testing, the information that will help interpret the results.

I am a little wary of the quick finger-prick test for total cholesterol used in work-site screenings and at health fairs and health clubs. Unless the technicians are well trained, the results of laboratory tests of the blood samples obtained by a finger-prick test can vary 30 mg/dl too high or too low. In addition, in nonmedical settings, there is more chance for unsanitary conditions that can cause infection. But knowledge of your cholesterol level is important to you, so if you decide to participate in a work-site or public screening program as a first step, check to be sure the technicians come from a reputable medical setting and are well trained and experienced in the methodology. Then, if there is any question about the results, talk it over with your own physician to determine what action is required.

HYDROGENATED FATS AND SERUM CHOLESTEROL

Earlier in this chapter I mentioned that the hydrogenation of polyunsaturated fats such as corn and soybean oils to make margarines for spreads and shortening for baked goods may produce a kind of fat that has undesirable effects on your cholesterol level. This possibility has been known for some time in animal research, but it has only recently been shown to be true for humans.

Although hydrogenation led only to about half the elevation in total serum cholesterol that resulted from saturated fat in this new

[11]Standing or sitting tends to elevate serum cholesterol, compared with lying down.

research, hydrogenation led to a relatively greater *increase* in LDL (the bad cholesterol) and a relatively greater *decrease* in HDL (the good cholesterol) compared with saturated fat. This produced a particularly unfortunate effect on that total/HDL ratio I spoke about in the preceding section. Recall that the higher the ratio, the more dangerous, since it indicates less of the potentially protective effect of HDL relative to the bad LDL.

The total/HDL ratio went up almost twice as much to hydrogenated fat as it did to saturated fat (22.6 percent versus 13 percent). [12]

Subjects in the research study ate more fat each day than the typical average American, who tends to range between 2 and 8 percent of calories from these potentially dangerous hydrogenated fatty acids, compared with 16 to 18 percent of calories in saturated fat. But with a potential danger from hydrogenated fats as well as saturated fats, the study confirms the desirability of following a low-fat diet. Please take notice: If you have been using more margarine, baked goods containing hydrogenated shortenings, and coffee whiteners made with hydrogenated vegetable oils rather than dairy products, under the assumption you were better off in so doing, you may be wrong and you would do well to cut back.

What about triglycerides?

Triglycerides are the form in which fat is carried in the bloodstream. Scientists are split on the importance of triglycerides in the development of heart disease. When a relationship is found in research, it tends to be stronger in women than in men. High levels (over 250 mg/dl) can be serious, especially when kidney disease and diabetes are present.

When people with perfectly normal triglyceride levels (around 100 mg/dl) switch to a high-carbohydrate, low-fat diet, which is obviously beneficial to their overall health, their triglycerides often go up slightly for a short period of time before returning to normal. No ill effects have ever been noted in such cases, to my knowledge, and the change is temporary. However, a certain rare form of hereditary hyperlipidemia (too much fat in the blood) can be aggravated by a high-carbohydrate diet. This condition is usually discovered early in life, so, if you are susceptible, you probably already know it and are under a doctor's or dietitian's care. There is some evidence,

[12]The fatty acids produced by hydrogenation have a strange atomic configuration and are called *trans* fatty acids. I'll discuss this in greater detail in Appendix A.

however, that even moderately high triglycerides (around 200 satu-rated) combined with low HDL levels (under 40 mg/dl) can present some danger.

We normally measure the baseline levels of fat in the bloodstream after an overnight fast. However, some researchers are beginning to think that it may be the total amount of fat and fat-like substances (lipids) in the bloodstream and *the speed with which the body removes them* **right after eating** that are most important in heart disease.

This is of interest to me because I remember the striking differ-ence, both in the fasting state and in the rate of lipid clearance after eating, in the serum of Type A individuals compared with Type B individuals in Dr. Meyer Friedman's laboratory. (Dr. Friedman is a co-originator of the Type A construct and remains a leading re-searcher in the field.) His Type A persons, perhaps because of their hurried and hostile behavior patterns or the stress they tend to expe-rience, had a much slower rate of lipid clearance after a high-fat meal, as well as a higher baseline state. Their blood serum looked absolutely milky. They also had a significantly higher incidence of heart disease. Other research shows that stress elevates lipid levels, and it may be through this route, as well as hypertension, that stress can increase the rate of heart disease.

The combination of a low-fat diet with exercise is one way to keep triglycerides under control and prevent the reduction of HDL, if not increase it, when you use a low-fat diet. Exercise also is a proven way to help deal with stress.

AND WHAT HAPPENED TO OAT BRAN?

In spite of the recent negative publicity, oat bran and other water-soluble fibers can have a beneficial effect on your cholesterol level. The negative results that gained so much attention were obtained in a study using people with baseline cholesterol levels below 200 mg/dl. Much less change, on the average, is to be expected in people who start low to begin with.[13]

If your cholesterol level is over 200 mg/dl, *there is simply too much strong research on the effect of water-soluble fibers on ELEVATED cholesterol levels to be ignored.*

---

[13]Slight reductions in cholesterol levels were obtained by people in this study who ate increased quantities of either soluble or insoluble fiber. The researchers concluded that eating more fiber of any kind leads to lower fat intake, and it's really the lower fat intake that leads to a lowering of cholesterol level, not any particular fiber.

But let me back up a moment and explain the difference between the two kinds of fiber that have been classified based on their reactions when mixed with water. There are actually many kinds of dietary fiber within each class and all of them seem to have at least some beneficial role in our diets.

Just as fats and oils are combinations of different fatty acids, grains, fruits, and vegetables almost always contain combinations of different fibers, but we tend to refer to these different foods with a label that reflects the predominant fiber.

Water-soluble fiber is, as implied, soluble in water and turns into a gel in your intestines. The gel may bind cholesterol in the bile and prevent its reabsorption from the intestines and its recirculation in the blood. Or the gel may prevent the absorption of dietary cholesterol in the first place. In both cases, serum cholesterol is lowered.

Oat, rice, and corn bran; rye and barley cereals; many fruits, including apples and citrus (especially the peel, which you can make into a candy—see the last recipe in Chapter 11); legumes; and certain vegetables such as carrots are high in water-soluble fiber. To get a major impact from a single source people have to eat prohibitive amounts and soon tire of it even if they don't suffer any uncomfortable digestive symptoms. For example, in one study where participants obtained a 20 percent reduction in cholesterol levels, they ate a cup of hot oat-bran cereal and *five* oat-bran muffins every day! You don't have to do this to obtain similar results. When you eat a low-fat diet and eat a variety of foods that can have a cholesterol-lowering impact, you can achieve a similar reduction without tiring of the method. Furthermore, you assure yourself of the additional nutrients that are contained in a wide variety of different foods.

So much attention has been paid to soluble fiber that we forget that all fiber appears to have beneficial effects. *Insoluble fibers* (found mainly in vegetables and wheat) are so called because, while they hold water and expand when exposed to it, they do not dissolve. Because of their bulk, they decrease transit time of food through the intestines. This can help prevent cancer, as well as diverticulosis, by lessening the time that food, feces, or any carcinogenic substances stay in the colon.

Americans, on the average, consume about 10 grams of fiber a day. The consensus among health professionals is that we should be eating from 20 to 35 grams a day, and there are many authorities who claim that a gradual increase to as much as 40 or even 50 grams would lead to a number of health benefits.

With respect to heart disease, I think you can obtain some additional benefit when you increase your soluble fiber intake *from a variety of sources,* especially if your cholesterol level is over 200 mg/dl at the start of the One Meal at a Time program. While the major impact will be from cutting saturated fat, increasing fiber can put the icing on the cake with another several points of cholesterol reduction.

WHAT DIETARY CHANGES LEAD TO A LOWER RISK OF HEART DISEASE?

Each of the following dietary changes has been shown to help reduce the risk of heart disease (and, as you will see in the next sections of this chapter, exactly the same advice will apply to other degenerative diseases).

Don't worry about the technical points in the following list. *The One Meal at a Time program will have you doing all the right things within four to seven weeks.* You will not be consumed with percentages, nor will you need to be counting anything when you finish. It becomes second nature. I'll give you the clues in **bold print** right now as I list the changes you need to make. I will go into the meal-by-meal details in Chapters 5 to 8.

1. Reduce saturated fat in the diet. I put this first, because it is the most important change. We need to get saturated fat below 10 percent of total calories. **We assure ourselves of reaching this goal by choosing lean cuts of meat and switching to low-fat or skim dairy products.**

2. Research shows that when people use more polyunsaturated and monounsaturated fats *in relationship to saturated fat* there is less heart disease. This will occur naturally when you take Step 1 above and reduce your saturated-fat intake. While polyunsaturated fats tend to reduce total cholesterol, including both LDL and HDL components, monounsaturated fats tend to reduce only the bad LDL, keeping the good HDL cholesterol high. **Olive, peanut, and canola oils are among the preferred, primarily**

monounsaturated oils to be used as fats for cooking and salads. If you use margarine at all, choose the softest kind—it contains fewer hydrogenated fatty acids.

3. Increase intake of water-soluble fibers. Since just about all grains except for wheat contain appreciable amounts of *water-soluble* fiber, as do legumes, most fruits, and many vegetables, and since *insoluble* fiber (the other kind, which is high in wheat and many vegetables) may be so important to cancer prevention, this is an easy recommendation to put in practice. **Replace the fat that you are going to eliminate from your diet by increasing your intake of breads, cereals, and all fruits and vegetables.**

4. *Certain polyunsaturated fatty acids, called omega-3 fatty acids, appear to have a unique role in helping to prevent heart disease.* These particular fatty acids may decrease the stickiness of blood and lower its ability to stick to the arterial walls. They also may reduce coagulability, lessening the likelihood of a blood clot in any arteries that may already have become narrowed as a result of atherosclerosis. In addition, omega-3 fatty acids may help prevent scarring of the arterial walls in the first place, and they may help lower blood pressure. I think this is a pretty compelling list of reasons to increase your consumption of foods that contain omega-3 fatty acids. It's very easy to do. They are found primarily in cold-water fish, and indeed, all over the world where people eat fish once or twice a week, there is less heart disease. **Eat fish once or twice a week, better twice. Fish high in omega-3 fatty acids include salmon, mackerel, bluefish, tuna, swordfish, menhaden, and herring.**[14]

5. Reduce the amount of cholesterol in the diet to less than 300 milligrams per day. (The average American consumes about 400 milligrams daily.) Cholesterol is found in both the lean and fatty tissues of meat, poultry, and fish, but only in the fat of dairy products. **Cholesterol in the diet goes down significantly when you choose lean cuts of meat, increase your number of meatless meals, and switch to low-fat or skim dairy products. Limit eggs to two or three per week.**

---

[14]No ill effects have ever been noted as a result of eating too much of the fish I have listed, but *many ill effects can result from the overconsumption of fish-oil capsules,* including liver disease. Do not take fish-oil capsules for the prevention or treatment of heart disease except under close medical supervision.

WHAT IS THE LIKELY EFFECT OF THE ONE MEAL AT A TIME PROGRAM ON ELEVATED CHOLESTEROL LEVELS AND HEART DISEASE?

Research from many laboratories all over the world shows that if your serum cholesterol level is elevated to start with, an average of about a 20 percent reduction can be achieved by the general dietary guidelines that I've just listed in the preceding section.

There will, of course, be some variability in the way different people respond to changes in diet. Nevertheless, speaking in terms of averages, for people with cholesterol levels initially around 250 mg/dl, following the above recommendations can result in a reduction of about 50 mg/dl. A 20 percent reduction in cholesterol level is likely to result in a decreased risk of heart disease of around 40 percent (about a 2 percent decrease for each 1 percent decrease in total cholesterol level).

If you are overweight to begin with, you are likely to see an even greater reduction in an elevated cholesterol level. If the total serum cholesterol is in the vicinity of 300 mg/dl at the start, reductions of 100 mg/dl, or over 30 percent, *without the use of drugs,* are quite common in overweight persons who lose weight on a low-fat diet.

The longer you stick with the program, the greater the decrease in risk.

For example, even if you obtain only a 10 percent reduction in your serum cholesterol, which starts out with a risk reduction of about 20 percent in the first few years, the risk reduction is likely to grow to 33 percent if you stick with the program for 10 years.

I've been concentrating on the direct association between serum cholesterol reduction and risk of heart disease. However, I want to emphasize that the figures I'm quoting are probably *conservative estimates of the benefits that are likely to occur.* Each of the dietary changes I'm suggesting has an additional risk reduction benefit that is not dependent on any reduction in your serum cholesterol level.

I'd like to digress for a moment and point out that similar beneficial effects accrue from many life-style changes. If you smoke cigarettes or are sedentary, quitting smoking or becoming active will lead to a continual lowering of your risk for heart disease and cancer as time goes on. No matter how many bad health habits you have, if they haven't already done their damage and you make the appropriate changes, the risks become lower with the passing of time. After a few years of healthy living, your future can look just about as bright as that for people who have had the best of health habits all their lives. But you musn't wait too long to start!

THE ROLE OF DRUGS IN THE TREATMENT OF HEART DISEASE

Drugs should always be a second line of defense.

All drugs have the potential for uncomfortable if not serious side effects. Many of the large-scale cholesterol-lowering studies used drugs, but the smaller studies that used diet alone obtained some of the best results in reducing serum cholesterol and risk of heart disease.

Since this book is not intended to offer medical treatment or advice, I will not discuss any of the medications that are available for lowering cholesterol or reducing blood pressure. That's a matter for you and your physician if your blood test yields a cholesterol level in the dangerous range, or if you suffer from any other risk factor and following the One Meal at a Time program does not solve the problem.

But here is a point to remember. Many physicians prescribe drugs because they don't believe that their patients will follow through on the life-style changes that would make drugs unnecessary. From past experience (if not with you, with other patients) they don't believe you will lose weight if you need to, cut out the fat in your diet, quit smoking, or start exercising regularly. Both patients and physicians share responsibility for this state of affairs.

Physicians often have the feeling that it's easier to pop a pill than it is to change behavior. It is certainly less labor intensive for them to write a prescription than to supply the information and counseling we might need to change bad habits and learn healthy new ones. I'm not talking here about prescriptions for antibiotics that are essential in times of infection, but about pain-killing and psychoactive drugs used for everything from tension headaches to anxiety, and about drugs sometimes prescribed for hypertension and cholesterol control. We, as patients, play into this scenario because we often doubt our ability to deal with the causes of our behavioral, psychological, or emotional problems. We pop pills instead of confronting the sources.

Just as your physician has a responsibility for your well-being, you have a responsibility in your relationship with your physician. Should your doctor seem eager to prescribe medications to help you reduce the risk factors for the diseases I'm talking about, you need to determine whether he or she does not trust you to make the changes in your life-style that could possibly accomplish the same purpose without those medications. Then it's up to you to convince your doctor you mean business.

I strongly suggest that you avoid niacin supplements in any form, but especially in the slow-release form, for the treatment of high cholesterol unless you are under a doctor's care. At dosages that can have an impact on serum cholesterol there is a serious risk of liver damage. Other gastrointestinal, neurological, and arthritic symptoms also have been reported. Because the long-term dangers of megadosing with niacin are so great, you need periodic checking if you take this vitamin to help control cholesterol. *Niacin is a drug when used at levels beyond your nutritional needs.*

THE ROLE OF FAT IN CANCER AND OTHER ILLNESSES

Before getting into the details on fat, fiber, cancer, and other illnesses, I want to reassure you on a very important point:

There is a basic consistency in the recommendations for a healthful diet. You don't need to drive yourself bananas trying to do special things for special purposes. *The dietary recommendations for reducing the risk of heart disease are almost exactly the ones that can have an impact on many degenerative diseases, including certain forms of cancer, hypertension, non-insulin-dependent diabetes, gallbladder disease, and obesity.* The One Meal at a Time program covers them all.

Here is a brief summary of the fat facts for cancer and certain other diseases.

CANCER
Too much fat in the diet, *any kind of fat,* is associated with colon, prostate, and ovarian cancer. Although the relationship to breast and

endometrial cancer has been controversial, a recent study showed almost twice the incidence of breast cancer in Chinese women eating a high-fat/high-calorie diet compared with those on a low-fat/low-calorie diet. This is a very convincing study indicating that *quantity* of fat was more important than *type* of fat, since the major part of their fat intake was from monounsaturated fat.[15]

Too much fat of any kind increases the risk of cancer.

Preventive measures. A reduction of about 35 percent in the incidence of all the cancers I've just listed would be obtained by reducing total fat in the diet to 25 percent of calories or even lower. It's for this reason that I have emphasized reducing total fat in the One Meal at a Time program, rather than focus only on saturated fat, which is the primary culprit in heart disease. When you follow the One Meal at a Time program, reducing total fat as I suggest, the required reduction in saturated fat occurs automatically, without paying conscious attention to it.

HYPERTENSION

Hypertension is a serious factor in heart disease and stroke. Obesity, almost always caused by too much fat in the diet, strongly increases your risk for hypertension. Even in the absence of overweight, however, both total fat and type of fat can affect your blood pressure. *A low-fat diet, especially when it's low in saturated fat, is associated with lower blood pressure.*

Preventive measures. The One Meal at a Time program brings total fat and saturated fat well below any dangerous level. In addition, research shows that using the monounsaturated fats I mentioned earlier (canola, peanut, and olive oils) in place of other fats may help you obtain a modest reduction in blood pressure should yours be on the high side.

---

[15]As this book went to press another important study appeared linking overconsumption of saturated fat in beef, pork, and lamb to colon cancer in women. Dairy products were not implicated. Additional details can be found in Appendix A.

DIABETES AND GALLBLADDER DISEASE

Both non-insulin-dependent diabetes and gallbladder disease are associated with obesity. However, very little research has been done on the direct relationship of fat in the diet as a causal factor in these two diseases. Nevertheless, insofar as weight gain is brought about by the overconsumption of fatty foods, there is, in my opinion, an indirect association.

Preventive measures. Reducing total fat in the diet and increasing complex carbohydrates and fiber lead to much better blood glucose control in non-insulin-dependent diabetes. With weight loss, correct diet, and exercise, as much as 80 percent of non-insulin-dependent diabetes might be brought under control without medication, or prevented in the first place. The prevention of obesity itself would help prevent gallbladder disease. *Beware of losing weight too quickly if you are overweight: Losing too quickly may aggravate and possibly initiate a certain form of gallstones.*

OBESITY

Where the diet can be closely controlled, as in animal research, high fat intake is clearly associated with the development of obesity. Animals switched from a diet containing 20 percent of calories in fat to one containing 40 percent double their body-fat content, even though total calories consumed remain equal. Little controlled research has been done with humans over long periods of time, but studies of several months' to a year's duration all show weight loss in overweight people when dietary fat is reduced. People of average weight show a change in body composition: The percentage of body fat goes down and the percentage of lean tissue goes up with a low-fat diet.

Preventive measures. A low-fat diet combined with exercise is the best approach to prevention and treatment of obesity. This is especially important for children since overweight children and adolescents are much more likely to be obese and hypertensive as adults and to develop atherosclerosis. The fat content of children's diets as early as age 2 should not exceed 30 percent of calories. Changes in diet should also be accompanied by cultivating the enjoyment of physical activity early in life. In adults, the creeping weight gain that often begins to occur in the late twenties and early thirties can be prevented by adhering to a low-fat diet and maintaining an active life-style.

THE ROLE OF DIETARY FIBER IN CANCER AND OTHER ILLNESSES

This section should more appropriately be titled "Effects of Carbohydrates, Legumes, Fruits, and Grains" since it's *foods* which are the sources of the nutrients that are vital to life and may offer protection against the degenerative diseases I've been talking about, and *not nutrients in isolation.*

It seems, however, as though every day a new study appears in which an *inference* is made to the protective effects of different fibers in heart disease, gastrointestinal cancers, gynecologic cancers, diabetes, hypertension, gallstones, and possibly other ills. But I need to point out that it's not the fiber *per se,* separate from the foods that it is found in, that has been proven to provide this protection: *It's the foods themselves which contain the fiber* **when these foods are eaten as regular parts of the daily diet.** Food producers (especially cereal manufacturers), pill producers, and the media tend to go beyond the data and tout inference as fact for news purposes, or for advertising and sales purposes when they have a particular brand of fiber cereal or pill to promote. Since no single fiber-containing cereal or fiber pill in and of itself has ever been shown to provide the benefits of a total diet high in fiber, the Food and Drug Administration is finally taking steps to curb misleading promotional activity in the marketplace.

But one thing *is* clear: Diets high in plant foods—that is, fruits, vegetables, legumes, and whole grains—are associated with less heart disease and less cancer, *including lung cancer,* as well as *all* the other diseases I have listed. *There is no doubt about this.* It's true in populations all over the world.

> **People who eat a lot of plant foods—bread, cereal, fruit, legumes, and vegetables—have less heart disease and cancer.**

When we try to pull out the essential protective dietary component in laboratory research, the results are confusing. The key ingredients seem to vary. Sometimes, as in the case of cancer, the key ingredient seems to be fiber, or vitamin A, or beta-carotene, or some other form of carotene, or vitamin E, or vitamin C, and so on. Each of these nutrients appears to be involved in one or another study with animals, but inconsistent results are obtained in experiments with humans. One reason for inconsistency is that our diets are much harder to control than animal diets. Perhaps even more important, there are many unknown substances in the foods we eat that may offer the protection, and not the known vitamins, minerals, or fiber, so we are not sure just where to look.

And while I'm on the topic of specific vitamins and minerals, it is important to point out that no evidence exists for the protective effects of taking supplemental vitamins and minerals, natural or artificially fabricated, in pill form, beyond the Recommended Dietary Allowances, for any of the life-threatening degenerative diseases I'm talking about. Of course, that's not to say that research in the future will fail to discover some positive relationships. At the present time, however, don't believe anyone who promises miraculous protection in an attempt to sell you any vitamin or mineral supplement. Your best protection is a nutritious diet!

An interesting illustration of our lack of knowledge as to the crucial protective substance in particular foods involves cruciferous vegetables. People who eat lots of foods in the cabbage family (broccoli, cauliflower, kale, mustard greens, cabbage of various kinds) seem to have less colon and rectal cancer. Evidence points to a nonnutritive chemical substance, but no one knows for sure at this time.

The whole issue concerning the health-promoting effects of fiber and plant foods is further confounded by the fact that people who eat a great deal of plant foods also tend to eat much less total fat, saturated fat in particular, and cholesterol. Of course, this only brings us all the way around to the beginning: *Cut the fat.*

THE BOTTOM LINE

I've tried to clarify a very complex set of issues in this chapter. But just in case there is any confusion about what needs to be done, let me give you a simple summary.

Here, in a nutshell, is what you need to do, *as you take the most important step of reducing the fat in your diet,* in order to maximize your potential for obtaining all the vitamins, minerals, fiber, and other unknown substances that are associated with good health:

First, *don't* focus on single nutrients or single foods in isolation. That's the way to throw your diet out of balance, turn yourself into a nervous wreck, and become obsessed with your diet instead of enjoying it.

Second, *do* focus on the *array* of foods that have been associated with good health. I'm talking about the entire group of plant foods— fruits, vegetables, legumes, and grains. Expand your horizons, try foods in all of these groups that you have never tried before, and vary your choices from day to day. This can be an exciting, creative adventure, which I hope you will experience as you learn attractive ways of preparing new dishes. Use the plant foods I've been talking about to replace some of the calories you will be subtracting when you cut out the *major* hazard in your diet, which is *too much fat.*

Finally, if you have, in the past, felt confused and frustrated by the overwhelming amount of complex nutrition advice that's available to you, and have despaired of ever making sense of it and being able to put it all into practice, stop bothering yourself about it—just go ahead and follow the One Meal at a Time program. It will take you step by step, one meal at a time and one day at a time, through the *practical* construction of a healthful low-fat diet. Within four to seven weeks you will understand what it takes and how to do it. Only then will you know the real meaning of "a healthful, low-fat diet" rather than a mess of words, rules, and guidelines. To paraphrase an old Chinese proverb: Words do not guarantee understanding—understanding is achieved only in the doing.

CHAPTER 3

WHAT IS THE ONE MEAL AT A TIME PROGRAM?

My ultimate goal is to show you how to eat.

I want to show you how to make a healthful diet so satisfying and so easy to implement that it will become second nature. I think you will be able to do this with the One Meal at a Time program. After you have learned what you need to know about choosing the foods you like to eat, there will be no records to keep and you will never in the future have to worry about counting anything. Not milligrams of cholesterol, not calories, not milligrams of sodium, not food exchanges, not even grams of fat, *not anything.*

It normally takes between four and seven weeks for people to learn how to design a new, more healthful diet with the One Meal at a Time program. The speed with which you move, and improve, depends on your personal preference—you will end up a winner no matter how fast you decide to go.

THE LEARNING PROCESS

The One Meal at a Time plan is based on some fundamental concepts that make learning to eat a healthful low-fat diet just about as easy and automatic as tying your shoelaces in the morning, driving a car, or reading the words you have just read. When you were first learning to do these things, however, they didn't happen overnight. They may not have felt particularly easy. Some of the things you do almost automatically today required weeks, months, or even years to accomplish.

Many of the things we do each day we learned to do in a series of steps, more or less graded to take us from the simple to the more complex. Intellectual skills, such as reading and arithmetic, as well as the more physical skills required in handwriting, sports, playing a musical instrument, or learning to drive a car, were all acquired over extended periods of time in step-by-step fashion. Of course, if you had good teachers and good learning programs, they made each step as simple and as painless as possible (which is something I also intend to do).

When it comes to reading and writing, or driving a car, most of us reach some level of competence and stop there. We don't need to get better at these skills to be successful in our work, nor do we need daily practice to maintain our competence. Playing tennis or a musical instrument is different. As any enthusiast will tell you, these activities require constant practice just to stay in shape.

The One Meal at a Time plan is much more like reading or driving a car than it is like playing tennis or a musical instrument. Once you know how to use the new nutritional knowledge you gain with the One Meal at a Time program, you don't have to think about it anymore. You just do it. Of course, we can always learn more and get better at things we like to do, so if reading this book excites your curiosity, you can continue to learn more about nutrition. You might even find more joy in cooking than ever before and want to read some other good cookbooks to enlarge your cooking repertoire. But once you have followed the One Meal at a Time program for four to seven weeks, you will have in your hands all the knowledge and skill you need to implement a healthful and enjoyable low-fat diet. You graduate!

Besides the step-by-step learning strategy that's basic to the One Meal at a Time plan, there is another, different kind of learning that plays a major role. It's a very satisfying, fun kind of learning which I'm sure you have experienced before. Just reflect for a moment: Some things you know *did not* involve step-by-step learning. They became understandable in a flash. You may have been struggling with a problem for some time when suddenly, out of the blue, the solution appeared.

When an insight appears in this manner, we say to ourselves "Aha!" and feel great. Psychologists have called such one-shot, single-trial learning experiences "aha experiences." Such insights almost always occur in areas where we have some background knowledge and are attempting to apply that knowledge, together with our intuition and imagination, to a new problem. Many of the greatest advances in mathematics and science have occurred in this way, but we all have experiences like this throughout our lives. Such insights often make doing things that were previously very difficult, very easy.

Both step-by-step learning and one-trial "aha" experiences play important roles in the One Meal at a Time plan.

As a step-by-step program, the One Meal at a Time plan makes putting a low-fat diet into practice surprisingly simple. First, unlike other nutritional programs, *you don't need to learn everything there is to know today,* all at once, before you can start the program. There is a single primary focus: We need to learn where the fat is in our foods, but we are going to do it *one meal at a time.* Second, *you don't have to change everything about your eating habits in one fell swoop.* Once again, it's *one meal at a time.* One meal at a time is manageable, both in the learning and in the doing.

But the one-shot deals, the "aha"s, are more fun. You are going to discover that there are wonderful low-fat substitutes for the unhealthful high-fat foods you have been eating up to now. As the saying goes: Knowledge will set you free. Immediately.

Perhaps one example will help you understand what I'm talking about. I'll use a food that most people feel can never find its way into a healthful diet.

Do you like chocolate? A typical chocolate bar has 240 calories and 14 grams of fat. Those 14 grams of fat contain 126 of the calories, or *53 percent,* of the total. Most people are surprised (and chocolate lovers relieved) to learn that Hershey's chocolate syrup and Smucker's chocolate fudge topping are almost completely fat free. The thick, rich-tasting Smucker's contains only 130 calories in a 2-tablespoon serving and only 1 gram of fat. That 1 gram of fat contains *only 9 calories, or just 7 percent* of the total. Which means, of course, that you don't have to give up the flavor of chocolate as you reduce the fat in your diet.

I will show you many comparisons of this kind—desserts, snacks, main dishes—and you will discover many more on your own as you study the Nutrient Counter at the back of this book. Each bit of knowledge will provide you with an insight you can act upon immediately—no further step-by-step learning required in these instances. You're done. And you will be just as happy with the low-fat substitutions as you were with the high-fat bombs. That's why you will be able to stick with this approach to a healthful low-fat diet.

There are, in addition, other benefits to the One Meal at a Time program.

You are likely to feel better than ever. If you suffer from any digestive problems related to the overconsumption of fat or the lack of fiber—for example, indigestion or general uneasiness after eating, or constipation—these symptoms are likely to disappear. The program is easy to follow. You will find *no* long list of tedious and often irrelevant "behavior modification" strategies that must be incorporated into your life forever. We are out to cut the fat and we go straight to the point. I think I can give you the nutritional information and exact skills you need to succeed.

Once you learn what you need to do, it will be as easy to follow the One Meal at a Time program as it is to follow your present diet. Maybe easier.

LEARNING TO USE THE ONE MEAL AT A TIME PLAN

If you were to keep an eating diary for a few weeks, writing down all your meals, I think you might be surprised at your limited food repertoire. Most people tend to repeat certain selections at each meal. If we eat breakfast (and I encourage you to), we eat three or four different breakfasts most of the time. We repeat perhaps five or six different lunches, and rotate something like 10 or 12 main courses for dinner. Even when eating out, most people visit a few favorite restaurants and repeatedly select from a limited number of preferred dishes. Of course, there are special occasions that may include unusual foods prepared in unusual ways, and most of us will make slight variations within the context of our preferred style of eating. But many of us are in something of a rut—we are not getting the wide variety of foods that would assure adequate nutrition, and we have settled into a dietary pattern that includes an unhealthy amount of fat.

To illustrate my point: A recent survey by the National Cancer Institute showed that on any given day, almost half of the adult population does not eat one single piece of fruit, 20 percent do not eat a vegetable, and more than 80 percent do not eat a single serving of a high-fiber bread or cereal. Other research shows that about half the people in this country consume 40 percent or more of their calories from fat. Indeed, over 45 million Americans eat in a fast-food restaurant every day, where the typical meal can contain 50 percent of its 1,100 to 1,200 calories from fat (cheeseburger, french fries, and a shake). We're talking 50 to 60 grams of fat *in a single meal,* which is all if not more than most of us should eat *in an entire day.* You can see the impossibility of including such a meal in a sensible daily eating plan. But you may be surprised, and delighted, to learn that an occasional high-fat meal *will not destroy the quality of your diet.* Although you might want to choose something other than a cheeseburger and fries for those special high-fat feasts, whatever you choose, the One Meal at a Time program is designed to include them in such a way that your diet, over time, will meet the healthful low-fat guidelines we set for it.

Those of us who must eat out a great deal may have special problems even when we don't normally frequent fast-food establishments. If you eat at many different restaurants, especially if you travel, and if you enjoy an international cuisine, you are going to have to learn how to order healthful dishes prepared in a variety of styles. I'll tell you how to obtain special orders on airlines and how to select from an international cuisine in restaurants in Chapter 7.

The One Meal at a Time program focuses on how to construct a set of healthful meals, one meal at a time. First, we deal with breakfast—that's the easiest meal to work with, and the most logical since it starts the day for most people. We will need several healthful breakfasts that you can live with most of the time. You also will want a few recipes for special occasions. Then we move on to lunch, dinner, and snacks.

Each chapter includes a section on eating out. I'll cover everything you need to know to deal with all your eating environments, especially with the people in charge of the food.

OUR PRIMARY GOAL IS TO REDUCE THE FAT IN OUR DIETS

There is, of course, much more to designing a sound diet than just keeping the fat within healthful boundaries. But fat in the diet is our greatest hazard, and fat reduction opens the door that makes the other considerations fall into place much more easily than any other change you can make. Watch and you will see.

Most health organizations have set a target for fat at 30 percent or less of total calories. Just about all authorities agree, however, that even greater health benefits would be obtained if we took the "or less" seriously, and aimed for 20 to 25 percent. The problem we face is twofold: Can we design a satisfying diet at under 30 percent fat, and, once designed, how easy will it be to follow?

I think I can show you how to solve both these problems with the One Meal at a Time plan. We are going to aim for an average of 25 percent fat. This allows for leeway on both sides.

If you wish to stick within American Heart Association guidelines at an average of 30 percent of calories from fat, by holding to 25 percent of calories from fat for five or six days a week, you will be able to hit one or two days as high as 40 percent fat, with as much as 500 or even 1,000 extra calories on these days. By sticking to 25 percent on most days, you will still hit an average of 30 percent or less when calculated on a weekly basis. I'll prove it to you later in the chapter.

If you wish to average my recommended 25 percent of calories from fat (rather than 30 percent), once again you can hit some days as high as 40 percent fat, with as much as 500 or even 1,000 extra calories, and then *compensate* over the next few days. That's the way I do it, and the One Meal at a Time program makes it easy. I'll show you how later in the chapter.

If for any reason you need to cut back even further because of an existing health condition, I'll show you how to reach any percentage of fat intake that's necessary—

But you cannot think in terms of percentages on a daily basis whatever you decide to do! It won't work.

The only way that works is the fat-gram approach.

Here's why.

Unless you are a human calculator, you cannot carry a running percentage count even for one day, not to mention a week at a time, for two reasons. First, the total calorie content per serving of the different foods we eat varies greatly. Second, the percentage fat in each food also varies, from zero to 100 percent.

Look at this simple breakfast, and consider what it would take to keep track of your fat intake over all your meals, every day, if you needed to do it in terms of percentages:

2 slices bread	13% fat	140 calories
1 tablespoon margarine	100% fat	100 calories
4 ounces orange juice	0% fat	40 calories
coffee, 1 tablespoon half-and-half	77% fat	20 calories

I think you can see the problem: This breakfast contains 300 calories, but what is the percentage of fat contained in that *total?* Here's what you would need to do if you had to figure percentages on a food-by-food, meal-by-meal basis.

First, multiply the total calories of each food by its percentage (converted to decimal form) to get the number of calories in fat for each food item.

Second, total those individual amounts.

Third, divide the total fat calories by total calories.

Are you dizzy? I'll do it, rounding to the nearest full calorie:

Percentage (as a fraction)		Total Calories		Total Fat Calories
0.13	×	140	=	18
1.00	×	100	=	100
0	×	40	=	0
0.77	×	20	=	15
		300		133

Dividing total fat calories by total calories, 133/300, gives 44 percent of calories from fat so far.

Forty-four percent of calories from fat! You may be surprised by this high percentage of fat in such a simple breakfast. It's not as ominous as it looks, as you will see in a moment.

My main point is that any approach that requires the constant calculation of percentages won't work. We need another, simple shorthand technique—and wouldn't it be preferable if the technique ultimately did not require counting!

THE FAT-GRAM APPROACH

Whether you decide to eat 20, 25, or 30 percent of your total calories as fat, it is far, far easier to set your daily target in terms of the weight of fat you eat each day, in grams, rather than worry about percentages on an ongoing basis. It works like this:

For the average woman, who eats around 1,800 calories total each day, my recommended goal of 25 percent fat would be 450 calories. We know that each gram of fat contains 9 calories' worth of energy. Dividing 450 by 9 we get 50 grams. That is, 50 grams of fat will provide 450 calories, or 25 percent of the usual total. *So we set 50 grams as our daily target, and learn the fat-gram counts of the foods we like to eat.*

For the average man eating around 2,200 calories per day, 550 would be 25 percent, and that amounts to around 60 grams, give or take a gram.

Now, let's take a look at the above example in terms of fat grams[1]:

bread	2 g (1 g per slice)
margarine	12 g per tablespoon
orange juice	0 g
1 tablespoon half-and-half	2 g

At this point you have had 16 of your 50 (or 60) grams of fat for the day. When you look at this amount of fat as part of your fat-gram total for a day, 44 percent of calories from fat in this one small meal is not quite so ominous as it first appeared since it's less than a third of the day's quota. However, by counting fat grams instead of percentages, you see immediately that you could cut out much of the fat by reducing the amount of margarine on the bread and using a bit of jelly instead. With only 1 teaspoon of margarine, the meal adds up to just 8 grams of fat, and that's just 16 percent of your fat-gram quota for the day.

In case you wish to control your fat intake at some other specific percentage of total calories, Table 3–1 provides you with the num-

---

[1]The amounts have been rounded to the nearest whole gram, which is the simple way that I recommend you do it. Round down for less than 0.5 gram, and up for 0.5 gram or more.

TABLE 3–1. FAT-GRAM TOTALS FOR DIFFERENT PERCENTAGES OF TOTAL CALORIES[a]

Total Calories	These Different Percentages of Total Calories in Fat				
	10%	15%	20%	25%	30%
	Equal These Figures in Terms of Fat Grams:				
1,200	13	20	27	33	40
1,300	14	22	29	36	43
1,400	16	23	31	39	47
1,500	17	25	33	42	50
1,600	18	27	36	44	53
1,700	19	28	38	47	57
1,800	20	30	40	50	60
1,900	21	32	42	53	63
2,000	22	33	44	56	67
2,100	23	35	47	58	70
2,200	24	37	49	61	73
2,300	26	38	51	64	77
2,400	27	40	53	67	80
2,500	28	42	56	69	83
2,600	29	43	58	72	87
2,700	30	45	60	75	90
2,800	31	47	62	78	93
2,900	32	48	64	81	97
3,000	33	50	67	83	100

[a]Highly active persons of normal weight may need to consume more than 2,400 calories a day to maintain their weight. At higher levels of calorie intake, 25 and 30 percent of calories as fat go over my recommended upper levels of 50 and 60 grams per day for women and men, respectively. My recommended levels were based on calorie intakes of 1,800 for women and 2,200 for men. Unless you are highly active (for example, running 10 or more miles a day) or working in extremely cold or hot weather day after day (near zero or 100 degrees), there is no need to exceed my recommended upper limit of 50 or 60 grams of fat per day. If you stick with these upper limits, you will achieve a lower, healthier percentage of fat in your diet even if you need as much as 2,700 or 3,000 calories a day to maintain your weight. The additional figures have been added to the table for reference.

ber of fat grams required for a variety of different total daily calorie levels. If you wish to get a precise in-between value, you can use the following formula:

$$\frac{\text{Total calorie intake} \times \text{Desired fat \%}}{9} = \text{Fat-gram goal.}$$

You must, of course, convert the desired fat percentage to a decimal, and the "9" in the formula refers to the calories in each gram of fat. For example, suppose you determine that you average 1,650 calories a day, and you decide you would like to aim for 20 percent fat in that daily total:

$$\frac{1,650 \times 0.20}{9} = 36.7, \text{ or roughly 37 grams of fat a day.}$$

IT IS VERY EASY TO LEARN THE FAT-GRAM CONTENT OF THE VARIOUS FOODS YOU EAT.

During the next four to seven weeks you will become aware of the fat content of the foods you normally eat in four simple ways:

1. By studying the extensive Nutrient Counter in Appendix B, which contains information on total calories, total and saturated fat, fiber, sodium, and cholesterol for approximately 2,000 different foods, combination dishes, and fast-food items.
2. By using my recipes, which contain similar nutritional information.
3. By following my suggested meal plans, which contain the fat-gram counts of all the recommended dishes that contain fat.
4. By studying the labels on the foods you buy at the grocery.

Within four to seven weeks you will have designed your meals and snacks to automatically come out very close to your target and you won't have to count fat grams anymore, or anything else for that matter.

If you have been a calorie-counting, percentage computer, you are going to breathe a real sigh of relief when you follow the One Meal at a Time plan—it's enormously easier.

ELEMENTS OF SOUND NUTRITION IN THE ONE MEAL AT A TIME PLAN

As I mentioned previously, there is more to the design of a nutritious diet than keeping fat within healthful boundaries. Let me review some recent dietary guidelines, targeted for everyone over the age of 2, agreed upon in 1990 by a conference of ten leading health organizations.[2] There are six primary recommendations:

[2]The ten health agencies included the American Cancer Society; the American Diabetes Association; the American Dietetic Association; the American Academy of Pediat-

1. Reduce consumption of fat, especially saturated fat, and cholesterol.
2. Eat a nutritionally adequate diet consisting of a variety of different foods.
3. Achieve and maintain a reasonable body weight.
4. Increase consumption of complex carbohydrates and fiber.
5. Reduce intake of sodium.
6. Consume alcohol in moderation, if at all. (Children, adolescents, and pregnant women should abstain.)

The committee also made some special recommendations for certain groups, such as women and children. Adolescents and young women should eat more high-calcium foods, such as low-fat dairy products. Children, adolescents, and women of childbearing age should eat more foods rich in iron, such as meat, fish, and fortified cereals, to avoid anemia. To avoid dental cavities, limit between-meal snacks containing sugar.

If you think for a moment about the six primary recommendations, it's obvious they assume that many, if not a majority of, Americans may not be getting an adequate diet: We don't get adequate variety, we eat too much fat and not enough complex carbohydrates and fiber, many of us are overweight, we eat too much sodium, and we perhaps drink too much alcohol. In other words, there would have been no need to make these recommendations if they did not apply to a great many of us and did not have serious implications for the health and economic well-being of our country because of health-care costs.

This set of recommendations is actually a landmark event in the field of nutrition. It represents the first time that all major professional and government organizations have been able to agree on these very important guidelines. Their basic purpose was to increase nutrition awareness and motivate us to do better.

Unfortunately—and perhaps you've noticed—these guidelines are very vague. They are actually far more watered down compared with what leading nutrition scientists would prefer to recommend. They had to be, evidently, or there would have been no consensus![3]

rics; the American Heart Association; the Centers for Disease Control; the National Cancer Institute; the Heart, Lung, and Blood Institute; the Department of Health and Human Services; and the U. S. Department of Agriculture.

[3]Several months after this committee meeting, the Departments of Agriculture and Health and Human Services of the federal government came out with the federal

But we must do better than generalities. Even if there is some debate remaining among the pros, someone has to translate such guideline expressions as "nutritionally adequate" and "variety" or "increase" (carbohydrates) and "reduce" (fat) into specific daily recommendations. If we are going to make healthful changes, we must have a *target* for each area in which recommendations can be made with any reasonable degree of certainty.

The targets must satisfy several requirements:

• They must be easily attainable, given the nature of the food supply in this country.
• They must present no danger.
• They must *not* entail undue sacrifice. Let's face it, if the process of reaching healthful targets doesn't feel good or taste good, we won't stick with that process.

With these three requirements first and foremost, I have translated the generalities of the six guidelines into six specific targets that are contained in the One Meal at a Time program. The program will show you how to put these specifics into practice on a meal-by-meal, day-by-day basis, so that you end up doing exactly what you need to do to preserve good health and help arrest or reverse risk factors for disease. Naturally, if you have a medical problem, or a special risk, you must confer with your doctor and get his or her permission to follow my plan. Your doctor may want to add some special instructions.

Here are the targets for the One Meal at a Time program, with a few words on how we will reach those targets. More will come as we deal with each meal, and with snacks.

---

nutrition policy statement for 1990. Unfortunately, this statement deviates from the committee statement and is even more vague and watered down than the government's recommendations for 1985! Health professionals from a number of consumer groups, including the Center for Science in the Public Interest, immediately criticized the government for what is evidently an effort to placate various commercial food interests. The recommendations that follow in this chapter are based on National Research Council (NRC) guidelines (which were published in 1989 after an examination of literally thousands of research studies) and on important studies published since then. They are not compromised by any commercial interest.

ONE MEAL AT A TIME TARGETS FOR EACH NUTRITION RECOMMENDATION

GUIDELINE 1. REDUCE CONSUMPTION OF FAT, ESPECIALLY SATURATED FAT, AND CHOLESTEROL

Fat is our greatest nutritional hazard and gets our primary attention. I suggest you start by aiming for an average of 25 percent fat on most days, realizing that there will be considerable variation from day to day. You will be amazed at how easy it is to implement a diet at this level of fat consumption once you examine my suggested meals and snacks, and begin to use my fat-gram approach. By choosing low-fat meat and dairy products and adding little or no fat during preparation, it is actually very easy to end up with between just 15 and 20 percent of your total calories as fat if you choose to. However, a quota of 25 percent is appropriate for most people. There is no need to aim lower unless you have an existing fat-related illness or the presence of specific risk factors.

At 25 percent of calories from fat, most women will have an upper limit of around 50 grams of fat per day, and men will be at around 60 grams. (You can adjust this for any calorie level by using the figures in Table 3–1.)

Do not go below 10 percent of calories from fat per day without discussing it with your physician. Fat is an essential nutrient. You cannot metabolize other nutrients in food or transport fat-soluble nutrients to your body cells without adequate fat in your diet. The first signs of too little fat are dry skin, a cracked lip, and gnawing hunger throughout the day. We begin to see these symptoms in some people when they get below 20 grams of fat per day, regardless of total calories.

GUIDELINE 2. EAT A NUTRITIONALLY ADEQUATE DIET CONSISTING OF A VARIETY OF DIFFERENT FOODS

The best way to assure adequate nutrition is to eat a wide variety of foods *within each food group:* breads and cereals, vegetables and fruits, protein foods (meat and meat substitutes, fish, and poultry), and dairy products. To assure wide variety, I will encourage you to experiment with different foods and fully explore your favorite supermarket. You need to find several kinds of breads, cereals, and muffins that you like, and begin to incorporate a variety of vegetables and fruits into your meals and snacks. I will give you some great ideas for preparing low-fat meats, fish, and poultry. If you haven't already done so, you will need to investigate low-fat dairy products, including low-fat frozen desserts.

To further help expand your horizons and achieve that variety as we work on each meal at a time, I will suggest different dishes from each of the food groups each day, and give you some delicious recipes.

Just in case you are unaware of another great benefit to choosing a wide variety of foods: It helps you avoid the concentration of natural and unnatural carcinogenic substances that are associated with any single food.

GUIDELINE 3. ACHIEVE AND MAINTAIN A REASONABLE BODY WEIGHT

If you need to lose weight, I will give you the T-Factor Diet principles, which have helped so many people lose weight and keep it off, in Chapter 10. You can lose weight easily by simply cutting back on the fat in your diet. There is no need to try to count or cut calories.

I also will help you discover a healthy "set point" for your weight and body fat. This can be extremely important to you since the weights recommended in standard weight tables may or may not be appropriate in the light of where your weight will naturally end up when you follow a healthful diet and activity program. These weights may be too high or too low! As for the percentage of body fat that's being recommended by many health authorities, the targets are often unsuitably low, and possibly unhealthy, for many people, especially women. *You need to know how to arrive at what's right for you.*

GUIDELINE 4. INCREASE CONSUMPTION OF COMPLEX CARBOHYDRATES AND FIBER

We have some minimum targets for increasing complex carbohydrates and fiber that are consistent with the recommendations of the Committee on Diet and Health of the National Research Council. You need a *minimum* of five servings of fruits and vegetables a day. (Recall that almost half of the population in the United States doesn't have a single serving of fruit each day and one out of five do not eat any vegetables—I hope this does not apply to you.) You also should have a *minimum* of six servings of bread or cereal foods—and you can include legumes (for example, kidney beans and other similar beans, chick-peas, lentils, and so on) in this category because of their starch and fiber content.

Of course, I am talking about averages over time when I state these minimums. Some days you may have more or less than five servings of fruits and vegetables and six servings of grains. And, of course, you can have double portions! You don't have to choose five or six different foods in each category every day. Generally speaking, however, aim for variety.

Now, *don't worry about the starch and the calories in this food group.* They are not likely to make you fat or prevent desired weight loss when you reduce the fat in your diet.

I want to emphasize that these are *minimum* targets. In the end, I think you will find that you can eat just about all the complex-carbohydrate foods you like—no counting, and no measuring of portions. If you are worried about your weight, remember this: Most overweight people cannot eat enough complex carbohydrates to maintain their weight. They lose weight automatically when they switch to a low-fat diet and replace some of the fatty foods with fruit, grains, and vegetables. *The reason is not hard to understand: A total of 11 servings of fruit, vegetables, and grain foods will usually total* **less** *than 600 calories.* **It's the fat in your food that makes you fat.**

GUIDELINE 5. REDUCE INTAKE OF SODIUM

Most of us consume several times the amount of sodium we need to stay healthy. About 15 percent of the population is sodium sensitive, and for people in that group, too much salt raises their blood pressure and is a definite health hazard. Leading health authorities feel that 6 grams of salt per day is a reasonable target (that will amount to about 2,400 milligrams of sodium), but that an intake within the range of 1,100–3,300 milligrams is safe for most healthy people.

One teaspoon of salt contains about 2,000 milligrams of sodium, and many foods contain considerable sodium in their natural state. The best way to reduce your intake of salt is the opposite of what many health professionals recommend. You are told not to add it at the table. However, research shows that when people add salt at the table *rather than use it in cooking,* they tend to reduce their intake by about 70 percent. Unfortunately, many foods cooked completely without salt fail to develop the full flavor of other seasonings. More on how to deal with this in Chapter 11.

You can reduce your need for salt by cutting it out for a week, and then adding it back in pinches. Sensitivity to salt increases the less you use! (The same goes for sugar.)

GUIDELINE 6. CONSUME ALCOHOL IN MODERATION, IF AT ALL
For those who consume alcohol, most authorities recommend no more than two drinks (equivalent to two beers, two small glasses of wine, or 2 ounces of 80-proof liquor) per day—that is, on any given day (no averaging!). While a small amount of alcohol may help prevent heart disease, the risks of alcohol in the population outweigh its benefits. Too many people cannot stop with two drinks. If you don't use alcohol, don't start; if you do, cut back if you consume more than two drinks per day. The first thing you will notice, after fighting your urge to drink more if you have been accustomed to, is that you will sleep better and feel more energetic when you get up in the morning. *Even two drinks at night, with dinner, can interfere with the quality of your sleep.*

YOU DON'T HAVE TO BE PERFECT

The quality of your diet is not determined by a single food, a single meal, or, for that matter, a single day. What matters is your average over time.

You don't have to be perfect to meet your long-term fat-gram goals and fall within the range of 25 to 30 percent of calories from fat. If you are a woman and follow my advice to average 50 grams of fat a day (which is 25 percent of calories from fat in a diet of 1,800 calories), you can splurge and eat 70 grams of fat on both Saturday and Sunday. When it comes to the nutritional value of your diet, you will not have "blown it." You will still end up with an average *below* 30 percent of calories from fat when you consider the week as a whole. See the example in Table 3–2. Men have similar leeway.

Of course, there are certain dangers in this! Extra fat grams mean extra calories, 9 per gram, and that could lead to weight gain. So we find in practice that just about everyone who has learned the fat-gram approach in the Vanderbilt program prefers to do as I do. *We compensate.* That is, if we go over our quota by a certain number of grams of fat on a given day, we simply cut back *below* that quota by an equal amount so that we end up at whatever target we have set for ourselves over time.

TABLE 3-2.   YOU DON'T HAVE TO BE PERFECT: EFFECT
OF EXCEEDING YOUR FAT-GRAM QUOTA TWO DAYS A
WEEK ON THE AVERAGE FAT INTAKE[a]

Day of the Week	Fat Grams	Calories	Number of Fat Calories	% Fat
Monday	50	1,800	450	25
Tuesday	50	1,800	450	25
Wednesday	50	1,800	450	25
Thursday	50	1,800	450	25
Friday	50	1,800	450	25
Saturday	70	1,980	630	32
Sunday	70	1,980	630	32
Totals for the week (with average %)	390	12,960	3,510	27

[a] For illustrative purposes, the diet for five days a week was hypothesized to contain exactly 1,800 calories and 50 grams of fat, or 25 percent of total calories as fat. In actual practice there would be some variability. You can see, however, that adding 20 grams of fat on two days, which might equal the extra fat found in two typical high-fat entrees, two high-fat desserts, or four high-fat snacks, does not result in a diet that is out of the range of 25 to 30 percent of calories from fat. It averages out to just 27 percent when calculated on a weekly basis.

This example should help make the point. Suppose you choose to aim for what I believe is a healthier 25 percent of calories from fat, rather than the Heart Association's 30 percent. Tracking fat grams makes it truly simple. If, on a given day, you go over what would normally equal 25 percent of calories by 10 or 20 grams, just cut below your fat-gram target by an equal amount afterwards. *If you go over by 20 grams, you don't need to compensate in one day. You can reduce your intake by 5 grams over four days. It is simple and convenient.* If your goal is 50 grams of fat a day, you can compensate gradually for 20 extra grams by eating 45 grams rather than 50 grams for that four-day period. *In addition to keeping you at 25 percent of calories in fat, compensation via the fat-gram approach leads to an automatic compensation in calories and prevents weight gain.*

Obviously, you can use this method of compensation for any desired target of fat intake. But you will not need to do any counting. I've used numbers in the previous examples only to illustrate the freedom and flexibility in the One Meal at a Time program. Within a few weeks your new knowledge about where the fat is in your food and your experience in using the program will make low-fat food choices second nature. As I have shown in my examples, you only need to make these choices most of the time. Perfection is not required. And please believe me—within a matter of weeks, counting anything, even for compensation, will be unnecessary. You will have a feeling for it "in your bones." That's why people say—

IT'S EASY AND IT WORKS

We ask participants to evaluate our program at Vanderbilt periodically. Some of the evaluation is done anonymously so that participants can say what they wish, without worrying about the group leaders' feelings. The most frequent comment about the One Meal at a Time approach is a simple one:

"The other programs I've tried are complicated and confusing. Taking my time, going meal by meal, took all the pressure off."

Others add comments such as "I can handle this," "This is something I can live with," or "It doesn't overwhelm you."

If you are responsible for planning and preparing the meals for your family, you don't need to worry about their acceptance of the changes you want to make. "I'm still preparing the same kinds of foods, only in lower-fat versions. My family didn't even notice."

If you are only on the eating end, and not the preparing end, of the meal chain in your family, the results are similar. It takes but a few weeks for the person who prepares the meals to get the hang of low-fat food selection and preparation. Everyone in the family will be able to change with you to a more healthful diet without feeling any deprivation or voicing any complaint.

You will find that the changes you make with the One Meal at a Time plan are much more likely to become permanent than with any other approach to improving your diet that you have tried in the past. In one of our work-site programs involving almost 500 people, 97 percent of the participants indicated in follow-up that concentrating on lowering the fat in their diets by following the fat-gram approach resulted in a permanent change in their eating habits.

You have a lot to look forward to when you follow the One Meal at a Time plan.

Within a matter of weeks, you are likely to note a change in the way you feel physically. People seem to feel more energetic on a low-fat diet, and many digestive problems associated with too much fat clear up. Because you feel better, you are going to like yourself better. The nutrient value of your diet is going to improve dramatically. If you have been eating a high-fat diet typical of the average American and switch to my One Meal at a Time plan, *you will be getting from 20 to 50 percent more of the various vitamins and minerals for every 1,000 calories you eat.*

If it will help motivate you, remember that loaded gun. Keep that extra bullet out of that empty chamber. To help you assess the results, go to your doctor and get a physical *before* you begin the One Meal at a Time plan. Then, monitor the risk factors: You are likely to see a drop in your cholesterol level and your blood pressure. Glucose tolerance should improve if you have a problem in that area. If you are overweight, you'll see the pounds start to melt away without cutting or counting calories. All these benefits happen naturally, and the worse off you are to start with, the greater the improvement.

So let's get on with the first step in the One Meal at a Time program.

CHAPTER 4

GEARING UP

Here are a few things you can do to make sure you breeze through the changes you are about to make with the One Meal at a Time program.

The first step is to establish the right frame of mind. Think of getting ready to change the way you eat as similar to getting ready to take a trip or go on a vacation. Although I once really did know a man who often bought himself a plane ticket on the spur of the moment and flew empty-handed to his destination, buying what he needed when he arrived, most of us make plans and pack a few things to take along. We need to do something similar when we change the way we eat. It does take a bit of planning and we may have to take a few things along.

Besides planning, there are several things we can do to stay motivated and make sure we have the support of family and friends. The next four suggestions are important for everyone.

TALK THE PROGRAM OVER WITH EVERYONE WHO WILL BE AFFECTED BY THE CHANGES YOU WANT TO MAKE

This is a key step. Are you alone among the people you live with and work with in your desire to improve your diet?

Unless you live and work alone and never eat a meal with anyone else, the changes you are about to make will have an impact on the people around you. They are likely to have reactions that will either help or hinder you, but they will rarely be simply neutral.

Make sure everyone understands the program and the reasons why you want to change. If they don't understand your explanation, have them read this book. If you are like most people, you are more likely to deviate from your best intentions when you are in the presence of others, and influenced by their food choices and suggestions, than in any other situation. The more you can do to get everyone on board, the better. Although I don't suggest you put it to them this way, you will be doing a valuable service to everyone you help change to a low-fat diet.

In the family, let others look at the recipes and help design the menus. It is often a good idea to have the children in the family begin to do some of the cooking, and to invent new recipes themselves. When people help make the change, rather than just going along for the ride, you have greater commitment.

If you frequently eat out in the company of others, especially co-workers so that it occurs on a regular basis, it is essential that they understand and, at the very least, not interfere with what you are trying to accomplish. Unless you brown-bag it daily, the choice of restaurant can be crucial.

CHECK OUT THE RESTAURANTS YOU WILL BE EATING IN BEFORE YOU START THE PROGRAM

Our research shows that people find it much easier to change their diets at home than when eating out. Although some people have problems with impulse eating or emotional eating, and these problems can be associated with obesity, most people who deviate from their best intentions do *not* do it for these reasons. They do it in a social setting, under the influence of their friends or the presence of high-fat foods that they no longer keep in their own homes.

Therefore, besides making your friends aware of what you are trying to do and gaining their cooperation, you need to scout around and find restaurants that will provide you with a selection of appetizing low-fat dishes. Fortunately, more and more restaurants are becoming aware of the changes that are taking place in consumer food preferences and are making an effort to create a larger selection of healthier foods. But do your scouting in advance; don't get caught after you start the program.

For the past two years I have been working with Shoney's, a Nashville-based chain of family restaurants, in the creation and promotion of low-fat meals. Shoney's is famous for their traditional American cooking, but they also have felt a responsibility to offer low-fat alternatives to their customers. Besides giving you some general principles to guide you in ordering when you eat out, I will use selections from Shoney's menus as specific examples of what to look for in any restaurant, wherever you may be, at each meal.

READ EACH CHAPTER WELL IN ADVANCE OF THE WEEK IN WHICH YOU WILL BE WORKING ON ANY PARTICULAR MEAL

Another important step. Each chapter has a shopping list, and you will want to choose recipes and menus. You need to have the principles that go along with each meal well under your belt and the shopping list in hand before you go for your groceries and design the series of breakfasts, lunches, dinners, and snacks that you will be working on during these next several weeks. Don't get caught having to make extra shopping trips or having to make a last-minute decision on what you are going to eat for dinner when it's already 5:30 in the afternoon!

Conscious effort is required while you are learning what you need to know to make the changes; in four to seven weeks these changes will become a part of you. Then, like driving a car, you will not need to be as conscious of each decision and action as you were during the learning process.

PHOTOCOPY THE FAT-GRAM DIARY BELOW OR BUY A POCKET NOTEPAD

Before the program becomes second nature and you are done with record keeping, you will need to keep a fat-gram record. Copy the fat-gram diary on the next page or buy a pocket notepad. Just write down your fat grams for the day during the next four to six weeks. By the time you have completed learning how to design each set of meals and selected your snack foods, you should find it easy to reach whatever fat-gram quota you have chosen. My suggested limits of 50 for women and 60 for men assume approximately 1,800 and 2,200 calories, respectively. If you eat more or less than this, or desire to aim for a different percentage of fat in your diet, you will need to choose a different fat-gram limit (see Table 3–1 in Chapter 3). However, unless you eat over 3,000 calories a day, 60 grams of fat will certainly provide all you need. So if you eat between 2,200 and 3,000 calories a day, by keeping 60 as your quota you will end up at an even lower and healthier percentage of fat in your diet than the 25 percent I have used as my target.

The previous directions are, in my opinion, essential. My next suggestions are optional. Many people skip them, but if you are curious, the knowledge they will provide can be surprising, satisfying, and motivating.

HOW MUCH FAT IS IN YOUR PRESENT DIET?

This step is educational and can lead to great personal commitment. It will also give you practice looking up foods in the Nutrient Counter (Appendix B) so that you will find it easy to use as you start the One Meal at a Time program.

Find out how much fat is in your diet now, before you begin. Keep a fat-gram record for a few days, and include one day in which you

FAT-GRAM DIARY

Food Item (quantity)	Grams of Total Fat	Grams of Saturated Fat (optional)	Calories (optional)	Comments

go out to eat and choose some of the dishes you have been choosing in the past. Look up the fat contents in the Nutrient Counter and keep a record on a copy of the fat-gram diary. Using the pocket notebook that I've recommended, which you can carry with you, is even more convenient. Write down each food and fat-gram content as you go through the day. Our primary interest is in the total fat content. Assuming that you eat the average number of calories that I have used for my calculations, are you over the upper limit of 50 grams a day for a woman or 60 for a man?

You will increase the educational value of this exercise if you also keep track of total calories. You can do it in the optional "calories" column of the fat-gram diary, or you can make a column in your notebook. This will allow you to calculate the percentage of total calories you eat as fat in case you eat more or less than my reference woman at 1,800 calories and reference man at 2,200 calories per day. Just multiply your fat-gram total for the day by 9. That will give you the number of calories in fat, which you can then divide by total calories to see the percentage of fat. If you find that you ate 1,800 calories one day, and had 50 grams of fat, then $9 \times 50 = 450$. When you divide 450 by 1,800 you get 0.25, which indicates that you have eaten 25 percent of your total calories in fat.

Here's an example from our follow-up research on a group of women surveyed between one and two years after completing the Vanderbilt program and using the fat-gram-counting approach we teach in the One Meal at a Time program to lose weight. According to their eating diaries, their average intake was 1,771 calories and 35 grams of fat per day. Therefore, $9 \times 35 = 315$ calories from fat, and $315/1,771 = 0.177$, or, rounding up, 18 percent of total calories as fat.

If you are a big meat eater, you might want to see how many grams of saturated fat you've been eating and add that to your record in the appropriate column of the fat-gram diary. The saturated-fat content of various foods also can be found in the Nutrient Counter in Appendix B. In the end, we want to keep saturated fat well under 10 percent of total calories. When you keep total fat at the levels I suggest, and follow my recommended meal plans, I think you will find that this happens without paying special attention to it.

The same women I used in the above example at follow-up were eating an average of 11 grams of saturated fat per day. Using the same approach that we used for total fat, we get the following: $9 \times$

11 = 99 calories from saturated fat, and 99/1,771 = 0.055, or, rounding up, 6 percent of total calories from saturated fat.

The women I'm using as examples had been out of the program for up to two years. For them, eating a low-fat diet had become second nature. They did not normally keep eating records any longer. For follow-up, they were instructed to keep an eating record for three days, including one weekend day. They were to give weights and measures (which they had been trained to do in the program) but not do any calculations. We used the Food Processor II computer program to analyze their diaries. Although I suspect that keeping the records may have made them even more conscious of choosing low-fat foods than they might ordinarily have been, I think you can see that there is plenty of room for upward deviations without getting over the healthy boundaries.

There are several noteworthy things about these findings that I hope will motivate you when you compare your own records if you choose to do this optional gearing-up step.

First, the follow-up subjects average well under 25 percent of calories in total fat. We have done a number of follow-up studies investigating total fat consumption when people use the fat-gram-counting approach to implementing a low-fat diet, and never has the percentage been over 22 percent of calories as fat.

Second, they are well under 10 percent of total calories in saturated fat. By following instructions to choose low-fat cuts of meat and low-fat dairy products, you are virtually assured of keeping within that 10 percent limit if your total fat intake is 25 percent or under. *You do not need to keep a saturated-fat count.* If you don't believe me, do a saturated-fat count once or twice, just to assure yourself once you have started the One Meal at a Time program.

Third, the follow-up subjects are no longer keeping eating diaries—a low-fat diet is second nature. For me, this is the most important finding of all. *It means people like the approach and are living with it.* If they didn't and couldn't, then we would not be able to see the important low-fat dietary achievements reflected in the first two findings.

If you decide to keep this pre-program record, you will find out how much fat you have been eating in your present diet. You can compare it with the follow-up data from our research subjects. That comparison may motivate you more than ever to make the One Meal at a Time changes. But if you hate keeping records as much as most people do (including me), just remember that once you learn where the fat is in your foods, and making low-fat selections becomes as natural as it is to people who have been through our program, you will be done with counting.

DO AN INVENTORY OF YOUR PANTRY AND REFRIGERATOR

What do you have in the house right now? What's the fat content?

Take a blank sheet of paper, make a list of the foods that you have in the house today, and write down their fat contents. Study the labels on packaged goods, and look up anything that doesn't have nutrition information on its label. Also look up the fat contents of any meats and snacks, any foods in the freezer, and so on. You may be surprised at the fat content of many of the foods you keep in the house.

No, I'm not going to tell you to throw all the high-fat foods in the garbage, or give them away! Of course, you can if you like, but as we go through the program, one meal at a time, starting with breakfast, you will have a chance to use what you have in the house now at other meals during the day. You will replace those foods with items from the shopping lists that appear at the ends of each of the next four chapters. There's one for breakfast, for lunch, for dinner, and for snacks.

Be prepared to customize your eating environment. In the end, you help ensure the permanent success of your nutritional changes by making sure your eating environment is designed to support your intentions, not sabotage them. When you purchase what I include on the shopping lists, you will be stocking your home with everything you need to follow the One Meal at a Time program. You will be creating a healthful eating environment. *Do not keep high-fat foods on hand at all times—they will tempt you to exceed your fat-gram quota.*

Perhaps it will help you get into the right frame of mind to think in terms of "everyday foods" and "occasional foods." The occasional foods are those you might include in a restaurant meal, have at a dinner at a friend's home, or bring to your own home for an occasional treat. Yes, birthday cake and ice cream, pizza with cheese and meat, a hamburger, fries (ugh), and a shake can, if you like, fit into a low-fat diet on an occasional basis, as I will illustrate in the nutritional analyses presented in Chapter 9. Meals like this cannot, however, comprise more than 10 or 20 percent of your diet. The best way to make sure they don't is not to include these foods in your everyday eating environment.

MUST YOU WORK ON EACH OF THE MEALS IN THE ORDER I SUGGEST?

No. You can take them in any order you like. I start with breakfast because it is the easiest and most natural place to start for most people. Although we work through the meals in the Vanderbilt program in the order I present them in the book, some people have found themselves focusing on dinner before lunch. Others get right to snacks immediately. As for the timing of particular meals, you can mix up the meals and times to suit your day. Some people prefer dinner at lunchtime, and a smaller meal at night. Many health professionals agree that it is better to eat the largest meal in the middle of the day. But each meal presents its challenges, so spend a good week on each.

No matter how you choose to approach it, I think you will find that the One Meal at a Time program is a culinary adventure. It's an enjoyable trip that gets people to their destination: a low-fat diet for a healthier, happier, longer life. Regardless of how you decide to proceed thereafter, start with breakfast and read the next chapter in plenty of time to plan your week so that you can get off to a good start.

CHAPTER 5

BREAKFAST: THE MOST IMPORTANT MEAL OF THE DAY?

Breakfast has an important role in a healthful diet. Breakfast literally "breaks" the "fast" that occurs between the evening and morning meals, fuels the body for morning activity, and helps meet daily vitamin and mineral requirements.

Unfortunately, many people skip breakfast, some because they don't feel comfortable eating first thing on arising. So, let me clarify some issues about this meal and our three-meal-a-day eating pattern.

First, while there is *much* to recommend having a healthful breakfast, it is not *essential*. However, if you skip breakfast, you ought to take special steps to compensate or your diet is likely to be less nutritious.

Second, the three-meal-a-day pattern itself is a rather modern convention. Nibbling many small meals throughout the day may be more like the human race has eaten for much of its history, and it may be the most healthful way.

Third, when it comes to losing weight, if you have been eating breakfast, you may find it easier to lose if you *temporarily* change your eating pattern and skip breakfast. However, if you have been skipping breakfast, as so many overweight people do, you may find it much easier to lose if you start eating breakfast. I'll discuss this recent finding in Chapter 10.

In the end, whether or not you have breakfast is a matter of choice. Many people have difficulty digesting food early in the day. The biological rhythms that prepare for eating after a night of sleep can change as a result of years of skipping breakfast. They also may be different as a result of genetic influences.

There are many benefits to starting the day with a good breakfast. After you have read this list, you will see why I encourage *everyone* to experiment with my suggestions. Compared with people who skip breakfast, people who start the day with a meal shortly after waking are likely to:

- Eat less fat in their diets
- Have lower cholesterol levels
- Eat less food at lunchtime
- Consume a significantly more nutritious diet
- Suffer less fatigue later in the day
- Be better problem solvers early in the day
- Eat less from 4 or 5 P.M. until bedtime
- Weigh less, especially if the meal is part of a pattern of eating five or more times a day, rather than three or fewer

I think that's an impressive list of reasons why people who omit breakfast should reconsider their habit. So I want everyone to try my suggestions *for at least two weeks.* If you have been skipping breakfast, it may take that long for your system to turn itself around and adapt to a change in eating habits. Your body prepares for getting up in the morning with changes in its hormone and endocrine systems that begin a few hours before rising. People who skip breakfast have bodies that are not physiologically prepared to receive food soon after they get up. If you have been skipping breakfast for any length of time, the physiological rhythms must be reset in order for you to adjust to eating after awakening.

You will know after two weeks whether you are one of the few people who don't adjust easily and don't end up feeling better when you eat a healthful breakfast. If this proves to be the case, one good approach is to brown-bag your breakfast for later in the morning. Another is to include breakfast foods later in the day as snacks.

CONTENTS OF A GOOD BREAKFAST

We tend to stay satisfied longest when our meals have all three major nutrients: carbohydrate, protein, and a little bit of fat. Carbohydrate foods containing starch and fiber fill us up because of their bulk, and protein and fat take longer to exit from the stomach. We probably obtain more nutrition when we eat combinations of different foods since nutrients, including vitamins and minerals, work together in our bodies.

There is absolutely no scientific basis to the claim that our bodies can digest only one kind of food at a time and that we should eat only certain foods in the morning and others later in the day. It's probably not doing you any harm if you feel good doing this, but the rationale is simply not true.

To construct a good assortment of breakfasts that we can rotate five or six days a week, we need to find an array of foods that we like, and stock our pantries and refrigerators. We'll need some hearty breads and muffins, some cereals, and, preferably, some fruit. While many people do not take well to fresh citrus fruit first thing in the morning, dried fruit is a good addition to a cereal. Eggs, fatty meats, and cheese are generally out, as is more than 1 teaspoon of margarine or butter on your bread or hot cereal. Each week you can, if you like, fit two or three higher-fat meals, including breakfast, into a low-fat diet. It won't hurt your overall average (see my menu analyses in Chapter 9). But save that high-fat breakfast for a special occasion, perhaps a Sunday brunch.

I think you will be surprised at how your tastes for breakfast foods change. Many people who have been eating a high-fat breakfast—for example, bacon or sausage and eggs, doughnuts or Danish—have become accustomed to vague digestive distress that lasts for a good part of the morning. They have a lingering and annoying aftertaste in their mouths, or their tummies rumble, or, worst of all, they have a sour stomach or heartburn. Is this true for you? If you have any one of these problems, *fat* is almost always the culprit. You are going to feel a whole lot better when you cut back on the fat in your breakfast.

A WORD ABOUT MILK AND MILK PRODUCTS

If you haven't already, you must try switching to low-fat or skim milk. Whole milk is a high-fat product, and, like butter, the fat is over 60 percent saturated. A glass of whole milk contains about 8 grams of fat, of which over 5 are saturated. If you are sensitive or allergic to milk, try yogurt or low-fat milk containing acidophilus or bifidum cultures. Some people feel that these cultures help them digest milk more easily. If you are one of the millions of Americans who cannot digest milk without unpleasant side effects, you may want to check with your physician or a registered dietitian about adding a special enzyme (lactase) to your milk to help your body break down the sugar in milk (lactose). Low-fat milks with lactase already added are available in many regions of the country.

If you choose to leave milk and milk products out of your diet, you will have to pay special attention to obtaining your calcium from other sources, such as green leafy vegetables and fish and animal products with soft, chewable bones. If omitting milk prevents you from eating dry cereal products, you are also missing an important avenue through which you can increase the overall nutritional value of your diet. Dry cereals generally are fortified with a number of vitamins and minerals, and my most recommended ones contain appreciable amounts of dietary fiber. One of my nutritionist friends with a milk allergy found that mixing his cereals with vanilla-flavored low-fat yogurt and different fresh fruits solved his problem. He eats a different mixture almost every day, which also responds to his need for variety.

FAT-GRAM TARGET FOR BREAKFAST

Most people like to ration their fat intake through the day, leaving the largest amount for their largest meal. This tends to be the evening meal. While it is a good idea to eat more of your food earlier in the day and have a light dinner, that's not convenient for most of us, including myself. It probably doesn't make a great deal of difference if dinner remains your largest meal, unless you overeat just before retiring. You are likely to suffer from wakefulness halfway through the night, as your stomach empties. In addition, a large, high-fat meal before bedtime is particularly dangerous if you have heart disease and obstructed arteries. That's because your fat-laden blood will flow more slowly during sleep. Let me emphasize once again that you are less likely to overeat at night if you eat a sound breakfast.

You may find that it's a good idea to aim for no more than one-quarter of your fat-gram total in your breakfast meal. If you are a woman with a fat-gram quota of 50, aim for 10 to 12; a man might aim for 15 of his 60-gram quota. Many people discover that they can design great breakfasts with between 5 and 10 grams of fat once they have found a preferred selection of cereals and breads. These are usually very low in fat. A breakfast containing under 10 grams of fat will give you more flexibility for the fat content of your other meals and snacks.

STOCKING THE PANTRY AND REFRIGERATOR

When you eat a breakfast consisting of bacon or sausage and a couple of fried or scrambled eggs, with two slices of toast, each with a teaspoon of butter or margarine, you are consuming about 35 grams of fat, a good deal of it saturated. Doughnuts, croissants, and Danish can contain up to 20 grams of fat each. While it is possible to eat a certain amount of these foods each week without exceeding an average of 30 percent fat for the entire week, frequent meals consisting of these foods can put you on a course straight to "heart-attack city." I hope that my suggestions and your changing tastes will make your desire for such high-fat breakfasts disappear.

We need some basic breakfasts, at or below 10 grams of fat, that we can live with five or six times a week. We also need some special recipes for the other days, just as easy to prepare and just as tasty as the "heart-attack specials," but with a fraction of the fat.

Here are some recommendations for the foods you will need for several "basic" breakfasts. Afterwards, I'll make some suggestions for special dishes—for example, pancakes and French toast—and for complete breakfast menus.

Although all the suggestions I am about to make are important to the success of the One Meal at a Time program, I want to place special emphasis on breads and cereals:

• HEARTY, SATISFYING BREADS AND MUFFINS THAT CAN BE ENJOYED WITHOUT ADDED FAT ARE CRITICAL FOR THE SUCCESS OF THE ONE MEAL AT A TIME PROGRAM.

• HAVING A VARIETY OF CEREALS THAT YOU ENJOY AS BREAKFAST FOODS AND SNACKS IS JUST AS IMPORTANT AS FINDING A SELECTION OF GOOD BREADS AND MUFFINS.

Breads Stock a selection of whole-grain or mixed-grain breads. Keep some extra in the freezer so you won't run out. Bagels, English muffins, and bran and other grain muffins with added fruit are satisfying, and raisin bread is a treat. Choose breads and muffins that contain from 1 to 4 grams of fat per serving. Recipes for homemade breads and muffins can be found in Chapter 11. After you have tried my recipes you will know how good hearty breads and muffins can taste. Then you can search out equivalents at local bakeries. Good bread, including raisin bread, and muffins need nothing on them. No butter, cheese, jelly—nothing. They are satisfying straight, with your favorite morning beverage. They also are good for nibbling as snacks.

Cereals Keep a large variety of dry, ready-to-eat cereals made from different whole and mixed grains, including wheat, oat, corn, barley, and rice, and rotate among them through the week. Choose dry cereals that contain 1–3 grams of fat, 3 or more grams of dietary fiber, and generally less than 250 milligrams of sodium per serving. You can blend a low-fiber cereal of your choice with a high-fiber cereal, such as 100 percent wheat-bran cereal. Oatmeal and oat bran are good choices for hot cereals. Among the cereals in my own pantry (I just looked to make sure) are Bran Flakes, Raisin Bran, Meuslix, Shredded Wheat, Grapenuts, Whole Wheat Total, Total Corn Flakes, Cheerios, Bran Buds, and All Bran. There are many others equally as good. The selection is large because my wife and I have different tastes, and we both like to sample new cereals as they come on the market. Cereals can serve as healthful low-fat snacks as well as breakfast foods. Keeping an interesting variety on hand will lessen the temptation to turn to higher-fat snacks.

Fruit You will need a selection of fruit for appetizers and for mixing with your cereals. Sliced bananas, peaches, nectarines, and plums are good with cereal, as are berries in season and dried fruit, such as raisins, prunes, and dates. For appetizers, choose fruit juice and halved citrus fruits, and melon in season. Fruit is virtually free of fat (except for avocados, and the Florida variety has half the fat of the California variety).

Dairy Choose low-fat or skim milk for cereals and as a beverage, low-fat cottage cheese, and no-fat or low-fat yogurt to mix with berries or cereals. Look for a fat content between zero and 2 grams per serving in these products.

Jam, etc. Keep a small supply of favorite jams, jellies, and preserves to use with your breads, pancakes, and French toast, in place of butter or margarine. Preserves with the best taste and texture, in my opinion, are made with either fruit juice or 100 percent sugar (no corn syrup), pectin for thickening, and possibly citrus juice or citric acid. (Jams, jellies, and preserves are fat free.)

Beverage Low-fat or skim milk, coffee, or tea. If you like milk or cream in your coffee or tea, be sure to count the fat grams—half-and-half has about 2 grams per tablespoon. Occasionally, if you are pressed for time, try one of the commercial breakfast mixes with low-fat or skim milk for a "complete" breakfast in a glass. These breakfast beverages may lack fiber, but they are fortified with vitamins and minerals.

What about eggs, breakfast meats, and butter or margarine?

If you are serious about keeping saturated fat under 10 percent of total calories and dietary cholesterol low, it is wise not to have more than two or possibly three eggs a week. I do not eat eggs except as ingredients in certain casseroles and muffins, where I use the whole egg. Eggs have almost 5 grams of fat each, and about 200 milligrams of cholesterol. My wife and I together use a dozen eggs every two or three months and I never order them when I eat breakfast out.

If you like breakfast meats, I suggest switching to Canadian bacon, or lean baked or boiled sliced ham. These can be had with only 1 gram of fat per serving (which is usually an ounce, but is sometimes three-quarters of an ounce). Check the labels on the prepared products, since some brands will have 5 or more grams per ounce. We do not use breakfast meats at all.

Pastrami and corned beef, which some people like for breakfast as well as for luncheon sandwiches, are now available in lean "deli" cuts. But be an informed shopper: When you see the claim "Less than 10 calories per serving," check the serving size. One local brand of sliced pastrami, which happens to taste quite good, can make the claim "only 10 calories per serving" by slicing so thin that a serving size weighs only one-third of an ounce, rather than the more customary and realistic three-quarters to one ounce. Why, the slices are so thin you can actually see light through them! Such practices make you question what an honest serving size really is in the first place.

Butter and margarine have about 4 grams of total fat per teaspoon (12 grams per tablespoon). Butter contains more saturated fat than margarine, and soft margarine is less hydrogenated than hard margarine. The reduced-calorie (reduced-fat) margarines generally contain 2–3 grams of total fat per teaspoon (they are blended with water for weight and volume). We don't use margarine. We do use butter, but only in special recipes and at dinner parties. Let's face it: Nothing tastes as good as butter in certain recipes. However, we have kept track and found that, including entertaining, we use about two pounds of butter per year.

BASIC BREAKFASTS

Here are some suggestions for your everyday, basic breakfasts. They are quick to prepare and satisfying. You can mix and match your own combinations, using fruit, a bread or cereal, and a beverage. Skip the citrus fruit if it upsets your stomach. Remember that if you choose a high-fiber bread or cereal, you are less likely to be hungry later in the morning, or to overeat at lunch. Having breakfast also tends to make you less likely to overeat at night.

I tend to prefer whole-grain breads, but I realize that not everyone will want to eat whole-grain breads at all times. Try mixed grains for variety. Both mixed- and whole-grain breads will supply more fiber and trace minerals than white bread, but if you like white bread occasionally, go ahead and have it. When you follow the One Meal at a Time program in all its aspects, you will be getting plenty of fiber, and the vitamins and minerals found in whole grains, elsewhere in your diet.

I have not included butter or margarine because I think you will soon learn that you don't need to use them with good breads. However, if you do use them, be sure to include in your records 4 grams of fat for each teaspoon.

In order to get a wide variety of grains and fruits, rotate among these different basic breakfasts from day to day. If you don't care to prepare hot cereal, just use the first three breakfasts or add a fourth of your own design. My low-fat special breakfasts mentioned in the following section also can be used every day.

When a recipe can be found in Chapter 11, the item will be set in **bold print**. (To locate these quickly, use the index to this book.)

Breakfast 1

Orange juice; ready-to-eat cereal with fruit (1–3 g fat); low-fat or skim milk (0–2 g fat per cup); slice of **Quick Honey-Wheat Bread** (or other whole- or mixed-grain) toast (1 g fat; jelly optional); beverage (2 g fat for 1 tablespoon half-and-half)

Total fat: 2–8 g

Breakfast 2

Melon or other fresh fruit; two slices favorite bread (see bread recipes in Chapter 11), bagel, or English muffin (1–2 g fat); jam or jelly (optional); low-fat or skim milk, 1 cup (0–2 g fat), or other beverage of your choice (2 g fat for 1 tablespoon half-and-half)

Total fat: 1–6 g

Breakfast 3

Fruit or juice; choice of muffin (3 g fat, see muffin recipes in Chapter 11) or 2 slices **Raisin-and-Cinnamon Bread** (2 g fat); coffee, tea, or milk (0–2 g)

Total fat: 2–5 g

Breakfast 4

Choice of fruit; hot cereal with cinnamon and raisins (2–4 g); toast (1 g per slice); jam (optional); coffee, tea, or milk (0–2 g)

Total fat: 3–7 g

Chapter 11 also contains a number of other recipes that are as easy to prepare as the ones I have just recommended. And there is nothing to prevent you from using leftovers from a low-fat dinner as breakfast!

NUTRIENT COMPARISON OF BASIC LOW-FAT AND TYPICAL HIGH-FAT BREAKFASTS

The breakfasts I have recommended are significantly lower in fat and higher in other essential nutrients than the typical high-fat American breakfast. For comparison, in Table 5–1 I present the nutritional analysis of Breakfast 1 above and a nutritional analysis of a breakfast consisting of two scrambled eggs in margarine, two slices of bacon, two slices of white toast with 2 teaspoons of butter, 4 ounces of orange juice, and coffee with 1 tablespoon of half-and-half. I think you will need little additional convincing.

TABLE 5–1.   COMPARATIVE NUTRITIONAL ANALYSES OF A HIGH-FAT BREAKFAST AND BREAKFAST 1[a]

Nutrient	Amount in High-Fat Breakfast	Amount in Low-Fat Breakfast[b]
Calories	717	535
Protein	26.2 g	19.1 g
Carbohydrates	81.7 g	117.0 g
Dietary fiber	2.57 g	9.17 g
Fat—total	33.4 g	4.68 g
Fat—saturated	13.4 g	2.1 g
Cholesterol	467 mg	10 mg
Vitamin A	357 RE	556 RE
Thiamine (B_1)	0.722 mg	0.910 mg
Riboflavin (B_2)	0.880 mg	1.02 mg
Pyridoxine (B_6)	0.382 mg	0.908 mg
Cobalamin (B_{12})	1.21 μg	2.44 μg
Folic acid	237 μg	305 μg
Pantothenic acid	2.33 mg	1.78 mg
Vitamin C	161 mg	160 mg
Vitamin E	1.94 mg	2.24 mg
Calcium	231 mg	402 mg
Copper	0.349 mg	0.663 mg
Iron	4.09 mg	10.4 mg
Magnesium	85.5 mg	176 mg
Phosphorus	406 mg	558 mg
Potassium	1,220 mg	1,691 mg
Selenium	46.2 μg	33.7 μg
Sodium	963 mg	589 mg
Zinc	2.41 mg	5.65 mg
Calories from protein:	14%	13%
Calories from carbohydrate:	45%	80%
Calories from fat:	41%	7%

[a] The low-fat breakfast consisted of 4 ounces of orange juice, ¾ cup of bran flakes, ½ cup of 1 percent milk, 1 slice of whole-wheat toast with 1 teaspoon of jelly, and coffee with 1 tablespoon of half-and-half. The high-fat breakfast consisted of 4 ounces of orange juice, 2 scrambled eggs cooked in 2 teaspoons of margarine, 2 slices of bacon, 2 slices of white toast with 2 teaspoons of butter, and coffee with 1 tablespoon of half-and-half.

[b] Even though it contains 182 fewer calories, the low-fat breakfast is significantly higher in almost all vitamins and minerals. It contains almost 30 fewer grams of fat and over 450 fewer milligrams of cholesterol. The most important nutrient comparisons are in **bold print**.

Special breakfasts. There were times in the distant past when a Sunday breakfast at our house was an even greater nutritional disaster than the comparison I just made. It included corned beef and pastrami on pumpernickel bread, with mustard *and* mayonnaise, bagels with smoked salmon and cream cheese, and sometimes another kind of smoked fish. We'd finish up with coffee cake or Danish. We have lost our taste for this kind of a meal, but, as you will see (Chapter 9), you can still have that occasional high-fat breakfast and get in under the wire.

However, why stuff yourself with 30–40 grams of fat when you can enjoy substitutes with fewer than 10 grams and end up without the discomfort of having overeaten for the rest of the day? Here are some suggestions.

MORE FESTIVE LOW-FAT BREAKFASTS

You will find low-fat but tasty versions of **French Toast** and **Basic Pancakes** in Chapter 11. Use powdered sugar and cinnamon with the French toast, or jam, fresh fruit, or your favorite pancake syrup with either of these recipes. They don't need butter or margarine. Because pancake syrups vary so greatly in flavor, it's worth scouting around until you find something special (such as pure maple syrup). It won't take long before you get used to eating both French toast and pancakes the way I suggest, sweetened if you like, but without the fat. *You can use all of my special recipes at any time in place of any of the bread or cereal products in the suggested basic breakfast menus.* I include them under this special heading because they take extra time to prepare.

If you like breakfast meats, remember to use Canadian bacon or low-fat boiled or baked ham in place of the fatty varieties. Add two slices (no more than 1 ounce each) of lean ham between three pancakes, and cover them with a good-quality pancake syrup. The lean ham will add only 2 grams of fat to your breakfast.

Turkey bacon is available in some supermarkets, and some packing companies are producing sausage with a reduced amount of fat. Check the labels for fat content. *Don't be misled by those fancy labels that proclaim "85 percent fat free."* It still means over 4 grams of fat per ounce, and possibly 8 to 10 grams of fat per serving. If you can get lean ground turkey, which is less than 10 percent fat, or ground beefalo (a hybrid cow and buffalo, which is even leaner), try my **Country Sausage.** It will contain only a quarter to half the fat of the packaged "low-fat" varieties.

To help round out your breakfast selections, I include in Chapter 11 recipes for over half a dozen different breads and muffins, for **Mock Danish** and **Corny Breakfast Cakes,** and for a couple of egg dishes.

See Table 5–2 for a summary of my suggestions for healthful low-fat breakfasts and some good low-fat substitutes for high-fat breakfast foods. You might like to make a few photocopies and put them in convenient places, such as on the refrigerator and in your pocket or purse.

TABLE 5–2.　BREAKFAST TIPS AND SUGGESTIONS

Whole-grain breads, English muffins, bagels, bran and fruit muffins, and raisin toast (1–3 g fat per serving) are delicious low-fat substitutes for croissants, doughnuts, pastries, sweet rolls, and biscuits (12–20 g fat per serving).

Commercial muffins can contain as much as 10 or more grams of fat each—make your own. Recipes on cereal boxes are well tested, but usually need only half the fat and half the number of eggs. Use low-fat milk in place of whole milk, or a mixture of milk and yogurt or milk and applesauce (about 3 g fat per serving).

Use a variety of ready-to-eat cereals (1–3 g fat per serving). Try mixing a high-fiber cereal with a preferred low-fiber cereal or a cereal that provides 100 percent of the Recommended Dietary Allowances.

"Sweeten" cereals with fresh or dried fruit.

Flavor hot cereals with a touch of cinnamon or nutmeg, and add dried fruit.

Use skim, ½ percent, or 1 percent milk (0–2 g fat per cup) instead of whole milk (8 g fat per cup).

Instead of butter or margarine (4 g fat per teaspoon) on bread, use jelly or jam (no fat) or reduced-fat spreads (2–3 g fat per teaspoon).

One egg contains 5 grams of fat. Boil or poach instead of frying or scrambling with fat. Use eggs sparingly, primarily in recipes.

Use Canadian bacon, turkey bacon, or extra-lean ham (1–2 g fat per ounce) instead of regular varieties. Substitute homemade sausage (with ground turkey breast or beefalo, 1–2 g fat per ounce) for commercially packed sausage (5–10 g fat per ounce).

In recipes that call for many eggs, try a combination of fresh eggs and frozen egg substitute. For example, in place of 6 eggs, use 1 egg, 1 cup frozen egg substitute, and 2 egg whites. This cuts the fat by 80 percent.

Cook eggs, pancakes, and French toast without added fat in a nonstick skillet or with nonstick cooking spray. A smidgen of fat may be added for flavor.

Top pancakes with fruit, yogurt, or a favorite pancake syrup.

Try blenderized low-fat cottage cheese or yogurt cheese as a spread on bagels or English muffins. Mix with either salsa, onions, sardines, canned salmon, or other foods and seasonings. (Make yogurt cheese by allowing no- or low-fat yogurt to drip through cheesecloth or coffee filters suspended over a bowl for 6–8 hours.)

For crunchiness on yogurt, hot cereals, or pancakes, use Grapenuts.

For bacon flavor, use imitation soy-based bacon bits with your eggs. For scrambled eggs, mix 1 egg with egg substitute in an amount suggested on the package.

When eating out, instruct your server to hold the butter or margarine on toast and pancakes. If you like, add a little at the table. Use jam, fruit, or syrup in place of fat.

When eating out, ask to have grits or cereals served without fat—or they might arrive drowning in it.

A "real" bacon or sausage and egg breakfast, or any other high-fat breakfast, can fit in an overall healthful low-fat eating pattern on occasion. Think in terms of your entire week and don't have more than two or three high-fat meals overall.

EATING BREAKFAST OUT ON THE ONE MEAL AT A TIME PROGRAM

Except when I'm traveling, I rarely eat breakfast away from home. When I do, I don't force myself to exist only on cereals or toast and coffee. At the same time, I know I will be busy with either interviews or a presentation later in the day, so I eat lightly. I choose muffins, fruit (such as half a grapefruit or melon), and coffee most of the time. If my preferred bran muffins aren't available, I order an unbuttered English muffin. I also have a fondness for buckwheat pancakes, which I order without butter.

If you have breakfast at a fast-food restaurant, check the Nutrient Counter in Appendix B for the fat contents of the various foods you can order at different chains. It's accurate as of this writing, but chains are constantly introducing new items. In general, watch out for the biscuits, croissants, and breakfast-meat sandwiches—they are typically loaded with fat. Some chains are introducing low- or no-fat muffins and tarts in response to public demand. They are also providing nutrient information on request, so ask! And most chains do have a selection of cereals. Ask for low-fat milk, if available.

Chains of family-style restaurants offer a wider selection than fast-food restaurants. Unfortunately, however, most chains make it difficult to order a low-fat breakfast. If you are lucky enough to have a Shoney's in your area, it's much easier. The Shoney's breakfast bar contains just about all of the foods I've suggested for my basic breakfasts. As for something special, Shoney's pancakes have less than half a gram of fat per pancake and their French toast has only 3 grams of fat per slice, which is pretty much as if you had used my own recipes at home. The chefs at Shoney's also can modify many menu items to your specifications, which is not usually possible at fast-food restaurants.

If you must eat most of your breakfast meals out, search your area for a restaurant that will serve the same kind of low-fat breakfasts that I have recommended for eating at home. If the restaurant offers a breakfast bar, and the breakfast bar has the customary array of high-fat foods, and if you are the kind of person who can't resist the sausage, eggs, hash browns, and Danish when they're right in front of your nose, *then don't go to the breakfast bar!*

I'm no longer tempted by these high-fat foods, so I choose the same bread or muffins and fruit from a breakfast bar that I would have ordered from my table. If this is hard for you to do, order from your table, even if your server just goes to get your order from the breakfast bar. I have found that in most instances you will be charged less for the individual items than if you had chosen the fixed-price "Breakfast Bar Special." If you are concerned, ask about the price in advance. Your server will figure it out for you both ways.

If eating breakfast out is infrequent—perhaps once a week—you might make this one of your higher-fat meals. However, if you are at all like most people who become accustomed to a lower-fat diet, you will note just how much better you feel when you skip greasy foods. Even on a high-fat day, you are likely to choose just one higher-fat item, not several.

Look for the following items on a breakfast bar. If the restaurant you frequent does not have them, ask the manager to begin including them in the future.

- A variety of ready-to-eat cereals, including average- and high-fiber varieties.
- A hot cereal, including grits, that is not swimming in fat.
- A selection of whole or sliced fruit, including melon and berries in season, in addition to a variety of juices.
- A nice variety of breads, bagels, rolls, and muffins, including whole-grain versions, with a nice selection of jams and jellies.
- If French toast and pancakes appear on the bar, they should not be covered with butter or margarine in their trays.
- If a breakfast meat is served, ask for inclusion of a low-fat ham or Canadian bacon.

• Low-fat milk for a beverage and for adding to your coffee in place of nondairy creamers (most are very high in saturated fat).

SUPPOSE I DON'T EVER BECOME ACCUSTOMED TO BREAKFAST?

People who eat breakfast tend to consume less fat in their diets and end up with what nutritionists call a "nutrient-dense" diet. That is, they get more bang for their buck—more vitamins and minerals per calorie of food consumed.

If you skip breakfast, you tend to miss out on a grain food (usually vitamin and mineral fortified), a low-fat calcium source (such as low-fat milk), and fruit. When figured over time, your diet is likely to be lower in vitamins A and C, iron, pyridoxine (B_6), zinc, magnesium, and copper, as well as calcium. Make up for this by choosing a cereal food for a snack, especially at bedtime. You are likely to find that you sleep better afterwards. Milk contains certain amino acids that encourage sound sleep. Eat the fruit you missed at breakfast as a mid-afternoon snack. If it replaces something higher in fat that you have been accustomed to eating, so much the better.

Adding foods back into your diet that you missed by skipping breakfast—using them to replace the higher-fat snacks that you now eat later in the day and before bedtime—will increase the nutrient density of your diet as well as reduce the fat directly. And, I repeat, you might first try to brown-bag your breakfast for later in the morning.

SUMMARY OF DIRECTIONS FOR BREAKFAST

Test out my suggestions for a healthful breakfast, experimenting with the breakfast menus and your own combinations for at least one week. If you have been skipping breakfast, you may need to take two weeks.

Don't pay particular attention to the other meals this week. However, you will be studying the Nutrient Counter in Appendix B, so if you find that making some low-fat modifications and substitutions will be easy at your other meals, go ahead and make them.

Make sure you have all the foods you will need to implement the

One Meal at a Time program for a healthful breakfast. Use the shopping list that follows.

If you eat breakfast out more than occasionally, find a restaurant that makes low-fat eating easy for you.

If you eat breakfast out with family or friends who tend to make choosing a good restaurant and healthful choices difficult, talk it over with them. I think you can arrange to find a restaurant where everyone can obtain what they want, and remember that you can have food prepared the way you want it in almost all sit-down restaurants, if you will only assert yourself.

Keep a daily record of your fat-gram count. You will see how your breakfast meal begins to stack up.

Look up the fat contents of the foods you eat during the rest of the day. Compare the fat contents of different possibilities for each meal and snack, such as the different cuts of meat, combination dishes, and desserts. Even without attempting any changes as yet, this information is an important first step in gaining all the knowledge you will need to make the kind of permanent change in your diet that we are aiming for during these next four to seven weeks.

Whatever you do, don't be in a hurry. This is the start of a change that will last a lifetime and help assure your good health. Take time to find the foods and breakfast menus you can live with. It's important to like what you are doing—and eating.

BREAKFAST SHOPPING LIST

Fruits	Breads and Grains
apples_____	whole-grain bread_____
applesauce_____	mixed-grain bread_____
apricots_____	raisin bread_____
bananas_____	bagels_____
berries_____	English muffins_____
grapefruit_____	bran or fruit muffins_____
melon_____	ready-to-eat cereals (variety)_____
oranges_____	whole grain_____
peaches_____	mixed grain_____
raisins_____	hot cereals_____
other dried fruit_____	oatmeal_____
fruit juices_____	oat bran_____
other_____	

Milk and Dairy Products

skim or low-fat milk_____

evaporated skim milk_____

nonfat yogurt_____

low-fat cottage cheese_____

low-fat sliced cheese_____

Meats and Eggs

Canadian bacon_____

eggs_____

egg substitute_____

ham, lean_____

Miscellaneous

all-purpose flour_____

whole-wheat flour_____

wheat germ_____

cornmeal_____

baking powder_____

baking soda_____

yeast, dry_____

sugar_____

brown sugar_____

honey_____

jelly or jam_____

pancake syrup_____

cinnamon_____

margarine_____

vegetable oil (canola)_____

nonstick cooking spray_____

coffee_____

tea_____

other_____

CHAPTER 6

LUNCH

Lunch at home is often a bore, and eating out every working day is a disaster for many people seeking to lower the fat content of their diets.

At home, it's up to you to create enough variety to avoid facing the same old cottage cheese or tuna fish. If you eat out every day of the week, remember that the low-fat choices in most restaurants are limited but the temptations aren't. Unless you can find a restaurant with a commitment to offering low-fat dishes, you must rotate among several different restaurants to increase variety. Otherwise you'll get tired of the limited choice and, more often than not, find yourself succumbing to a high-fat dish.

If you are going to be successful in maintaining a low-fat lunch most of the time, you are going to have to be creative about variety. That's because we are much more easily bored by low-fat foods—they are not as enticing as high-fat foods. Although this is not true of everyone, it is true of most: Soup and a salad for lunch are not as appealing as cheeseburger, fries, and a shake. If my particular examples of high-fat items are not your favorites, I'm sure you can think of something in the high-fat line that would keep you reordering, day after day, many times beyond your soup-and-salad limit.

Human beings are not alone in their preference for high-fat foods. Given a choice, most omnivorous animals are likely to choose (and overeat on) high-fat foods rather than low-fat foods.

So to repeat, both at home and out, to remain faithful to a low-fat diet we need a larger selection of foods, with interesting textures and seasonings, to compensate for the loss of fat.

The key to your success lies in easy preparation at home, and easy access in restaurants. Let me show you how to accomplish this.

LOW-FAT LUNCHES AT (OR FROM) HOME

Although we don't need everything available at once, we need variety and convenience. Here's a list of foods and dishes that make for satisfying low-fat lunches. Most of them are easily taken to work as well, in the proverbial brown bag:

- Lean luncheon meats
- Hearty breads for sandwiches
- A variety of sandwich spreads and other fillings
- Tasty condiments for those sandwiches
- A variety of salad and sandwich greens, and other vegetables for nibbling
- Interesting dressings for those salads
- Dips for those vegetables
- A selection of broth-based soups, hot and cold
- Crackers and other crunchies to accompany those soups
- Fruit for accompaniment and dessert

Notice: I haven't even mentioned canned tuna and cottage cheese! Or, for that matter, leftovers from the night before, which can take us out of the ordinary realm of luncheon choices.

We have half the battle won when we become aware that our choices may be much more numerous than we thought. The other half of the battle is won when we find a way to make selecting and preparing these choices interesting, quick, and easy.

Here's how. Have on hand an assortment of the following:

Lean meats	Sliced breast of turkey or lean ham. Many brands are available at 1 gram of fat per ounce (usually a slice). Deli beef is usually lean, but check with the butcher. All the leftover meat dishes from dinner (see Chapter 7) will be lean. *Avoid salami and bologna:* They usually have 6 to 8 grams of fat per ounce.
Hearty breads	Have at least two good breads, a whole or mixed grain and a rye or pumpernickel, for toast and sandwiches. Or use rolls, English muffins, or bagels. Substitute a baked potato with low-fat trimmings for a sandwich occasionally, or use flour or corn tortillas.
Spreads	Make tasty spreads from different bases: Try beans, canned fish, cottage cheese, or tofu. For more details see below and browse in Chapter 11.
Fish	Sardines, canned salmon, and canned tuna make excellent sandwich fillings. See my suggestions for seasonings and salad-style fillings in Chapter 11.
Salad makings	Once or twice a week, cut up a selection of crunchy vegetables and store them in a covered plastic container in the refrigerator. I suggest carrots, sweet green and red peppers, celery, radishes, cabbage—anything that will keep for several days. This makes them easily available for salads at both lunch and dinner and for snacks. Don't include greens that will wilt (and don't buy more salad greens and lettuce than you can eat in a few days; these spoil rather rapidly). Combine fresh or leftover vegetables with pasta for a pasta salad (see **Summer Pasta Salad** in Chapter 11). Sardines, canned tuna, and canned salmon make excellent salad components (and see **Shrimpy Tomato Aspic** in Chapter 11).
Dressings	Low-fat commercial dressings are fine if you like them. However, I like to make my own, using an olive-oil base and different vinegars for variety. See my salad dressing recipes in Chapter 11. Helmann's (Best Foods) makes an excellent low-fat mayonnaise with about half the fat of their regular kind, but I still prefer the full flavor and texture of the "real" variety in *smaller* quantities.
Condiments	*Condiments can make or break a low-fat diet.* Herbs and spices, especially hot spices, can compensate for a reduction in fat and salt. Keep a variety of salsas, mustards, herbs, and spices around to liven up your fillings, spreads, and salads. You will find over a dozen different brands and styles of salsas and mustards at your supermarket—have at least three of

each on hand for variety. Mix mustard or salsa with a small amount of mayonnaise (1 *teaspoon*) for a sandwich dressing. Recipes and other suggestions can be found in Chapter 11.

Dips   Fresh vegetable strips are tasty enough without additions, but some good dips make them interesting day after day. Spreads and some sandwich fillings also can be used as dips. See Chapter 11 for recipes.

Soups   Incredibly good homemade soups take only a few minutes to prepare. You won't believe how satisfying and filling soup can be, with or without a sandwich or salad. You'll find more details below and in the recipe chapter. If you don't have the time for homemade soup, there are good broth-based canned varieties and dry mixes available in the supermarket (but they won't compare with what you can do yourself). Soup as a first course at lunch can be an aid to weight loss.

Crackers   Whole-wheat saltines, Norwegian flatbread, Venus no-salt crackers, breadsticks, no-salt pretzels, and oyster crackers.

Fruit   Finish lunch with whole fruit or an assortment of melon, pineapple chunks, grapes, or berries in season. Cut up a selection of fruit once or twice a week and store it in a plastic container in the refrigerator. Keep fruit from turning color by adding lemon juice. You can also blend softer fruit (bananas, berries, peaches) with yogurt for a tasty shake.

Leftovers   All the dinner courses in the One Meal at a Time plan (see Chapter 7) make excellent leftovers for the next day's lunch. They're good for brown-bagging, too. Some are best reheated but many can be eaten cold as part of a sandwich or made into salads.

BASIC LUNCHEON SUGGESTIONS

We need to design four or five basic lunches that, with some variations from day to day, you can live with most of the time when you are eating at home. Soups, sandwiches, and salads form the core of these lunches, together with leftovers. Just to show you how easy it is, here is an overview of how I go about preparing soups, salads, and sandwiches when I'm eating lunch at home. The details will be found with specific recipes in Chapter 11. Remember, these are your basic, easy, everyday luncheon suggestions. Later in this chapter I will suggest low-fat recipes that take more preparation, for special occasions. You can also fit a higher-fat lunch into your plan once or twice a week if you wish—I'll illustrate in Chapter 9.

Soups start with homemade stock, or a can of stewed tomatoes, or water and bouillon cubes. I add sliced carrots, celery, and onion, and sliced potatoes or some brown rice right at the start if one of these is my choice of starchy vegetable or grain that day. If it's macaroni, I add that about 15 minutes before the soup is done. Seasonings include fresh ground pepper and one or more herbs, such as thyme, basil, marjoram, tarragon, rosemary, or parsley. If I have leftover chicken or fish, that can be added, too. The same goes for leftover vegetables, or greens that no longer look appealing for salads. Potatoes and spinach all by themselves make a good soup when added to a bouillon base. I simmer my mixture for 45 minutes to an hour. It's so good I always make at least a double portion. You can turn your concoction into a low-fat "cream" soup by adding dried milk powder. While a salad is nice with soup, these soups are so nutritious that toast or crackers are all you need to round out this lunch.

Since we almost always have chopped fresh vegetables and sliced fruit in the refrigerator, I can quickly make a salad with or without added greens and tomatoes. I'll occasionally make tuna or salmon salad, with a little mayonnaise, Lea & Perrins' white wine Worcestershire, and some chopped olives, onions, and celery. Pasta and leftover chicken or fish also make good cold salad ingredients.

Sandwiches are a snap. One of my favorites is open-faced, with just sliced tomatoes on whole-grain bread spread with salsa. On rare occasions I will add a teaspoon of mayonnaise. Cottage cheese is made interesting, as a spread or salad component, by adding cajun seasonings, onion or garlic powder, or a salt-free seasoning such as one of Mrs. Dash's many varieties. Cottage cheese also is good with fresh fruit or jelly. I have two favorite spreads: One is cottage cheese blended by hand with sardines or canned clams (drained), minced red onion, and some black and cayenne pepper (see **Norwegian Cottage Cheese** in Chapter 11). You can substitute anchovies for sardines if you are not making a special effort to reduce your salt intake. Another favorite spread is blended in a food processor from a can of red kidney beans (drained), ketchup, salsa, onion, and black and cayenne pepper (see **Mexican Bean Spread** in Chapter 11).

Both of these spreads serve equally well as dips for vegetables or toasted pita or bagel chips. Of course, there is always sliced turkey and ham, and if you choose the lean varieties you will have no trouble sticking within your fat-gram quota. However, if you wish to keep your saturated-fat intake down, you may want to skip meat for lunch most of the time. I do.

Some assortment, isn't it?

In the menus that follow, when I call for assorted fresh vegetables, just make a selection of sticks or slices of red or green bell pepper, carrots, celery, radishes, sliced tomatoes, cucumbers, summer squash, zucchini, Bermuda onion, scallions—whatever you like. Vary your choice from day to day.

I include an estimated total fat count for each lunch, assuming servings of average cafeteria size where I haven't spelled them out. *Values in parentheses for individual items are rounded, as are the totals, so please check out your true count when you implement my suggestions by looking up the fat contents of the foods according to the size of your portion in the Nutrient Counter in Appendix B.*

Although I just indicate "beverage" on these menus, you need to remember that skim or low-fat milk is usually recommended because it is one of the best sources of calcium. If you don't drink milk, you need to include one or more of the following every day in one of your meals in place of it, or you are likely to fall quite far below the RDA for calcium:

- Cottage cheese
- Fish with soft bones such as sardines or canned salmon
- No- or low-fat yogurt
- Salad greens such as spinach leaves (not lettuce) or other cooked greens (see Chapter 11 for recommendations)
- Nonfat dried milk in your soup recipes

Although I always suggest fruit for dessert, consider frozen yogurt when you want a sweet dessert other than fruit. If you can't find the no-fat kind, the packaged low-fat versions sold in supermarkets usually contain only 1–3 grams of fat per ½ cup. Frozen yogurt will help satisfy that calcium requirement as well. Sherbet and ices are good no-fat alternatives, too, but only milk sherbet will contain calcium.

When a recipe can be found in Chapter 11, the item will be set in **bold print**. (To locate these quickly, use the index to this book.)

Lunch 1

Mexican Bean Spread (1 g fat) or canned low-fat refried beans (2 g fat) served on a toasted bagel (1–2 g fat) or 2 flour or corn tortillas (2–5 g fat); salsa for seasoning; assorted raw vegetables; choice of fruit; beverage

Total fat: 4–9 g

Lunch 2

Italian Tuna Salad (6 g fat) served on lettuce or salad greens with assorted fresh vegetables; whole-wheat crackers (2–4 g fat); choice of fruit; beverage (Italian Tuna Salad also can be served as a sandwich)

Total fat: 8–10 g

Lunch 3

Soup Supreme (1 g fat) (or other broth-based canned or dry soup mix) served with your choice of crackers or toast (2–4 g fat); tossed vegetable salad with **Herb Dressing** or other dressing of your choice (2–3 g fat); choice of fruit; beverage

Total fat: 5–8 g

Lunch 4

Sliced turkey breast or lean ham (2 oz., 2 g fat) on multigrain roll or 2 slices rye bread (2–4 g fat) with choice of condiment or dressing—cranberry sauce and bean sprouts, or 1 teaspoon each mustard and mayonnaise (4 g fat), sliced tomato, lettuce leaves; pretzel sticks (1 oz., 1 g fat); choice of fruit; beverage

Total fat: 5–11 g

THE FOLLOWING FOUR LUNCHES HAVE A HIGHER CALCIUM CONTENT. THEY ARE MEANT FOR EVERYONE, OF COURSE, BUT ARE ESPECIALLY RECOMMENDED FOR PERSONS WHO DON'T DRINK MILK BUT DO USE OTHER DAIRY PRODUCTS:

Lunch 5

Norwegian Cottage Cheese (6 g fat) served on toast, bagel, or whole-grain crackers (2–4 g fat); assorted raw vegetables; choice of fruit; beverage

Total fat: 8–10 g

Lunch 6
Nonfat or low-fat yogurt with berries, banana, or other favorite fruit, mixed in a blender (0–2 g fat); assorted raw vegetables; whole-wheat crackers or pretzel sticks (2–4 g fat); beverage
Total fat: 2–6 g

Lunch 7
Salmon-Herb Spread (6 g fat) served on toast, bagel, or whole-grain crackers (2–4 g fat); assorted raw vegetables; choice of fruit; beverage
Total fat: 8–10 g

Lunch 8
Baked potato served with ½ cup low-fat cottage cheese (2–4 g fat) sprinkled with diced green onions and (optional) Cajun seasoning; tossed salad with low-fat dressing (2 g fat); choice of fruit; beverage
Total fat: 4–6 g

Here are the makings for one of my favorite sandwiches. I haven't included it among my recommended lunches because there are so many people who don't like plain sardines as much as I do. I include sardines and canned salmon quite frequently in my diet because, except for adding it to my cereal, I don't drink milk.

Sardine sandwich. Two large slices of dark pumpernickel bread, spread liberally with Grey Poupon mustard, 2 ounces of canned sardines, drained, squeeze of fresh lemon, thinly sliced tomato, and either a few bean sprouts or a leaf of romaine (9 g fat).

SPECIAL LOW-FAT LUNCHES
These lunches require a little more preparation, but they are still low in fat.

Lunch Special 1
Shrimp-Feta-Pasta Salad (5 g fat); breadsticks (2–4 g fat); choice of fruit; beverage
Total fat: 7–9 g

Lunch Special 2
Sweet-'n'-Savory Chicken Salad (2 g fat) served on leafy greens; whole-grain roll or triangle toast (2 g fat); choice of fruit; beverage
Total fat: 4 g

Lunch Special 3
Shrimpy Tomato Aspic (1 g fat); whole-grain crackers (2–4 g fat); choice of fruit; beverage
Total fat: 3–5 g

Lunch Special 4
Easy Bean Burritos for Two (2 burritos, 12 g fat); assorted raw vegetables; choice of fruit; beverage
Total fat: 12 g

Lunch Special 5
Collard Soup (6 g fat); whole-grain crackers or breadsticks (2–4 g fat); choice of fruit; beverage
Total fat: 8–10 g

WHERE'S THE BEEF, OR HOW OFTEN CAN I EAT A HIGH-FAT LUNCH?

Depending on your degree of indulgence at a given time, it's possible to fit some higher-fat choices at lunch into an overall low-fat eating plan. However, I try to avoid the high-fat lunches and save the major portion of my fat quota for the evening meal. I normally save meats such as beef or pork for dinner because it's difficult to eat a low-fat diet, especially one low in saturated fat, and include these meats on more than an occasional basis. I never order casseroles or sauces made with a high-fat dairy product. Sauces and casseroles containing more than a dab (and I really mean a dab) of butter, cream, or cheese have not been enticing to me for many years. The recipes included in the One Meal at a Time plan show you how to make creamy-tasting sauces and casseroles with a fraction of the usual fat content.

As for fried foods—forget them, regardless of the fat used in cooking. Frying changes fine, healthful foods like poultry, potatoes, and vegetables into junk foods: Foods normally low in fat suddenly triple their calories, of which two-thirds or more now come from fat.

Once again, let me emphasize two important ideas. First, you don't have to be perfect. Second, think in terms of "everyday foods" and "occasional foods." It's possible to include some high-fat dishes a couple of times a week and still be eating a healthful low-fat diet over time. The higher-fat dessert or the bar of candy should be thought of as an "occasional" food, eaten only once or twice a week.

To put it another way, *do not do a little bit of cheating every day!* Research shows that that's not likely to work. Over time, it will add up to more than what we might call *controlled cheating.* By thinking in terms of "occasional" foods, you can plan on including a higher-fat choice or two, once or twice a week. Planning in this way can help keep you satisfied without going over the limits that you will most certainly exceed with "just a little bit of this and a little bit of that" every day.

While you are learning where the fat is in your food, keep a fat-gram count every day and you will find out for yourself just how many times you can deviate from your basic low-fat eating plan and still, on the average, meet the goals you have set for yourself.

See Table 6–1, following the next section, for a summary of my suggestions for healthy low-fat lunches.

EATING LUNCH OUT ON THE ONE MEAL AT A TIME PROGRAM

Although it's getting easier and easier to find tasty low-fat foods in every kind of restaurant, there's no question about it: You are likely to find it much easier to manage a low-fat diet at home, after you have controlled your home eating environment, than to manage a low-fat diet eating out on a frequent basis. The temptations on the menu are ever present, and the dessert tray may be brought and settled on the table without a word of warning. And your luncheon companions may undercut your resolve unless they are of a similar mind.

To facilitate your success, you need to do some of the following (which I'll discuss in greater detail below):

- Find one or more restaurants that offer a good variety of low-fat selections.
- Discuss with your server (or the manager if necessary) your desire to have your favorite dishes prepared the way you want them, if you plan to eat at that restaurant often.
- If you eat lunch only at fast-food restaurants, you will be limited, and not likely to stick with those limitations day after day (check the Nutrient Counter in Appendix B for the selections in different fast-food establishments with the lowest fat).

- Just about all restaurants that prepare foods to order will make anything on the menu without added fat (except for the casseroles and dishes that by their nature are fatty—for examples, lobster Newburg); just ask.
- Order all dressings and sauces on the side.
- Save the higher-fat meal for a special occasion, out on the town, rather than cheat a little every day.

More and more restaurants are responding to the growing interest in eating a more healthful diet. Some are doing much more than a token response, and I suggest you search out one of these for most of your workday lunches, if not for the entire family for weekends and dinners, too.

Shoney's, the chain that I have been working with, has put a major emphasis on developing a variety of low-fat choices that can keep any appetite interested over a long period. Besides baked and char-broiled fish, shrimp, and chicken, there are light versions of lasagna and spaghetti. They serve turkey and ham sandwiches with low-fat mayonnaise or mustard. There is always a low-fat soup, averaging 2 grams of fat per bowl. It's actually possible to get soup, salad, and fruit from an extensive salad bar at about 3 grams of fat for the entire meal if you choose their low-fat salad dressing. A luncheon-size baked potato can be had with toppings coming in at about 12 grams of fat. All milk at company-owned stores is low-fat.

Even if you can't find a restaurant with choices similar to those offered by Shoney's, you can exert a major influence wherever you plan to eat on a frequent basis by asking for foods prepared as I have just described. Key words are *baked, broiled* (or *charbroiled*), *poached,* and *steamed.* Survey the menu and ask if whatever is being offered can be prepared for you in one of these ways. When I decided to lose 70 pounds back in 1963 there was only one little grill around the university where I could choose from the menu and have foods pre-pared the way I wanted. Once the owner understood my needs, I had no trouble ordering and I ate there almost every weekday.

Fast-food restaurants are also responding to the interest in eating a more healthful diet, but because of the way they pre-package and pre-prepare food, it is almost impossible for the cook to modify the standard offerings. You simply have to avoid the popular cheese-burger, fries, and shake (which together can total over 50 grams of fat) and go for the lowest-fat items available. Just about all fast-food restaurants will make a nutritional analysis pamphlet available to you if you ask. Normally, sliced turkey or grilled breast of chicken will be among the lowest-fat items, if available, but in some chains the added dressing can make the fat-gram count even of a roast chicken sandwich rather astronomical—20 grams or more! A fish sandwich cannot always be trusted, either. It may be deep fried and served with a high-fat dressing. Sometimes a plain hamburger with ketchup (not the regular mayonnaise-based dressing) is really the lowest-fat item on the menu. Check the Nutrient Counter in Appendix B for the latest information that was available to me at the time of publication for a number of fast-food chains.

If you must eat lunch away from home, don't forget the brown bag.

Except when I must eat a business lunch at a restaurant, I always brown-bag it when I go to my office. I can package almost any lunch I might eat at home to go, but I discovered that the major problem is taking the time to prepare it. If you wait until you are late for work and rushing to get out of the house, all can be lost.

That is, unless you grab for the luncheon meat and some bread (which I sometimes do), and keep nonperishable seasonings at the office. Of course, if there is a refrigerator at your office, keep a small selection of low-fat foods on hand. If there is a microwave oven, you can bring reheatable leftovers and soups in microwaveable containers.

Try making things that require extensive preparation—such as spreads and some of the salad mixtures—the night before.

Some of my friends keep bread, crackers, and fruit at the office just in case they are caught without something to eat and hunger strikes. I, too, like to keep the breadstuffs handy at the office, but I prefer to carry fresh fruit from home.

Finally, just as for breakfast, *take your time.* Work at lunch for at least a week. Take longer if it means finding a selection of restaurants or settling on a routine for preparing brown-bag lunches. Once you have the luncheon problem licked, you're halfway there!

TABLE 6–1.   LUNCH TIPS AND SUGGESTIONS

Whole-grain breads, bagels, English muffins, or whole-grain rolls are best for sandwiches (1–2 g fat). Croissants contain 12–20 grams of fat each.

For zesty low-fat condiments or sandwich spreads, experiment with a variety of mustards or salsas (no fat) in place of mayonnaise (11 grams per tablespoon).

Choose turkey or lean ham (1–2 g fat per ounce) as sandwich meats rather than high-fat cold cuts like bologna or salami (6–8 g fat per ounce).

Broth-based soups like chicken noodle, minestrone, and vegetable (2–3 g fat per cup) contain at least 80 percent less fat than cream- or cheese-based soups.

Use pretzels or breadsticks (1 g fat per ounce) as crunchy accompaniments to sandwiches instead of potato or nacho chips (10 g fat per ounce).

Skip the cheese on sandwiches (8–10 g fat per ounce) or use a reduced-fat variety.

Choose lower-fat crackers (and preferably whole grain), saltines, flatbread, melba toast, matzoh, oyster crackers, or graham crackers instead of higher-fat snack crackers.

For brown-bag treats, choose lower-fat cookies like fig bars, gingersnaps, animal crackers, graham crackers, and cereal-marshmallow bars.

Cut up raw vegetables and store in water in an airtight plastic container in the refrigerator. They will stay fresh and crispy for lunches, snacks, or cooking.

Keep a supply of canned tuna (water packed), salmon, sardines, clams, and crabmeat. Try them with different condiments, low-fat dressings, or as sandwich spreads.

Mix cottage cheese with dry soup mix, Cajun seasoning, salsa, clams, or any of your preferred herbs or seasonings.

At the salad bar, fill up on vegetables, garbanzo beans, and fruit. Use only small amounts of meats, cheese, eggs, and mayonnaise-based salads.

Add regular salad dressing with discretion (7 g fat per tablespoon) or try the low-fat commercial dressings.

LUNCH SHOPPING LIST

Fruits

apples_____

bananas_____

berries_____

grapes_____

melon_____

nectarines/tangerines_____

oranges_____

peaches_____

pears_____

pineapple_____

plums_____

raisins_____

other dried fruit_____

other fruit_____

fruit juices_____

Vegetables

alfalfa sprouts_____

beans, dried_____

beans, refried, canned_____

beans, garbanzo_____

bell peppers_____

broccoli_____

carrots_____

cauliflower_____

celery_____

cucumber_____

green onions_____

lettuce_____

onions_____

potatoes_____

squash (summer, zucchini)____

tomatoes_____

Bread and Grains

whole-grain bread_____

mixed-grain bread_____

rye or pumpernickel_____

bagels_____

English muffins_____

pita bread_____

sandwich rolls_____

corn or flour tortillas_____

breadsticks_____

croutons_____

pretzels_____

saltines, whole wheat_____

other crackers_____

pasta, noodles_____

Milk and Dairy Products

skim or low-fat milk_____

nonfat yogurt_____

nonfat dry milk_____

low-fat cottage cheese_____

low-fat sliced cheese_____

other cheese_____

Meats, Fish, Poultry

clams, canned_____

ham, lean_____

roast beef, lean_____

salmon, canned_____

sardines, canned_____

tuna, canned in water_____

turkey breast, sliced_____

Miscellaneous

ketchup_____

cranberry sauce_____

dressings (no- or low-cal)_____

mayonnaise (reduced fat)_____

mustards_____

salsa_____

soups (broth based)_____

broth or bouillon_____

coffee_____

tea_____

soda or seltzer_____

seasonings, spices_____

other_____

CHAPTER 7

DINNER

Of all the meals you eat at home, the evening meal is probably the one that takes the most creativity. It's usually the largest meal of the day, so there are several different foods to prepare. If several people are eating together, there may be different tastes to satisfy. However, changing to a low-fat style of cooking is relatively easy once you discover the array of foods that are available and understand some general principles.

I think you can be well on your way to managing your evening meals in a week, but plan on taking two if you want to sample more of my fantastic recipes. After that, you can go on and experiment with creating your own. You might enjoy doing what I sometimes do—study the cookbooks written by the great chefs of the world and figure out how to alter interesting recipes when they are too high in fat. You will find that you almost always can cut the fat by at least 50 percent. With the careful addition of other liquids (for example, broth instead of fat) and thickeners (a little extra cornstarch or flour to low-fat milk in place of cream), you can still preserve the flavor and much of the texture that make these recipes great.

Your first step is to consider the dishes you customarily prepare for dinner. If you are like most people, you rotate your evening meals around 10 to 12 different main courses, simply prepared, occasionally with small variations. People who work outside the home are often especially concerned with ease and speed of preparation—we don't have a great amount of time to spend making dinner on most weekdays.

Besides our basic everyday 10 to 12, we need some festive recipes for special events. Even though we can deviate from our low-fat meals on occasion without defeating our objective, it would be much to our advantage if these festive recipes were also low in fat.

Here are the basic requirements for success:

- First and foremost, if any new recipe is going to become part of your standard repertoire, then everyone who shares the dish must like it. Not many people want to cook several different meals for different members of the family.
- We need to cover the full range of foods you like to eat as your main course: basic meat, poultry, fish, pasta, casseroles, and combination dishes, such as beans and rice.
- We need ways to make the starches and other vegetables interesting and satisfying, with herbs, spices, and only limited amounts of fat.
- We want some appetizers, soups, salads, breadstuffs, and of course desserts.
- The ingredients should be easy to obtain and the recipes fun to prepare.
- As a rule, the evening meal should contain a maximum of between 20 and 30 grams of fat for women who are not out to lose weight (assuming that you have restricted your intake to approximately 20 grams earlier in the day and are aiming at a quota of 40 to 50 grams). Men, with a fat-gram quota of about 60 per day, should simply use larger portions; there is no need for different preparation or different foods.

SOME GENERAL PRINCIPLES

There are two key words here: *choice* and *style.*

When it comes to *choice* of foods, you know exactly what to buy for the dozen or so meals you like to eat at the present time. But in choosing foods such as beef, pork, and poultry, you may be selecting cuts that have twice the fat, or even more, than lean cuts, which can be just as tender and tasty. You also may be making unnecessarily fat-laden choices for appetizers, soups, and desserts.

As for *style* of cooking, unless your recipes have been specifically designed to be low in fat, almost all of them that call for fatty ingredients may contain 50 to 75 percent *more added* fat than they actually need.

My dinner menus and recipes are designed to show you how to make good choices among low-fat foods and to make you an expert in a low-fat style of cooking.

First, here is some important background information.

Let's deal with the choice of meats, fish, poultry, and dairy products. I'll talk in terms of a typical 3.5-ounce serving, which is the serving size you will see in most nutrient counters. In order for you to translate the percentages that you see on packaging when the fat is not stated in grams, remember that 3.5 ounces equals 100 grams almost exactly. Thus, any food labeled 10 percent fat will have 10 grams of fat per 3.5-ounce, or 100-gram, serving, and so on. This knowledge can be important in making a good choice of meat from the supermarket butcher shop, where only the percentage of fat or lean, and not grams, may be mentioned. Perhaps the new labeling regulations will help clarify this situation, but in one market the ground beef or turkey may say "not less than 88 percent lean," while in another market it may say "not more than 12 percent fat." It's up to you to calculate the grams per ounce or per serving.

In the following discussion, I round the figures for clarity and contrast. When you are keeping records, look up the more exact figures in the Nutrient Counter in Appendix B.

BEEF

Fatty roasts and steaks will have from 20 to 30 grams of fat per 3.5-ounce serving, cooked. Thus they run between 20 and 30 percent fat content, by weight. Fatty steaks include ribeye, T-bone, sirloin, New York strip, and porterhouse, while fatty roasts include blade, chuck, rib, and brisket.

Lean roasts and steaks, with visible fat trimmed, will all run between 6 and 9 grams of fat for a 3.5-ounce serving, cooked. These lean meats are thus only about 6 to 9 percent fat, by weight. Lean steaks include flank, club, tenderloin, and London broil (round steak), and lean roasts include eye of round, round, and sirloin tip. Rump tends to fall in between the lean and fatty cuts, with about 15 grams of fat per serving.

Of course, if you could trim *all* the visible fat from the fatty meats, you might cut the fat by half or more, but most people do not trim that well! It takes patience and a very sharp knife. Besides, no matter how well you trim, you are still left with the fat that runs throughout the muscle. It shows up as the fine ivory-colored strands, or marbling. While food scientists can do it in a laboratory for analysis, the average person (including myself) will not want to develop the skill or take the time to trim a chuck or other fatty roast or a ribeye or other fatty steak to the point where it is as devoid of fat as the more naturally lean cuts.

Remember: Fat left on meat during cooking melts and permeates the lean tissue, doubling the fat content of the meat you end up eating.

When it comes to hamburger, there are as yet no standards set by law that regulate labeling in the supermarket. Although the Department of Agriculture and other branches of the government are working on rules and legislation, at the present time "lean" in some stores may be under 10 percent fat whereas in others it may be 15 percent fat. I was in one supermarket where the "lean" was 20 percent fat! I suggest you look for lean that is no more than 10–12 percent fat. Regular hamburger is usually *at least* 22 percent fat, but in some stores it may be as high as 30 percent. *Ground chuck is not lean!* It is often just as high in fat as regular hamburger. Ground round is leaner, but you have to ask the butcher about the fat content. It may be considerably higher than 10 percent. If you have a microwave oven, you can remove much of the fat from hamburger by shaping it in the form of a doughnut, placing it in a microwave-safe plastic colander which in turn is placed on top of a microwave-safe plate to catch the fat, and heating it on high for about two minutes (time will vary depending on the wattage of your oven). If your oven does not have a turntable, rotate once during heating.

In some areas of the country it is possible to purchase beefalo—a cross between a cow and a bison. Beefalo is naturally lean, with only 1 to 2 grams of fat per ounce, and almost no cholesterol. It's very delicate in flavor and very tender. Because it is so much higher in lean tissue relative to fat by weight, it tends to be a little watery in texture (muscle is 60 to 70 percent water; fat tissue is about 80 percent fat, only 20 percent water). Although it takes a little more care in preparation, try it if it is available.

PORK AND HAM

If you like pork (and I have some particularly fine recipes for a pork tenderloin and pork scallopine), keep in mind that the tenderloin is the only naturally lean part of the pig. Well trimmed, it will run about 5 grams of fat per 3.5-ounce serving, or just about 5 percent fat. Some producers trim the loin roast so well that it, too, can be very lean—only about 10 percent fat. (A loin is not the same as a tenderloin. It comes from a different part of the pig and, untrimmed, contains 20 to 30 percent fat.) If you choose the loin, examine the packaged product carefully for the amount of visible fat. You will see fairly thick ribbons or layers of fat on the outside of the meat if it has not been well trimmed. To be sure of the fat content, you have to inquire. In some cases the butcher in the shop can tell you, but in others you will have to write or call the processing company. If the loin looks too fatty, ask the butcher to save you the trouble by trimming it for you and then repackaging it. My butcher never charges extra for this—but I'll never forget my surprise the first time he did this for me. It came back half the size!

Just recently, pork with much less saturated fat has been developed. I haven't seen it in Nashville, but I am sure it will be well advertised and labeled as it gets introduced in new markets.

Many packagers of ham have already responded to the interest in reducing fat in the diet with very lean baked and boiled ham. It contains only 1 gram of fat per ounce, or about 3.5 grams per 3.5-ounce serving. When you buy ham, examine the label to be sure you are picking the lean variety. Packages of lean ham may advertise the fat contents boldly on the front, since they can claim to be 95 or 96 percent "lean" or "fat free."

If you prepare a ham butt or shank yourself, and trim it well, you can get it down to about 10 grams of fat per 3.5-ounce serving. Left untrimmed, these cuts may contain twice as much fat or more.

POULTRY

Here are a few rules of thumb for the fat content of chicken and turkey:

Slightly more than half the fat is in and around the skin.

Dark meat has about twice the fat of white meat.

Frying doubles the fat content.

Coating with flour and frying will triple the fat content because the flour holds fat.

Batter-dipping and frying can increase the fat content five- or six-fold. Batter is even better at holding fat than flour.

White meat without skin has about 1 gram of fat per ounce, or 3.5 grams of fat per 3.5-ounce serving.

Dark meat without skin has about 2 grams of fat per ounce, or about 7 grams of fat per 3.5-ounce serving.

You can calculate the fat contents for servings of different sizes based on these figures.

WATCH OUT WHEN BUYING GROUND TURKEY!

Ground turkey has become very popular as a result of our growing awareness of its low fat content. However, many producers throw in as much fat as they dare to, and still hope to get away with it. Whereas the breast of turkey, at 3.5 grams of fat per 3.5 ounces, is only about 3.5 percent fat, ground turkey with 15 percent fat or more is common. That's because the skin and the fat beneath the skin may be included when the meat is ground. Read the label of the pre-packaged brands, and ask the butcher about the fat content of the store-packaged variety. Ground turkey need be no more than 5 percent fat, so look for packages that say "95 percent lean."

Since the skin and fat make the poultry more juicy and tasty, I have concentrated on finding ways of preparing it that can compensate for the fat reduction in my recipes.

SATURATED FAT AND CHOLESTEROL IN MEAT AND POULTRY

To be exact, you must look up the figures for saturated fat and cholesterol for each kind and cut of meat and poultry.

I have, however, a few other rules of thumb that will help you keep quite good track of your saturated fat, and fairly good track of your cholesterol:

Beef fat is about 40 percent saturated.

Pork fat is about 35 percent saturated.

Poultry fat is about 30 percent saturated.

Thus, if you multiply the total fat-gram content of beef, pork, or poultry in any fat counter by 0.4, 0.35, or 0.3, respectively, you will be quite close to the true saturated-fat content of those meats. The rest of the fat is primarily monounsaturated.

Here are a few examples:

A fatty rib roast has 30 grams of fat per 3.5-ounce serving. Using my rule of thumb and multiplying by 0.40, you get roughly 12 grams of saturated fat per serving.

An eye of round, well trimmed, has 6.5 grams of fat per 3.5-ounce serving. At 40 percent saturated, that's only about 2.6 grams of saturated fat per serving. *By choosing a lean cut, you have reduced your intake of total fat and saturated fat by over three-quarters.*

But you can do even better with poultry.

A similar size serving of white-meat chicken or turkey would have only 3 grams of fat per 3.5-ounce serving, of which only about 30 percent is saturated. *Thus, by eating chicken or turkey, you are down to about 1 gram of saturated fat per serving.*

This is worth thinking about:

A single small portion of a fatty cut of beef can bring us very close to the upper limit of saturated-fat intake if our goal is to keep saturated fat below 10 percent of total calories. We get about 115 calories of saturated fat in a single serving of a fatty roast, which is dangerously close to 10 percent of calories—that is, 160 to 180 for someone eating 1,600 to 1,800 calories per day.

Switch to the lean roast that I recommend and you get only about 23 calories of saturated fat, or just one-fifth the amount contained in the fatty cut. You do even better with white meat of poultry—only about 9 calories in saturated fat.

Is it any wonder nutritionists put so much emphasis on switching a good part of your meat intake to poultry in place of red meat, and on choosing the lean cuts of beef when you do eat meat? As you will see in a moment, you are even farther ahead on the saturated-fat count when you substitute fish.

Cholesterol tends to run from about 50 milligrams per serving to almost 100 milligrams, in the muscle parts of both meat and poultry. (Organ meats, such as heart and liver, can be from two to eight times higher, so they ought to be used sparingly if not avoided completely.) Cholesterol is evenly distributed throughout the meat, so, ounce per ounce, lean cuts have as much cholesterol as fatty cuts. If you figure about 75 milligrams for every 3.5-ounce serving of meat or poultry, your rough count will be fairly accurate over time.

FISH

The fat contained in fish does not pose the same kind of health problem as fat found in meat. While too much fat of any kind may compound a weight problem, *even the most fatty fish tend to have only as much fat as the leanest meats.* In the case of the cold-water fish, such as salmon, mackerel, bluefish, and tuna, the omega-3 fatty acids that comprise a large part of the fat content seem to have a protective effect with respect to heart disease.

Light-colored, flaky, delicately flavored varieties of fish such as flounder, pike, haddock, snapper, and grouper run around 1 to 2 grams of fat for a 3.5-ounce serving. The fatty varieties such as salmon and tuna may run about 7 grams per 3.5-ounce serving. If you like fish steaks, swordfish has about half the fat compared with salmon and tuna, and halibut is almost as lean as the light fillets.

Contrary to what many people think, there is some saturated fat and cholesterol in fish. However, saturated fat comprises only about 20 to 25 percent of the total fat content. The rest is made up primarily of monounsaturated and polyunsaturated fatty acids. Thus you get less than 0.5 gram of saturated fat per 3.5 ounces of the less fatty fish, and only about 1.5 grams per 3.5 ounces of the fatty varieties.

The cholesterol content tends to run between 50 and 75 milligrams per 3.5-ounce serving, except for shellfish, which contain about 125 milligrams.

Because the consumption of fish is so clearly related to a lower rate of heart disease around the world, we should be eating more of it as we decrease our consumption of other animal products. I will show you a variety of ways to make fish really tasty. I have a special reason to be proud of my fish recipes, and a fond memory of how I learned.

For many years, every fish dish I ever made was a failure. My fish dishes were either too dry, too fishy tasting, or simply lacking in flavor. I thought I could never make fish well, and we had stopped preparing it in our home. But one afternoon, while on vacation and driving along a street in Miami with a commodore of the New York Yacht Club who had a second home in that city, I mentioned my ineptitude. He made a U-turn immediately, right in the middle of traffic, scaring the living daylights out of me and the other passengers in the car, and drove straight to his favorite fish market. That night he showed me how to prepare three varieties of fish—and I have been at it ever since.

A NOTE ON FAT CONTENT AND CALORIES

Ounce per ounce, gram per gram, the higher the fat content, the higher the calories. The increase tends to be disproportionate because fat contains 9 calories per gram and both carbohydrate and protein contain only 4. Thus, when you increase fat just 1 gram, replacing a gram of protein in meat, you gain 5 calories. Obviously the converse is true: Replace a gram of fat with a gram of protein (or carbohydrate) and you lose 5 calories. Table 7–1 contains some surprising comparisons *among equal-weight, 3.5-ounce servings* of a few examples of the meat and fish I have just been comparing. *Just look at how the total calories go down when you replace the fat with lean tissue in equal amounts of meat, poultry, and fish.* It's no wonder that people who cut the fat in their diets lose weight.

As you study the Nutrient Counter in Appendix B you will discover many more interesting comparisons among the different meat, poultry, and fish cuts and dishes in total and saturated fat, and in calories. In general, the values in Table 7–1 are representative of the difference between the fatty and lean cuts of meat and the fatty and lean varieties of fish and poultry.

I'm making all these comparisons and doing all this counting for informational purposes only. Just follow the One Meal at a Time program and let the correct choices of foods become second nature.

TABLE 7–1. COMPARISON OF FAT CONTENTS AND CALORIES IN 3.5-OUNCE PORTIONS OF MEAT AND FISH (COOKED)

Food[a]	Total Fat (grams)	Saturated Fat (grams)	Calories
Beef			
Prime rib roast	30.0	12.7	367
Sirloin steak	18.7	7.7	278
Eye of round	6.5	2.5	183
Pork			
Loin chop	22.5	8.8	314
Tenderloin	4.8	1.6	155
Poultry			
Chicken (batter, fried)	17.4	4.6	289
Turkey, dark with skin	11.5	3.5	221
Turkey, white meat only	3.2	1.0	157
Fish			
Salmon steak	7.4	2.0	182
Swordfish steak	4.0	1.1	118
Grouper	1.3	0.4	87

[a]You can reduce the fat and calories in the fatty cuts considerably by trimming well, but much of the fat is found marbled among the muscle strands and cannot be removed easily.

I promised you no need to count once you've learned where the fat is in your food, and no counting there need be! In Chapter 9 I present an analysis of the nutritional value of the One Meal at a Time menus combined over a two-week period. Just put them all together, any combination you like, and you come out where you need to be—no counting.[1]

PASTA, COMBINATION DISHES, AND STIR-FRY

The more you switch from animal products to pastas, combination dishes, and stir-fry meals, the lower your fat intake will become.

Over the years, pasta has become a mainstay at our house. We have experimented with different sauces, and, for our tastes, we have absolutely perfected a number of different ones: clam, meat, turkey, and vegetable. If you know how to get the fat out of the meat before cooking, you can reduce the fat content in your meat sauces by half or more, with no loss of flavor.

We have searched our supermarkets and health-food stores and found a variety of interesting pastas. We sometimes mix the regular, enriched-flour variety with whole wheat, spinach, Jerusalem artichoke, or any other variety that looks inviting. Some whole-wheat spaghettis are pretty mealy. You may have to try several different brands to find one you like.

Besides spaghetti with sauce, we have excellent recipes for spinach lasagna and cannelloni in Chapter 11.

As the design of tasty low-fat recipes became more important in helping people in the Vanderbilt program and in my own writing, I began to experiment with bean recipes—beans and rice or pasta, and chiles. You won't believe how good a meatless, virtually fat-free bean dish can be. If you are worried about the aftereffects of eating a large helping of beans as a main course, your system will likely adapt if you make beans a regular part of your diet. You may also have to experiment with different varieties of beans. Much of the extra gas in the system is formed by the microorganisms in your intestines associated with the digestion of beans; the kind and numbers of them can change as you change your diet. However, certain kinds of beans can remain a problem for some people. Some people adapt to limas,

[1]I present a more detailed discussion of the percentage of total calories as fat and the percentage of total fat as saturated fat in meat and fish in Appendix A.

but not to pintos, and vice versa. I have a number of tasty bean recipes and I normally use a combination of three or more different beans in a recipe because I like the different colors.

I have an all-time favorite greens casserole that can be used as a main or side dish. You can substitute any of your favorite greens in this recipe. It's another dish that we make in double quantities, so that we can feast on it for two or three days.

Finally, stir-fry dishes. You don't need a wok; I don't like to use one over an electric stove, anyway. We use a several-layered, thick-bottomed, stainless-steel frying pan that heats evenly, and throw in anything that's handy in the way of vegetables. You can add chopped or sliced meat, chicken or fish, fresh or leftover.

Except for the greens casserole, all of the dishes I've just described have minimal fat. Increased use of meals described in this section is the key to a really low-fat diet. Play around with my recipes until they suit your individual tastes and those of your family.

BASIC CONVENIENT MEAL PLANS FOR ONE MEAL AT A TIME DINNERS

I am going to show you a total of 14 dinner menus based mostly on simple, basic recipes. I include a few that I call "special" because, well, they are special. They are so good, I want very much for you to try them. They take only a little more work, and you might want to use them on a weekend or for company.

You can be very flexible on the One Meal at a Time program as long as you don't overdo the beef or pork as main courses. I like to keep beef and/or pork down to a maximum of twice a week (total for both), and in practice we rarely have beef or pork more than once. We have chicken once or twice, fish once or twice, and pasta, stir-fry, and beans and rice an average of once each week. I say *average,* because when it comes to pasta and bean dishes, I make gobs and gobs—enough for two or three days! Once you taste my recipes, I think you will do the same. If you don't like to eat the same dish two days in a row, my recipes will keep for several days in the refrigerator, and for months in the freezer.

To start you off, and introduce my approach to preparing lean meat, I include a beef and a pork recipe each week. The rest of the days contain fish, poultry, pasta, a casserole or a stir-fry, and a combination dish. Although you can meet One Meal at a Time program guidelines with beef or pork twice a week, as soon as you see how good my other recipes taste, I think you will want to limit your choice of either beef or pork to just once a week and replace the second serving with a recipe that contains less saturated fat.

Between the suggestions I give you below and my other recipes in Chapter 11, I am, of course, giving you a large pool from which to choose what will ultimately become your favorite basic 10 or 12 recipes. Since all of my recommendations are so good, perhaps you will end up enlarging your repertoire beyond the usual limits.

If you don't think you will like my specific suggestions, you can substitute!
There are three ways to substitute:

1. Choose another recipe from the same category of food from Chapter 11—for example, one fish dish for another, one beef or pork dish for another, and so on.
2. Prepare one of your own favorites from the same category of food, but with minimal fat, using my guidelines in Table 7–2.
3. Select from any category that is lower in fat, especially saturated fat. From high to low, go down from beef, to pork, then chicken, fish, pasta, stir-fry, or a combination dish (these last three are usually equally low in fat).

TABLE 7–2.   DINNER TIPS AND SUGGESTIONS FOR YOUR OWN RECIPES

Three ways to lower the fat content of your regular, family-favorite recipes:
  1. Substitute lower-fat ingredients.
  2. Alter the basic method of preparation.
  3. Reduce the amount of fat added.

For example:

1. Lean cuts of meat like flank or round steak, *well-trimmed* sirloin, London broil, or pork tenderloin have only one-quarter to one-third the fat of ribeyes or chuck. If you don't trim well before cooking, the melted fat seeps between the lean muscle fibers and doubles that fat content of the cooked lean meat.

To tenderize lean meats, marinate for several hours with wine, soy sauce, or fruit juice (anything slightly acidic) and seasonings.

Choose extra-lean ground beef, ground round, or ground turkey (1–3 g fat per ounce) rather than regular ground beef (10 g fat per ounce).

2. Use lower-fat preparation methods like baking, roasting, broiling, grilling, poaching, steaming, or boiling rather than frying or cooking in fat. Frying can increase the fat content from two to six times, depending upon the use of flour or batter.

3. Unless specifically designed as low-fat recipes, use only one-third to one-half of the fat called for.

To help you implement these three basic approaches:

Flavor vegetables with herbs and seasonings rather than added fat. If you generally add meat fat to beans or vegetables, use an ounce or two of lean ham for meaty flavor.

Stock these low-fat kitchen essentials: nonstick vegetable spray, broth or stock, nonfat yogurt, canned evaporated skim milk, and an assortment of seasonings and spices.

Sauté vegetables in a nonstick skillet with cooking spray, broth, or wine rather than oil or butter.

When using shredded cheese (8–10 g fat per ¼ cup) in a recipe or casserole, use less of a stronger cheese like sharp cheddar.

Blend low-fat cottage cheese with a touch of lemon juice for a creamy baked potato topping.

Substitute canned evaporated skim milk or skim milk with nonfat dry milk added for recipes that call for cream or whole milk.

Plan a meatless meal one or two nights a week. Try legumes and rice or pasta with a vegetable sauce.

"Oven"-fry instead of frying in fat—spray a baking dish with vegetable spray and bake at a high temperature, turning at least once. Dip fish or chicken in milk or egg whites and coat with seasoned breadcrumbs.

When a recipe calls for canned cream soup, substitute at least one can with an equal volume of evaporated skim milk with cornstarch or flour added as a thickener.

Basic everyday, low-fat desserts include fresh fruit, angel cake, low-fat cookies, low-fat puddings, frozen yogurt, ice milk, and sherbet.

In the menus that follow, I have alternated among the main-dish categories I've just mentioned in an arbitrary order that you can feel free to change. I start with pasta, using a red clam sauce, just to convince you that you can make a fantastic spaghetti sauce with hardly any fat. I have never had a better red clam sauce than this one. In fact, I have never had a better spaghetti sauce of any kind, period. But if you don't like clams, choose another sauce from Chapter 11. They are all excellent.

You can also substitute one vegetable for another, one dessert for another, and so on, but remember: Eat a wide variety of different foods. I have kept vegetable preparation simple in the menus by usually just calling for them "plain"; that is, prepare the specified vegetable by steaming, in a microwave, or using a little water in a saucepan. If you have time to fuss a bit, try any of my vegetable recipes (Chapter 11) in place of what is called for in the sample meal plan. Suit your own preferences for what goes well together. Make yellow and green vegetables, plus different varieties from the cabbage family (broccoli, cauliflower, kale, mustard greens, brussels sprouts, and green, red, and Chinese cabbage), mainstays of your diet. Have some raw vegetables as salad every day.

Do not limit yourself to the same two or three vegetables over and over, day after day. If you do, you may be cheating yourself of the complete nutritional value that I have included with the variety contained in the following menus. You can, of course, have some form of lettuce and tomato every day if you like them in your salads, but don't limit yourself only to these vegetables.

I know desserts are an important part of the dinner meal for most people. I like to focus on fresh fruit, but I include a number of suggestions (and recipes in Chapter 11) for satisfying low-fat sweets in my menus. If you like a sweet to finish your evening meal, feel free to add a no-fat or very low-fat treat in those menus where we have chosen to omit it. We have had people in the Vanderbilt program who finish every evening meal with no-fat or low-fat frozen yogurt (0–3 grams of fat per ½ cup), which they use to replace the 12–20 grams of fat they used to eat in ice cream. Frozen yogurt will pose no danger to a low-fat diet unless you polish it off by the quart. However, in my own case, I prefer to snack on popcorn after dinner, rather than include a sweet dessert.

Recipes set in **bold print** will be found in Chapter 11. The fat-gram contents are calculated on standard-size portions, as indicated in the recipes. Fractions of a gram, 0.5 or higher, are rounded up. All of the meals are designed so that you can, if you wish, almost always add a teaspoon of butter or margarine as spread or seasoning (4 grams of total fat per teaspoon) and still fall within my recommendations for your fat-gram quota. In addition, as I mentioned above, the fat contents of the meals are low enough for you to substitute frozen yogurt or a low-fat dessert from Chapter 11 for whatever dessert I've suggested on the menu. If you do add the fat or substitute a dessert slightly higher in fat content, be sure to include it in your daily total as you learn to use the One Meal at a Time program. By the time you reach the end of the course, you will know just how much you can add at each meal and still stay within your fat-gram quota and meet your percentage fat goal over the long run.

Dinner 14 is my "Graduation Menu." It contains some of my

favorite, special recipes, including **Oysters Rockefeller** and **Pork Scallopine in Lemon, Dill, and Fennel Sauce.** Invite your friends over to celebrate, and prove to them that not only is following a low-fat diet good for your health, it tastes good, too. (Both the oysters and the scallopine are complemented with a glass of dry white wine. I recommend a sauvignon blanc, which is also an excellent wine for using in the pork recipe.)

Dinner 1

Pasta with **Red Clam Sauce** (5 g fat); tossed salad; no- or low-cal dressing (2 tablespoons = 0–3 g fat); **No-Knead Herb Bread** (3 g fat per slice); seasonal fruit; 2 **Gingerbread Cookies** (1 g fat each); beverage

Total fat: 10–13 g

Dinner 2

Flank steak with **Simple Beef Marinade** (9 g fat); baked potato; green beans and water chestnuts; tossed salad; no- or low-cal dressing (2 tablespoons = 0–3 g fat); slice of whole-grain bread (1 g fat); citrus fruit cup; beverage

Total fat: 10–13 g

Dinner 3

Fish Fillet in Lemon-Tarragon Sauce (5 g fat); ½ baked acorn squash with 1 teaspoon butter or margarine (4 g fat); brussels sprouts or other green vegetable; fresh fruit salad; **Herb-Bran Muffin** (4 g fat); beverage

Total fat: 13 g

Dinner 4

Champ Beans (1 g fat) with ½ cup brown or wild rice (1 g fat); broccoli; tossed salad; no- or low-cal dressing (2 tablespoons = 0–3 g fat); 2-inch hard roll (2 g fat); nonfat or low-fat frozen yogurt with berries (0–3 g fat per ½ cup); beverage

Total fat: 4–10 g

Dinner 5

Barbecued Chicken (6 g fat); corn on the cob; asparagus; tossed salad; no- or low-cal dressing (2 tablespoons = 0–3 g fat); slice of whole-grain bread (1 g fat); **Fruit Crisp** (4 g fat per serving); beverage

Total fat: 11–14 g

Dinner 6
Roast Pork Tenderloin (6 g fat); baked sweet potato; cauliflower; tossed salad; no- or low-cal dressing (2 tablespoons = 0–3 g fat); slice of whole-grain bread (1 g fat); beverage
Total fat: 7–10 g

Dinner 7
Turkey or Chicken Divan (10 g fat); **Glazed Orange-Spice Carrots**; ½ cup brown rice (1 g fat); 2-inch hard roll (2 g fat); angel cake with fudge topping (1/12th cake with 2 tablespoons sauce = 1 g fat); beverage
Total fat: 14 g

Dinner 8
Pasta with **Thick and Zesty Spaghetti Sauce** (10 g fat per serving); zucchini; tossed salad; no- or low-cal dressing (2 tablespoons = 0–3 g fat); Italian bread (1 g fat per slice); fresh fruit of choice; 2 fig-bar cookies (2 g fat); beverage
Total fat: 13–16 g

Dinner 9
Teriyaki Beef Stir-fry (12 g fat per serving); ½ cup brown or wild rice (1 g fat); tossed salad; no- or low-cal dressing (2 tablespoons = 0–3 g fat); 2-inch hard roll (2 g fat); fresh fruit cup; beverage
Total fat: 15–18 g

Dinner 10
Royal Indian Salmon (8 g fat); steamed new potatoes; **Greens Casserole** (6 g fat per serving); tossed salad; no- or low-cal dressing (2 tablespoons = 0–3 g fat); slice of whole-grain bread (1 g fat); **Pineapple-Orange Frozen Yogurt** (0–2 g fat per ½ cup); beverage
Total fat: 15–20 g

Dinner 11
Easy Vegetarian Chili Texas Style (2 g fat); ½ cup brown or wild rice (1 g fat); asparagus or other green vegetable; **Crusty Buttermilk Cornbread** (1 g fat); citrus fruit cup; beverage
Total fat: 4 g

Dinner 12
Chicken Cacciatore (5 g fat); 1 cup pasta (1 g fat); green beans; tossed salad; no- or low-cal dressing (2 tablespoons = 0–3 g fat); Italian bread (1 g fat per slice); angel cake with berries; beverage
Total fat: 7–10 g

Dinner 13
Dijon Swordfish (11 g fat); **Beets to Beat All** (2 g fat); ½ cup brown rice (1 g fat); slice of whole-grain bread (1 g fat); tossed salad; no- or low-cal dressing (2 tablespoons = 0–3 g fat); **Baked Apple** (1 g fat each); beverage
Total fat: 16–19 g

Dinner 14
Oysters Rockefeller (5 g fat); **Pork Scallopine in Lemon, Dill, and Fennel Sauce** (10 g fat); green peas; **Cauliflower with Crumb Topping** (2 g fat); tossed salad; no- or low-cal dressing (2 tablespoons = 0–3 g fat); fresh fruit; beverage
Total fat: 17–20 g

FROZEN DINNERS

I have tried several brands of frozen entrees and complete dinners. Unfortunately, no brand has turned out to be consistently good, in my opinion. Often the vegetables have a rubbery consistency. Frequently the sauces are sweetened too much for my taste. Even more often, they are too salty. I hate to read the labels because many of the ingredients don't sound like food at all. Except to taste-test, I have *never* bought a frozen entree or dinner because I liked it!

Nevertheless, I realize that sometimes it may be more convenient to throw a frozen dinner in the oven or microwave than to cook something yourself. Many food processors have introduced low-fat brands of frozen foods recently. You are going to have to experiment for yourself to find the flavors and textures you like. Your major consideration should be to keep the fat grams equivalent to the meal you might make yourself. This usually means about 20 or less. Second, look to keep the cholesterol down and sodium at or below about 1,000 milligrams. With respect to sodium, it is possible to find some reasonably good frozen entrees and dinners at only 500 or 600 milligrams. You must read the labels.

To round out the nutritional value of a frozen-food dinner, add a vegetable salad and fruit for dessert if you have not had fruit with your other meals or as a snack. By and large, these additions will make the meal as nutritious as one of my own suggested menus.

EATING DINNER OUT ON THE ONE MEAL AT A TIME PROGRAM

I want to start by repeating the advice I gave you in the preceding chapter:

It is much better to eat a high-fat meal only once or twice a week than to "cheat" a little every day.

Cheating a little every day will tend to add up to much more fat in the end than the occasional high-fat meal. Thus, if you eat out only once or twice a week, you can save your high-fat meal for a restaurant treat. However, I strongly suggest that instead of a high-fat "meal" you think only of a high-fat "dish" as a special treat within the meal. That is, if you can't resist the duck, or the lobster Newburg, which you might never think of making at home, choose only low-fat items for appetizer and dessert.

I emphasize this point about your occasional high-fat meal under eating out because research shows that restaurant meals tend to be higher in fat content and lower in nutrient value than home-cooked meals. In addition, our own research in the Weight Management Program at Vanderbilt shows that people learn to manage their "at-home" meals much more easily than their restaurant meals. The restaurant environment puts too many high-fat choices at your fingertips, and the social situation tends to encourage ordering these high-fat dishes.

So your degree of vigilance is, in part, a function of how often you eat out. *If you eat out every day, you need to make careful choices at least 80 percent of the time.*

But don't be your own worst enemy! When it comes to eating out, my own experience as well as national surveys show that almost all restaurants that prepare food to order, regardless of ethnic style, will modify many of their offerings according to your desires. You create your own problems when you are too embarrassed to ask.

Since my tastes have changed so much as a result of many years of low-fat eating, I don't like to order fried foods, fatty roasts or steaks, or foods prepared with rich sauces. It's been years since I ordered veal stuffed with cheese and ham, or a food made with a butter or cream sauce. (Sometimes I order the sauce on the side to taste it. If I like it and can't figure out how it got its flavor, I ask. Then I go home to develop a low-fat version.)

First of all, I usually go to restaurants where they serve a wide variety of fish, poultry, and lean meat dishes, excellent salads, or interesting pasta dishes. The menu I mentioned for Shoney's at lunch (which is also available in dinner portions) is a good example of what I look for. In restaurants that offer this kind of variety, I am confident that I can get what I want. I usually have an idea of what I might like to eat before I get there, but I'm always flexible when I go to a restaurant that continually varies its menu.

While you are learning how to use the One Meal at a Time program, you might want to have a fat "budget" in mind; keep track of what you have been eating during the day, and save up a little surplus for dinner. *Do not skip meals.* Skipping meals frequently leads to overeating later in the day, whether you're at home or in a restaurant. Eat lightly earlier in the day and in the end you may not have to balance the books afterwards. Of course, as I explained earlier, if you go over your total by 10 or 20 grams of fat, just cut back by a certain amount each of the succeeding days until you are back to your desired average over time.

Second, if I'm in an unfamiliar restaurant, I go down the list of offerings paying particular attention to the fish and poultry, and ask how they are made. I then ask if the dish I might prefer can be lightly brushed with oil for grilling or broiling, or baked, poached, or steamed without any fat. I have never been in a restaurant that would not grill or broil whatever fish they were offering that evening. I ask if the sauce can come on the side. I ask about the ingredients in the pastas.

If I'm going to have an appetizer and I am in my lean mode, I ask which ones are the least fatty. If the server doesn't know, I ask him to go ask the chef! Avoid creamy things, mayonnaise-based dressings, and pâtés. And I prefer broth-based soups.

As for desserts, sometimes, but rarely, two of us will split a high-fat cake or pastry. But watch out when you order a single dessert, with an extra plate and fork, to be split between two people. One of the restaurants here in Nashville receives so many requests of this kind for its deservedly famous chocolate cakes and pastries that it doubles the price (and increases the portion slightly) when you order a single to be split two ways!

My questions and requests sometimes have unusual consequences. I once was entertaining a visiting professor at dinner and selected a fish with a marinara sauce, thinking it would be the least fatty of the various sauces offered at the French restaurant where we were dining. The waiter, who recognized me, came back after submitting my order to inform me that the chef added cream to his marinara sauce. Was that okay? I said no, and to ask the chef if he would please make mine without the cream. He did. It turned out very, very well. Later, the waiter came back and said the chef had decided, on the basis of what he had prepared for me, to delete the cream in his marinara sauce in the future. See if you can't have the same influence at your favorite restaurants.

Whether or not you have weight loss in mind, it's a good idea to be a little more active physically on days you eat out. Not only does physical activity help maintain desirable weight, but it can encourage your body to produce more "good" HDL cholesterol after you eat (see Chapters 2 and 13).

I almost never use butter or margarine with bread or rolls. I say "almost never" because several months ago I had the opportunity to sample a great 1966 vintage French burgundy wine. Burgundy is superb with hot French bread, sweet butter, and Roquefort cheese. What a treat! But that was the last time (for the cheese, as well).

I think you will find that good hot dinner breads and rolls do not require butter; if weight management is an issue, you may even want to skip them altogether, and be sure the server takes them from the table. If you must have something in your mouth at all times, and I used to be that way in restaurants, sip on iced water or iced tea.

TIPS FOR SELECTING FOODS PREPARED IN DIFFERENT ETHNIC STYLES

In view of my opinion that there is room for just about anything, cooked any way at all, when it is put only occasionally into an otherwise low-fat diet, I'm simply going to indicate which items are higher in fat, and which lower, to help you make informed choices in different kinds of restaurants. Here is a list of what to *try* (√) and what to *avoid* (∅) in various ethnic cuisines when you are in your low-fat mode.

Italian

Try:

✓ Pastas served with tomato-based sauces that do not contain meat. Marinara, pizzaida, and pomodoro sauces are good choices. Clam or calamari sauces are also a tasty, lower-fat alternative to meat or cream sauces.

✓ Baked or broiled chicken (without skin), veal cutlet, or fish dishes topped with meatless tomato-based sauces and minimal or no cheese. For example, chicken piccata or cacciatore.

✓ Seafood sautéed in wine rather than oil—for example, scampi al vino blanco (shrimp sautéed in white wine sauce).

✓ Minestrone, consommé with pastina, or cioppino (seafood soup) as an appetizer or for lunch.

✓ Fresh Italian bread without butter rather than garlic bread.

✓ Italian ices.

Avoid:

∅ Antipasto salad, Italian sausage, Alfredo and other cream sauces, cheese-cake, and dishes made with lots of high-fat cheese, meat, or oil (meat lasagne, manicotti, parmigiana, cannelloni, pesto).

As for pizza, try:

✓ Vegetable toppings, hold the meats. Traditional pizza toppings such as pepperoni and sausage are loaded with saturated fat. The meat actually cooks atop the pizza with all the grease being absorbed into the sauce and crust—and a little into the cardboard box (notice the difference in the grease in the bottom of pizza boxes that held a meat pizza versus a vegetable one!).

✓ If you must have meat, order Canadian bacon or ham.

✓ Extra sauce, easy on the cheese.

Avoid:

∅ High-fat meats (pepperoni, sausage, ground beef) and extra cheese.

Mexican

Try:

✓ Salsa, salsa verde, picante, or taco sauce as a topping or dip rather than guacamole or sour cream.

√ Black bean soup or gazpacho as an appetizer or for lunch. Hold the sour cream.

√ Tortillas or soft tacos (unfried) filled with chicken, seafood, or vegetables. Refried beans in a restaurant are generally loaded with lard. Good choices would be chicken or seafood burritos or enchiladas (go easy on the cheese).

√ Chili con carne (chili with meat) and soft flour tortillas on the side with a dinner salad.

√ Side orders of soft flour tortillas, black beans, or Mexican rice.

√ Seafood or chicken in tomato-based or vegetable sauces—for example, camarones de hacha (shrimp in tomato coriander sauce) or arroz con pollo (boneless chicken breast with rice).

√ Keep it simple and order à la carte—combination dinners are usually served with refried beans, sour cream, guacamole, cheese, and fried foods.

√ Fresh pineapple or baked bananas for dessert.

Avoid:

⊘ Sour cream, guacamole, fried items like chimichangas, tostadas, and tortilla chips, and items with lots of cheese or fatty meats.

Chinese

Try:

√ Chicken in tin foil as an appetizer.

√ Steamed dumplings (Peking raviolis).

√ Since many Chinese restaurants make menu items to order, use the opportunity to ask questions and make requests with respect to preparation method and use of fats.

√ Steamed vegetables, lean meats, chicken, tofu, and seafood dishes in a light wine sauce.

√ Steamed rice instead of fried rice.

√ Stir-fried (specify to your server "as little oil as possible") vegetables, lean meats, chicken, tofu, and seafood dishes. Some examples would be moo goo gai pan chicken, shrimp with snow pea pods, boned chicken or lobster cantonese, chicken chow mein over steamed rice, or moo shu chicken, shrimp, or vegetables.

√ Ask if shrimp, scallops, or chicken can be substituted for pork or beef in menu entrees.

√ Ask if chicken can be substituted for duck in menu entrees.

√ Wonton or other clear, broth-based soups.

√ For dessert, try fresh pineapple chunks or a fruit bowl with a fortune cookie.

Avoid:

⊘ Fried items like fried rice, "crispy" beef, batter-dipped items, spareribs, egg foo young, and chow mein noodles.

Japanese

Try:

✓ Clear soups, like miso soup, as an appetizer.
✓ Sushi and sashimi.
✓ Hibachi chicken or lean beef.
✓ Steamed, grilled, or broiled meats, chicken, or fish—teriyaki style is a good choice.
✓ Ask if shrimp, scallops, or chicken can be substituted for pork or beef in menu entrees.
✓ Mandarin orange sections, sherbet, and fresh fruit are low-fat dessert selections.

Avoid:

⊘ Fried bean curd, tempura, other foods battered and fried, agemono, and katsu dishes.

French

Try:

✓ Consommé or other broth-based soup as an appetizer.
✓ Steamed, poached, roasted, or grilled fish or chicken—for example, coq au vin (chicken in wine), pot-au-feu (stewed chicken), bouillabaisse (fish stew), or poached quenelles (steamed fish dumplings).
✓ Dishes served "en papillote" (steamed in a paper envelope).
✓ Steamed or sautéed (in wine, broth, or tomato sauce) vegetables served à la carte rather than vegetables served with hollandaise, butter, or cream sauces. Ratatouille is a lower-fat vegetable dish.
✓ If you choose to have a higher-fat entree, ask if an appetizer-size portion or a half portion is available.
✓ Sherbet, fresh fruit, or pears in wine sauce for dessert.

Avoid:

⊘ Fatty sauces like hollandaise, béarnaise, béchamel, beurre blanc, veloute, and Mornay; "au gratin" or "en casserole" items; items in a pastry shell; croissants; and quiche.

Indian-Pakistani

Try:

√ Mulligatawny or lentil (Dahl rasam) soup.
√ Chapati (unleavened bread) and nan (leavened bread) are preferable bread choices as many Indian bread items are fried.
√ Items prepared without frying or added ghee (clarified butter).
√ A curry dish made with chicken, lobster, shrimp, lentils, or vegetables.
√ Order plain rice or use a rice dish as a main entree.
√ Mango or papaya slices or Indian fruit cocktail as dessert.

Avoid:

⊘ Fried breads, coconut soup, and coconut cream.

Middle Eastern–Greek

Try:

√ Skim-milk yogurt and cucumber soup.
√ As an entree, choose grilled or baked items like shish kebab, baked fish with tomatoes and rice, or oven-braised chicken with kumquats.
√ Pita bread.
√ Fruit compote or poached apples for dessert rather than baklava, kataif, or rice pudding.

Avoid:

⊘ Pastries and items rich in cheese or eggs.

TIPS FOR AIRLINE TRAVEL

One of the airlines' best-kept secrets has to do with the ordering of special meals. Most airlines have a variety of special meals to suit the needs of travelers on special diets. In addition to kosher, low-sodium, and low-cholesterol meals, they almost always can serve fruit plates at any meal, and cold seafood plates for lunch or dinner. Sometimes you can special-order baked chicken, baked fish, or even a steak fillet regardless of what the standard lunch or dinner will offer on your flight.

For breakfast you can usually special-order cereal, low-fat milk, and fruit in place of eggs and sausage. If that's not available, pancakes will have less fat than the egg dish, and usually taste better, in my opinion.

When you make reservations, or the day before you fly, call the airline and ask what special plates will be available on your flight. You almost always need to give them 24 hours' notice. I do a great deal of traveling and never order anything other than the fruit plate (with cottage cheese) or the cold fish plate for lunch or dinner. In my experience, the cold fish plate is generally superior to any of the standard airline meals, so you sacrifice nothing except the fat when you special-order this dish. Try it.

Of course, if all else fails, carry your own brown bag. I have never had to do this for lunch or dinner, but I frequently do carry something for a snack (see Chapter 8).

So there you have it. Of all the meals, the dinner meal is the one with which you should take the most time. I hope you will experiment with all of my dinner recipes. They are basic. As you work with them, you may find that there are some alterations in seasoning that might make them more agreeable to your tastes. With your own recipes, you now know two basic principles: Choose the lean cuts of meat and use a minimum of added fat in preparation. In Table 11-1 in Chapter 11, I will give you a list of the herbs and spices that will help you liven up all foods as you cut back on fat.

DINNER SHOPPING LIST

Fruits

apples_____

bananas_____

berries_____

grapefruit_____ _____

grapes_____

melon_____

nectarines/tangerines_____

oranges_____

peaches_____

pears_____

pineapple_____

plums_____

raisins_____

other dried fruit_____

other fruit_____

fruit juices_____

Vegetables

acorn squash_____

beans, dried_____

beans, refried, canned_____

beets_____

bell peppers_____

broccoli_____

carrots_____

cauliflower_____

celery_____

cucumber_____

green beans_____

green onions_____

lettuce_____

mushrooms_____

onions_____

potatoes (baking, new)_____

spinach (fresh or frozen)_____

other greens_____

squash (summer, zucchini)_____

sweet potatoes_____

tomatoes_____

water chestnuts_____

Bread and Grains

whole-grain bread_____

mixed-grain bread_____

Italian, French bread_____

whole-grain rolls_____

corn or flour tortillas_____

noodles, macaroni_____

rice (brown, wild)_____

spaghetti, other pasta_____

croutons_____

Milk and Dairy Products

skim or low-fat milk_____

buttermilk_____

nonfat yogurt_____

low-fat cottage cheese_____

cheese, sharp cheddar_____

cheese, mozzarella (skim)_____

cheese, Parmesan_____

cheese, ricotta (skim)_____

evaporated skim milk_____

ice milk_____

frozen yogurt_____

butter_____

Meat, Fish, Poultry

beef, lean (flank, tenderloin, London
    broil)_____

beef, roast (sirloin tip)_____

beef, ground (extra lean)_____

chicken breasts_____

clams, canned_____

fish fillets_____

ground turkey_____

pork tenderloin_____

other_____

Miscellaneous

all-purpose flour_____

whole-wheat flour_____

cornmeal_____

yeast, dry_____

sugar_____

lemon juice_____

barbecue sauce_____

ketchup_____

dressing, no- or low-cal_____

vinegar_____

broth or bouillon_____

tomato sauce, paste_____

tomatoes, whole (canned)_____

garlic (fresh, powdered)_____

other seasonings, spices_____

margarine_____

vegetable oil (canola)_____

nonstick cooking spray_____

chocolate syrup_____

angel food cake_____

fig bars_____

gingersnaps_____

sherbet_____

other_____

CHAPTER 8

SNACKS

Have you ever checked the nutrition information label on the back of a bag of potato chips or those bite-size cheese crackers? On a can of peanuts or a bag of chocolate-chip cookies?

If you have, it will come as no surprise to you that as much as 40 percent and sometimes more of a day's total fat intake for many people is eaten in snack foods. On the average, potato chips and cheese snacks have about 10 or 11 grams of fat per ounce. And that's hardly a palmful! Peanuts have 9 grams per 2 tablespoons—I'm talking *level* tablespoons, not rounded. If you like peanuts, when was the last time you stopped after eating just 2 tablespoons? And that chocolate-chip cookie—a regular-size packaged variety contains almost 5 grams of fat per cookie.

If you happen to be a person who does like fatty snacks, don't despair. You're in for some surprises when it comes to finding healthful replacements. For all the fatty snacks I have mentioned there are a variety of foods with similar tastes and textures, but without the fat. They really do exist!

You can learn all about them in a matter of minutes. It's pretty

138

much one of those "one-shot deals" I spoke about in Chapter 3. For example, if you like crunchy, salty snacks, and are not salt sensitive, pretzels have only 1 gram of fat per ounce, which is only one-tenth the fat content in potato chips and cheese snacks. If you are concerned with salt intake, there are both low-sodium and salt-free pretzels on the market. If they are not available in your area, you can do what my wife does—scrape some of the salt off the regular varieties before eating.

I have listed some alternative snack selections in Table 8–1. You will find many others by examining the Nutrient Counter in Appendix B. As I said, you can learn all you need to know about snack choices in a few minutes, *but then you must learn how to put that knowledge to work so that you can actually carry out your intentions to switch.* That may require a few extra steps.

TABLE 8–1.   TIPS FOR LOW-FAT SNACKING

Fresh and dried fruit are the best sweet snacks. They should be among your first choices for sweets.

Vegetables such as carrot and celery sticks, sweet peppers, and summer squash are excellent crunchy choices.

Here are some suggestions for substituting low-fat for similar high-fat foods (fat content in parentheses).

Instead of:	Choose:
Chocolate candy (13–14 g)	Life Savers, jelly beans, gumdrops, lemon drops (no fat)
Potato chips, cheese snacks, nacho crackers (10–14 g)	Pretzels, pita chips, rice cakes, bagels (0–1 g)
Regular and premium ice cream (12–20 g)	Nonfat and low-fat frozen yogurt (0–3 g)
Nuts, including peanuts (10–14 g)	Popcorn (with oil), Cracker Jacks (2 g per cup)
Chocolate-chip or other fatty cookies (4–6 g each)	Gingersnaps, fig bars (0.5–1 g each)
Croissants, butter rolls (10–20 g)	Whole-grain rolls, bagel, pita bread (1–4 g)
Danish, doughnuts, pies, frosted cakes (10–20 g)	Raisin bread and rolls, angel food cake and fudge sauce (1–3 g)

HOW TO PUT YOUR KNOWLEDGE TO WORK

Our choice of snacks is probably more directly under the influence of environmental forces than any other food choice. That's because snacking is often a spur-of-the-moment activity and, instead of choosing anything that might take time to prepare, we reach for whatever is available. This allows our eating environment to dictate what we will eat.

Let me give you an illustration. I do a great many radio and TV interviews. I check out the snack machines at every station in order to make a point during my interviews. Usually I find as many as 30 high-fat candy bars, cookies, cakes, and salty snacks and not a single low-fat selection in their machines. At best I find gum or Life Savers. Why?

You know the answer. The machines are stocked with what sells. Just as in the story I told in Footnote 1 in Chapter 1, high-fat snacks disappear and low-fat snacks remain when they are made available together. Snack vendors will remove low-volume items (low-fat snacks) and replace them with high-volume items (high-fat snacks). During my interview, I ask my interviewer if he or she has ever had the urge to snack and made a trip down to the machine. The answer is almost always yes. So the points I want to make are easy: You can only eat what's available, and if low-fat items happen to be available, they don't appeal as much as the high-fat ones. If they are not available, they may have been at one time and since removed. Which leads me to—

FIRST PRINCIPLE

Avoid temptation. In your own home, keep *only* low-fat snacks *as a general rule.* If your tastes are at all like mine, it's much easier to avoid than to resist!

I mean by this statement that a decision not to purchase and store foods that don't fit into your *everyday* eating plan makes it easy to follow a low-fat diet. You can't eat what isn't there. But if you always have on hand, in sight and within arm's reach, the foods that can turn you on, in the end you will succumb. And I am really serious when I use the expression "turn you on," because the sight or smell of artfully seasoned high-fat foods will lead to an increase in salivation, gastric secretion, and insulin level. The body is getting ready to eat, and that call to readiness is not under your conscious control. As I said earlier, it's a biological, not a moral issue. You may be able to resist the urge to indulge yourself for a time, but in the end the instinctual call to "eat, eat!" will prevail.

I'm talking about general rules for everyday eating. When you think it's time for that *occasional* high-fat treat, buy exactly what you want for a single snack (or dessert, or other dish). If you buy more than that, occasional foods will soon become everyday foods and you're back eating a high-fat diet. I suspect that with snacks more than with any other aspect of your diet you must watch out for "a little cheating" every day. But "controlled cheating" once or twice a week *can* fit into the One Meal at a Time program without defeating your objective. Check out the nutritional analysis in Chapter 9 that includes some high-fat choices within a two-week period for a demonstration of what I mean.

Study Table 8–1 and see what selection of low-fat snacks might replace your present high-fat varieties. Keep them available and you will not feel deprived. I just checked my kitchen to see what we had in the house, and here is the list, in the approximate order of my preference. As you can see, many of these foods can be (and are) eaten at regular meals:

Fruit—including apples, oranges, grapefruit, cantaloupe, watermelon, raisins, and dates (in the last two days we finished the fresh peaches, nectarines, and pineapple and we have not replenished them as yet).

Pretzels, several varieties of low-fat crackers, pumpernickel, whole-wheat bread, raisin bread, and raisin rolls (good bread is excellent as a snack, toasted, with or without condiments such as salsa or jelly).

Popcorn, which is a frequent nighttime snack. Try it with nutritional yeast, curry powder, or garlic powder and you will need very little if any salt on it. I don't think you need force yourself to eat air-blown popcorn if it doesn't appeal to you. I like mine popped with olive oil or, for a special treat, avocado oil. The latter gives it a special mild, nutty flavor. Made with oil, using 2 tablespoons in a 12-cup popper, popcorn tends to be less than the 2 grams of fat per cup listed in the nutritional analysis because some of the oil sticks to the popper.

Cereal, which is often the very last snack we might eat at night. We always have several varieties on hand.

Finally, whenever we want to take the time, we make our own spicy pita bread or bagel chips for a special snack treat. Split and cut the pita bread into bite-size triangles, or slice the bagel into four thin strips (in the same direction you would slice for toasting), sprinkle with Cajun seasonings, spray if you like with a bit of vegetable spray, and bake for two minutes in a preheated oven at 475 degrees. You will never be tempted by potato chips or other fatty crunchy snacks after tasting these.

You may have noticed that there are no carrot and celery sticks in my personal list (they are recommended in Table 8–1). Many nutritionists suggest you use vegetables for snacks, but I don't care for them that way. I prefer carrots and celery in salads or cooked (steamed or microwaved) as a side dish at dinner.

SECOND PRINCIPLE

Be prepared! Now I'm talking about your office if you work outside the home, or if you travel. Carry something with you for your mid-morning or mid-afternoon snack. Or keep your own personal supply where you work. Don't get caught at the mercy of *your* office's snack machine.

If you travel frequently on commercial airlines, well, those little packages of peanuts that are supposed to keep you satisfied between meals (and may sometimes be all you get to eat for most of the day if your schedule gets messed up) hold half an ounce and contain 7 grams of fat and 85 calories. How many times have you stopped with eating just one package? Once again, carry something. If for some reason you aren't able to pack anything more healthful, you are much better off resorting to peppermints and Life Savers than to peanuts when it comes to avoiding fat.

When traveling many hours by car or bus I recommend a loaf of hearty, chewy bread and a selection of fruit. You will feel much better for eating bulky things that take a lot of chewing rather than fat-laden candies. Hard candy is a possibility, but many people tell me that they can finish an extraordinary amount of Life Savers and lemon drops in eight hours of driving, so I would limit the amount of this kind of food on a trip. Besides, sucking hard candy all day long is not good for your teeth.

IS SNACKING GOOD FOR PEOPLE?

I think it's unfortunate that some health professionals still recommend "three square meals" and no snacking. The habit of eating three meals a day is probably a fairly recent development in the history of the human race. Eating lightly several times a day may be more in line with the body's natural needs.

Our bodies can adapt to all kinds of eating patterns, of course. However, there is considerable research accumulating to show that it's probably healthier to eat many small meals than to eat just two or three times a day, especially if that limited pattern includes a large meal at night. A nibbling pattern is associated with lower weight, lower serum cholesterol, and better blood glucose control.

But note the tremendous difference in the fat content between the high- and low-fat selections in Table 8–1 and you will see how easy it is to take in 40 percent or more of a day's total fat and end up with a high-fat diet by eating fatty snacks. Just three servings of high-fat snacks can add up to as much as 50 or 60 grams of fat. You can eat twice as much of the low-fat alternatives and you are still likely to total less than 10 grams of fat. The low-fat choices will also contain 350 to 450 fewer calories!

Follow my snack suggestions and you will be increasing the nutrient value of your diet immensely. With three snacks a day chosen from a variety of breads, grains, cereals, and fruits you go a long way toward meeting the goals for increasing complex-carbohydrate foods that I discussed in Chapter 3. You also are likely to gain a couple of other immediate benefits: You will feel more alert and energetic all day long, and you won't be hungry.

SNACKS SHOPPING LIST

Fruits		melon_____
apples_____		nectarines/tangerines_____
berries_____		oranges_____
bananas_____		peaches_____
grapefruit_____		pears_____
grapes_____		pineapple_____

plums_____

raisins_____

other dried fruit_____

fruit juices_____

other fruits_____

Vegetables

bell peppers_____

broccoli_____

carrots_____

cauliflower_____

celery_____

cucumber_____

green onions_____

mushrooms_____

onions_____

radishes_____

squash (summer, zucchini)_____

tomatoes_____

Breads and Grains

whole-grain breads_____

mixed-grain breads_____

raisin bread_____

bagels_____

English muffins_____

pita bread_____

ready-to-eat cereals_____

corn or flour tortillas_____

breadsticks_____

crackers, whole grain_____

graham crackers_____

popcorn_____

pretzels_____

rice or popcorn cakes_____

Milk and Dairy Products

skim or low-fat milk_____

nonfat yogurt_____

low-fat cottage cheese_____

ice milk_____

frozen yogurt_____

Miscellaneous

angel food cake_____

chocolate syrup_____

fig bars_____

gingersnaps_____

hard candy, Life Savers_____

jelly beans_____

marshmallows_____

peanut butter_____

salsa_____

sherbet_____

soups, broth based_____

other_____

CHAPTER 9

PUTTING IT ALL TOGETHER

If you've been following my advice, rotating among the different breakfasts, lunches, and dinners and adding a variety of grains, cereals, and fruit as snacks, *you've been eating a very healthful diet.* So I hope congratulations are in order (or will be if you have jumped ahead to this chapter and are about to begin the One Meal at a Time program).

To determine the nutritional value of the One Meal at a Time program, we selected for our menus:

- All the standard and several of the special breakfasts and lunches from Chapters 5 and 6
- All 14 of my suggested dinners in Chapter 7
- Plus 3 added snacks a day, choosing a variety of my suggested snacks from Chapter 8

We then analyzed the diet over a 14-day period, using the Food Processor II Nutrition and Diet Analysis System.

In addition, whenever called for in the menus, we used the recipes in Chapter 11. In choosing from the alternatives in the suggested

individual-meal menus in Chapters 5–7 (such as no- or low-fat dressing), *we assumed most people would tend to use some of the higher-fat alternatives instead of the no-fat alternatives.*

We added 1 tablespoon of extra fat each day, which I indicated was
available, at your discretion, for spread, flavoring, or salad dressing.
(For purposes of analysis, we used margarine. Butter would be
somewhat higher in saturated fat.)

We used 1 percent low-fat milk, rather than skim, assuming that low-
fat milk probably would be preferable for most people.

We mixed up our cereals, using Shredded Wheat, Raisin Bran,
Cheerios, and sometimes a mixture of 100 percent bran and Total.
We assumed a mixed-grain bread, rather than whole-grain bread,
since most people probably don't limit themselves exclusively to
whole-grain breads.

We used canola oil for our recipe analyses, but the substitution of
other monounsaturated or polyunsaturated vegetable oils of your
choice will not make a significant difference in the amount of saturated fat in your diet, considering the limited amount of oil that's
used in cooking. (The calories will be the same whatever oil you
use.)

*Optional items in the recipes are not included in the analyses, and no salt is
added beyond what's called for in our recipes.* If you add salt to vegetables, popcorn, or other items, your totals for sodium will be higher
than those in the following reports.

Before giving you the verdict on the nutritional quality of the One
Meal at a Time program, I want to point out that we did not try to
design a perfect day to put our recommendations in the best possible
light, as do some other books on diet and nutrition. It's easy to
design a perfect day, but, obviously, people aren't going to eat the
same thing every day. Although any given week or two may be quite
similar to any other week or two, in real life we don't eat the precise
selection of foods that will come out perfectly in a 24-hour nutritional analysis.

Back in Chapter 3, and in Chapters 5–8, I gave you general principles for constructing a nutritious diet, and examples of *meals* that will
fit these principles *over time.* We followed the same general principles
that we want you to follow in designing your own diet to design the
menus we put into our computer analysis. I will review those principles after making our report. To design two weeks' worth of daily
menus, we simply rotated around my suggested *individual-meal*

menus, and added a variety of snacks. The two weeks of menus that we used are presented at the end of this chapter. If you like, you can use these as a guide in designing your own menus. But your diet must suit your own tastes and convenience.

THE VERDICT

Table 9–1 presents our computerized nutritional analysis of the One Meal at a Time program over a 14-day period. Note in particular that, averaged over time, the daily intake is:

Total fat	=	42.1 g
Saturated fat	=	11.2 g
Cholesterol	=	147 mg
Calories	=	1,827
Fiber	=	35.0 g
Sodium	=	2,785 mg

Recall that my primary purpose in designing the meal plans was to end up with approximately 40 grams of fat per day *to allow leeway for a little bit more fat within the 50-gram quota that will be appropriate for most women who are not interested in losing weight.* In other words, if you like your popcorn popped with oil, rather than air-blown, or if you prefer a regular salad dressing rather than a low-fat version, there is room for a tablespoonful, and you will not exceed your quota. And, of course, the larger portions suggested for men will bring them closer to the 50- to 60-gram range.

At 42.1 grams of fat per day, total fat is 20 percent of calories. This is intentional. It leaves, within the quota of 25 percent of calories from fat, room for adding some butter or margarine to vegetables or popping corn in oil, and for eating out, since restaurant meals tend to contain more fat than home-cooked meals.

At 11.2 grams of saturated fat the diet contains 5 percent of calories from saturated fat. Once again, there is leeway for adding a little fat according to your preferences and for eating out, without the likelihood of exceeding 10 percent of total calories from saturated fat. (If you choose to use 1 tablespoon of butter per day in place of margarine, saturated fat will increase to an average of 15.1 grams per day, which is still only 7 percent of total calories.)

TABLE 9–1. NUTRIENT ANALYSIS OF THE
ONE MEAL AT A TIME PROGRAM[a]

Nutrient	Amount	%RDA	Nutrient	Amount	%RDA
Calories	1,827		Pyridoxine (B$_6$)	2.60 mg	130%
Protein	88.7 g		Cobalamin (B$_{12}$)	9.01 μg	300%
Carbohydrates	283 g		Folic acid	464 μg	116%
Dietary fiber	35.0 g		Pantothenic acid	9.40 mg	134%
Fat—total	42.1 g		Vitamin C	274 mg	457%
Fat—saturated	11.2 g		Vitamin E	15.3 mg	192%
Fat—monounsaturated	14.9 g		Calcium	1,102 mg	138%
Fat—polyunsaturated	13.7 g		Copper	2.13 mg	—[b]
Cholesterol	147 mg		Iron	20.0 mg	111%
Vitamin A—					
carotene	940 RE		Magnesium	410 mg	136%
Vitamin A—					
pre-formed	655 RE		Phosphorus	1,937 mg	242%
Vitamin A—total	1,599 RE	200%	Potassium	4,333 mg	116%
Thiamine (B$_1$)	2.42 mg	241%	Selenium	150 μg	120%
Riboflavin	2.73 mg	226%	Sodium	2,785 mg	127%
Niacin (B$_3$)	27.9 mg	210%	Zinc	15.0 mg	100%

Calories from protein: 19%
Calories from carbohydrates: 61%
Calories from fats: 20%

[a]This analysis was performed using the Food Processor II Nutrition and Diet Analysis System. The food items analyzed are all those contained in the menus for two weeks presented at the end of this chapter, using some of the higher-fat alternatives (for example, low-fat instead of no-fat dressing) and 1 tablespoon of added margarine per day.

[b]A range of 1.5 to 3.0 mg is given by the Food and Nutrition Board as an estimated safe and adequate average daily intake for copper.

Cholesterol, at 147 milligrams, is well below the recommended 300 milligrams, and below the stricter guideline of 100 milligrams per 1,000 calories suggested by some authorities.

Fiber is a healthful 35.0 grams.

All other nutrients are at or above 100 percent of the RDAs recommended by the National Research Council.

SO YOU'RE NOT PERFECT! WHAT HAPPENS?

I told you there was room for an occasional high-fat meal, snack, or dessert. To prove it, we substituted at random a few doozies:

1. A large hamburger, an order of French fries, and a large chocolate milk shake for one lunch
2. A slice of birthday cake with a scoop of ice cream for a snack
3. Three pieces of pizza (typical restaurant variety with meat and cheese) and a salad with 2 tablespoons of regular salad dressing for a dinner
4. And, believe it or not, a high-fat breakfast of scrambled eggs in butter, two slices of bacon, two pieces of toast and butter, and coffee with half-and-half[1] for one of the regular low-fat breakfasts

As I told you, the quality of your diet is not evaluated properly by a single meal or on a single-day basis—it's evaluated properly over time. As can be seen in Table 9–2, when you look at the One Meal at a Time plan with these high-fat substitutions over a 14-day period, you get an average of:

Total fat	=	51.6 g
Saturated fat	=	15.1 g
Cholesterol	=	198 mg
Calories	=	1,954
Fiber	=	34.3 g
Sodium	=	2,960 mg

Even with these high-fat substitutions, which I hope you will find unnecessary to make, you remain at 23 percent of total calories from fat, with only 7 percent from saturated fat.

IT'S EASY TO STICK WITH THE GUIDELINES

You don't need to follow the mealtime suggestions I made in Chapters 5–7 to the letter, and choose precisely the same snacks as we entered in our computer analysis, to be sure that you are eating a nutritious diet.

Although we use all 14 of my suggested dinners, all standard

---

[1] We used butter rather than margarine to demonstrate that its occasional use will not raise total saturated fat over 10 percent of calories (15.1 grams equals 136 calories, which is about equal to 7 percent of the daily average of 1,954 calories).

TABLE 9–2.   NUTRIENT ANALYSIS OF THE ONE MEAL AT A TIME PROGRAM WITH ADDED HIGH-FAT MEALS AND ONE SNACK[a]

Nutrient	Amount	%RDA	Nutrient	Amount	%RDA
Calories	1,954		Pyridoxine (B_6)	2.56 mg	128%
Protein	92.0 g		Cobalamin (B_{12})	6.42 µg	214%
Carbohydrates	290 g		Folic acid	453 µg	113%
Dietary fiber	34.3 g		Pantothenic acid	9.33 mg	133%
Fat—total	51.6 g		Vitamin C	259 mg	431%
Fat—saturated	15.1 g		Vitamin E	15.8 mg	198%
Fat—monounsaturated	18.4 g		Calcium	1,135 mg	142%
Fat—polyunsaturated	14.7 g		Copper	2.01 mg	—[b]
Cholesterol	198 mg		Iron	19.6 mg	109%
Vitamin A—					
carotene	919 RE		Magnesium	401 mg	134%
Vitamin A—					
pre-formed	668 RE		Phosphorus	1,939 mg	242%
Vitamin A—total	1,608 RE	201%	Potassium	4,234 mg	113%
Thiamine (B_1)	2.45 mg	244%	Selenium	145 µg	116%
Riboflavin	2.82 mg	234%	Sodium	2,960 mg	135%
Niacin (B_3)	28.4 mg	214%	Zinc	15.2 mg	101%

Calories from protein: 18%
Calories from carbohydrates: 58%
Calories from fats: 23%
(Total calories do not equal 100% because of rounding.)

[a]A total of four high-fat dishes (two per week), including a breakfast, lunch, dinner, and snack, were substituted for other meals and a snack in the menus presented for Weeks 1 and 2 at the end of this chapter. The analysis was performed using the Food Processor II Nutrition and Diet Analysis System. See the main text for details.

[b]A range of 1.5 to 3.0 mg is given by the Food and Nutrition Board as an estimated safe and adequate average daily intake for copper.

breakfasts and lunches and some of the special ones as well, and a variety of fruits and grains for snacks, *we achieve the outstanding nutritional quality of the One Meal at a Time program by following the general principles I laid out for you earlier in this book.* I want to repeat them for emphasis because you can expect to do as well if you:

1. Choose only lean meats and low-fat or skim dairy products, most of the time.
2. Round out your meals with plenty of vegetables and starches, and

finish with fruit, frozen yogurt, or desserts similar to my recipes in Chapter 11.

3. Use fruit and only low-fat grain foods for snacks, most of the time.

As for each meal, we use the following *general* guidelines:

1. Breakfasts usually contain some grain food, fruit, and milk (or a milk product); eggs or a meat product are eaten only once or twice a week.

2. Lunches focus on salads, soups, spreads, and lean deli meats (when included) for sandwiches, and end with a choice of fruit.

3. Dinners (or the main meal of the day) focus on fish and poultry for animal products, and limit beef to once a week and pork to once a week (or twice for either without the other); they use combination dishes such as beans and a grain, stir-fries, and pasta two or three times a week, plenty of different vegetables and starches, and a low-fat dessert, such as frozen yogurt, fruit, or baked goods that are similar to my recipes in Chapter 11.

4. Snacks are generally grain products or fruit.

Our analysis assumes that you will use low-fat milk and other dairy products and average two servings a day, over time. If you don't drink milk and don't use other milk products, you will need plenty of greens, occasional animal products with chewable bones, and possibly calcium supplementation to meet your calcium requirements.

The best assurance of adequate nutrition is to eat a wide variety of different foods from each of the food groups:

- Milk and other dairy products (low-fat ones, of course)
- Grains, breads, and cereal products
- Vegetables and fruits
- Fish and low-fat meats and poultry

If you follow these principles, even if you happen to choose foods that are somewhat less nutritious than others within each food group, you are still likely to exceed the safe, lower boundary for the RDA set for each nutrient by the Food and Nutrition Board. That lower boundary is 67 percent of the amount needed to reach 100 percent. The amount required to meet 100 percent was set high enough to ensure the health of persons who might have somewhat less ability to absorb or utilize the various nutrients than the average person. Indeed, compared with the United States, other countries have set lower requirements for many nutrients.

However, if for any reason you must limit your selection of foods from any of these groups, you should consult a registered dietitian for advice on how to construct a healthful diet from a limited variety of foods. You also may need vitamin and mineral supplementation, which obviously is not needed by healthy people when they follow the One Meal at a Time program, as shown by the nutritional analysis in this chapter.

I want to write a special word of warning to vegetarians: I have had the diets of a number of vegetarian students in my health-promotion classes analyzed as part of class assignments for all students. They tend to fall below 67 percent of the RDAs for the B-complex vitamins, iron, and certain other minerals. They are low in calcium when the students don't drink milk. *The omission of animal products does not guarantee an increase in the nutritional value of your diet!*

One of the most interesting and educational ways to find out the nutritional value of your diet is to keep track of your meals and do your own analysis. This is made simple if you own a home computer and are willing to invest in a nutritional analysis program. In the Vanderbilt program we use the Food Processor II Nutrition and Diet Analysis System, which is available from ESHA Research, P.O. Box 13028, Salem, OR 97309 (telephone: 503-585-6242). This is a professional nutritional analysis program that sells for $295 as of this writing, but it does the work of programs selling for several times more. It's available in IBM or Apple format, and in both 3.5-inch and 5.25-inch disk size. As you can see from Tables 9–1 and 9–2, it analyzes the diet for 30 nutrients, including different fat and vitamin A components. By the time this book is published, ESHA expects to have a less expensive computer analysis program available for the average consumer, and it may be able to offer individual dietary analysis by mail, at a reasonable price, for those who do not wish to purchase a computer program.

A smaller but still helpful program that provides information on fat grams, calories, protein, carbohydrate, and cholesterol for many common foods, and offers you suggestions for alternative lower-fat choices when such are available, is the Executive Diet Helper, from Ohio Distinctive Software, 1078-G Merrimar Circle North, P.O. Box 20201, Columbus, OH 43220. Although this program does not provide information on vitamins and minerals, it is fun to use and a great value at only $3 plus $3 shipping and handling, for a total of $6. If you don't wish to make a great investment until you see how much use you might make of a computer nutrition program, and how much more information you would like to have available, the Executive Diet Helper is an excellent way to start. The company produces a Menu Planner as well, also priced at $3, which will help you design daily menus for different dietary requirements—for example, diabetes, heart disease, vegetarian, children's diets, and so on. You can order both programs for a total of $9 (send check or money order, and specify 5.25 or 3.5 diskette size).

ONE MEAL AT A TIME MENUS[2]

WEEK 1

DAY 1

BREAKFAST
1 ounce ready-to-eat cereal (1–3 g fat); ½ cup sliced, fresh peaches; 1 cup skim or low-fat milk (0–3 g fat); 1 slice mixed-grain toast (1 g fat); 1 teaspoon jelly or jam (optional); coffee or tea
Total fat: 2–7 g

MID-MORNING SNACK
½ cinnamon-raisin bagel (1 g fat)
Total fat: 1 g

[2]A nutritional analysis requires that we include serving sizes. Your diet will approximate the values we obtained if you simply think in terms of cafeteria-size portions. The only real need for measurement lies in the choice of foods that contain fat. Pay attention to the serving size of fatty foods while you are learning to use the program. Correct choice, without measuring anything, will become second nature within four to seven weeks.

The line "Total fat for day" at the conclusion of the day's menus shows the range of fat intake depending on whether you choose the low- or high-fat alternatives in the menus.

The line "Nutrient analysis with 1 tablespoon margarine added" shows the values should you add that amount of fat to the daily menu for spread or seasoning. (If you prefer butter in place of margarine, total fat remains the same, but saturated fat increases by 5 grams per day and cholesterol by 30 milligrams per day.)

To reduce your daily fat intake—for example, to lose weight—choose the low-fat alternatives in the menus, and do not add more fat to exceed whatever quota you have chosen for yourself within the range of 20 to 40 grams per day for women, and 30 to 60 grams for men.

Recipes set in **bold print** are found in Chapter 11.

LUNCH
Turkey-cranberry sandwich: 2 ounces sliced turkey for sandwich (1–2 g fat), ¼ cup cranberry sauce, ¼ cup alfalfa sprouts, 2 slices mixed-grain bread (2 g fat); 1 ounce pretzels (1 g fat); 1 orange; beverage
Total fat: 4–5 g

MID-AFTERNOON SNACK
1 pear
Total fat: 0

DINNER
1 serving pasta with **Red Clam Sauce** (5 g fat); tossed salad; no- or low-cal dressing (2 tablespoons = 0–3 g fat); 1 slice **No-Knead Herb Bread** (3 g fat); ¼ honeydew melon or other seasonal fruit; 2 **Gingerbread Cookies** (1 g fat each); beverage
Total fat: 11–14 g

EVENING SNACK
2 graham crackers (1 g fat); 1 cup skim or low-fat milk (0–3 g fat)
Total fat: 1–4 g

Total fat for Day 1: 20–32 g
Nutrient analysis with 1 tablespoon margarine added: **38.0 g total fat** (18%); 9.12 g saturated fat; 105 mg cholesterol; 1,916 calories; 32 g fiber; 2,555 mg sodium

DAY 2

BREAKFAST
1 cup sliced, fresh strawberries; **Apricot Muffin** (3 g fat); 1 cup nonfat or low-fat yogurt or skim or low-fat milk (0–3 g fat); coffee or tea
Total fat: 3–6 g

MID-MORNING SNACK
2 rice cakes; 1 teaspoon jelly or jam
Total fat: 0

LUNCH
½ cup **Mexican Bean Spread** or canned refried beans (1–2 g fat); toasted bagel (1 g fat) or 2 flour or corn tortillas (2–5 g fat); 1–2 cups assorted **raw** vegetables; ½ cup seedless grapes; beverage
Total fat: 2–7 g

AFTERNOON SNACK
½ cup frozen yogurt (0–3 g fat)
                    Total fat: 0–3 g

DINNER
3 ounces flank steak in **Simple Beef Marinade** (9 g fat); medium
baked potato; 1 cup green beans with water chestnuts; tossed salad;
no- or low-cal dressing (2 tablespoons = 0–3 g fat); 1 slice mixed-
grain bread (1 g fat); 1 cup citrus fruit mixture; beverage
                    Total fat: 10–13 g

EVENING SNACK
4 cups air-popped popcorn (2 g fat)
                    Total fat: 2 g

                    Total fat for Day 2: 17–31 g
Nutrient analysis with 1 tablespoon margarine added: **33.6 g total fat**
(17%); 8.26 g saturated fat; 100 mg cholesterol; 1,731 calories; 42
g fiber; 2,434 mg sodium

DAY 3

BREAKFAST
1 ounce Shredded Wheat or other ready-to-eat cereal (1–3 g fat); ½
cup fresh berries; 1 cup skim or low-fat milk (0–3 g fat); 1 slice
whole-grain toast (1 g fat); 1 teaspoon jelly or jam (optional); coffee
or tea
                    Total fat: 2–7 g

MID-MORNING SNACK
1 banana
                    Total fat: 0

LUNCH
1 cup **Shrimp-Feta-Pasta Salad** (5 g fat); 1 ounce breadsticks or
whole-grain crackers (2–4 g fat); 1 apple; beverage
                    Total fat: 7–9 g

AFTERNOON SNACK
1 ounce pretzels (1 g fat)
                    Total fat: 1 g

DINNER
1 serving **Fish Fillets in Lemon-Tarragon Sauce** (5 g fat); ½ baked
acorn squash with 1 teaspoon margarine (4 g fat); 1 cup brussels

sprouts or other green vegetable; 1 cup fresh fruit salad; **Herb-Bran Muffin** (4 g fat); beverage
Total fat: 13 g

EVENING SNACK
1 slice cinnamon-raisin toast (1 g fat); 1 teaspoon jelly or jam (optional); 1 cup nonfat or low-fat yogurt (0–2 g fat)
Total fat: 1–3 g

Total fat for Day 3: 24–33 g
Nutrient analysis with 1 tablespoon margarine added: **42.0 g total fat** (20%); 11.3 g saturated fat; 201 mg cholesterol; 1,855 calories; 36 g fiber; 2,266 mg sodium

DAY 4

BREAKFAST
½ cup orange juice; 2 slices commercial cinnamon-raisin bread or **Raisin-and-Cinnamon Bread** (2–3 g fat); 1 teaspoon jelly or jam (optional); 1 cup skim or low-fat milk (0–3 g fat); coffee or tea
Total fat: 2–6 g

MID-MORNING SNACK
1 apple
Total fat: 0

LUNCH
1 cup **Fresh Vegetable Soup** or other broth-based soup (2–3 g fat); **Herb-Bran Muffin** (4 g fat); 1 cup assorted raw vegetables; 1 pear; beverage
Total fat: 6–7 g

AFTERNOON SNACK
2 fig-bar cookies (2 g fat)
Total fat: 2 g

DINNER
1 serving **Champ Beans** (1 g fat); ½ cup brown or wild rice (1 g fat); 1 cup broccoli; tossed salad; no- or low-cal dressing (2 tablespoons = 0–3 g fat); 1 serving **Crusty Buttermilk Cornbread** (1 g fat); ½ cup frozen yogurt with berries (0–3 g fat); beverage
Total fat: 3–9 g

EVENING SNACK
1 ounce ready-to-eat cereal (1–3 g fat); 1 cup skim or low-fat milk
(0–3 g fat)
Total fat: 1–6 g

Total fat for Day 4: 14–29 g
Nutrient analysis with 1 tablespoon margarine added: **37.5 g total fat**
(19%); 10.9 g saturated fat; 84 mg cholesterol; 1,852 calories; 46 g
fiber; 2,776 mg sodium

DAY 5

BREAKFAST
1 serving **Family-Favorite Oatmeal** (3 g fat); 1 slice mixed-grain
toast (1 g fat); 1 teaspoon jelly or jam (optional); 1 cup skim or
low-fat milk (0–3 g fat); coffee or tea
Total fat: 4–7 g

MID-MORNING SNACK
¼ honeydew melon or other seasonal fruit
Total fat: 0

LUNCH
Chef salad: assorted raw vegetables, 2 ounces lean ham or turkey
breast, ½ ounce shredded cheese, ¼ cup croutons (7–9 g fat); no-
or low-cal dressing (2 tablespoons = 0–3 g fat); 1 slice mixed-grain
bread (1 g fat); ½ cup pineapple slices or other fruit; beverage
Total fat: 8–13 g

AFTERNOON SNACK
2 rice cakes or popcorn cakes (0–1 g fat); salsa (optional)
Total fat: 0–1 g

DINNER
1 serving **Barbecued Chicken** (6 g fat); 1 ear corn on the cob; 1 cup
asparagus or other green vegetable; tossed salad; no- or low-cal
dressing (2 tablespoons = 0–3 g fat); 1 slice mixed-grain bread (1 g
fat); 1 serving **Fruit Crisp** (4 g fat); beverage
Total fat: 13–16 g

EVENING SNACK
2 graham crackers (1 g fat); 1 cup nonfat or low-fat yogurt (0–2 g
fat)
Total fat: 1–3 g

Total fat for Day 5: 26–40 g

Nutrient analysis with 1 tablespoon margarine added: **42.9 g total fat** (22%); 12.2 g saturated fat; 143 mg cholesterol; 1,699 calories; 28 g fiber; 2,789 mg sodium

DAY 6

BREAKFAST
4 **Basic Pancakes** (8 g fat); 1 ounce Canadian bacon (2 g fat); ½ cup fresh fruit topping; syrup (optional); 1 cup skim or low-fat milk (0–3 g fat); other beverage
Total fat: 10–13 g

MID-MORNING SNACK
1 ounce dried apricots
Total fat: 0

LUNCH
2 ounces sliced chicken (or ½ serving leftover Barbecued Chicken) (3 g fat); 1 whole-grain sandwich roll (2–3 g fat); lettuce and tomato slices; 1 ounce pretzels (1 g fat); 1 orange; beverage
Total fat: 6–7 g

AFTERNOON SNACK
½ cup frozen yogurt (0–3 g fat)
Total fat: 0–3 g

DINNER
3 ounces **Roast Pork Tenderloin** (4 g fat); medium baked sweet potato; 1 cup cauliflower; tossed salad; no- or low-cal dressing (2 tablespoons = 0–3 g fat); 1 slice mixed-grain bread (1 g fat); beverage
Total fat: 5–8 g

EVENING SNACK
1 slice raisin toast (1 g fat); 1 cup skim or low-fat milk (0–3 g fat)
Total fat: 1–4 g

Total fat for Day 6: 22–35 g
Nutrient analysis with 1 tablespoon margarine added: **43 g total fat** (22%); 12.1 g saturated fat; 218 mg cholesterol; 1,806 calories; 24 g fiber; 2,775 mg sodium

DAY 7

BREAKFAST
1 ounce Cheerios or other ready-to-eat cereal (1–3 g fat); ½ sliced banana; 1 cup skim or low-fat milk (0–3 g fat); 1 slice mixed-grain toast (1 g fat); 1 teaspoon jelly or jam (optional); coffee or tea
Total fat: 2–7 g

MID-MORNING SNACK
1 tangerine or nectarine
Total fat: 0

LUNCH
¼ cup **Salmon-Herb Spread** (6 g fat); 2 slices mixed-grain bread or bagel (1–2 g fat); 1 cup assorted raw vegetables; 1 cup watermelon or other seasonal fruit; beverage
Total fat: 7–8 g

AFTERNOON SNACK
1 ounce pita or bagel chips (1–2 g fat)
Total fat: 1–2 g

DINNER
1 serving **Turkey or Chicken Divan** (10 g fat); ½ cup **Glazed Orange-Spice Carrots;** ½ cup brown rice (1 g fat); 1 2-inch-diameter whole-grain dinner roll (2 g fat); ½ cup fresh fruit salad; ¹⁄₁₂th angel cake with 2 tablespoons fudge topping (1 g fat); beverage
Total fat: 14 g

EVENING SNACK
2 graham crackers (1 g fat); ½ cup apple juice
Total fat: 1 g

Total fat for Day 7: 25–32 g
Nutrient analysis with 1 tablespoon margarine added: **41.5 g total fat** (19%); 11.2 g saturated fat; 96 mg cholesterol; 1,872 calories; 26 g fiber; 3,083 mg sodium

Daily averages for Week 1 as listed without added margarine: **28.8 g total fat** (15%); 8.81 g saturated fat; 135 mg cholesterol; 1,717 calories; 34 g fiber; 2,515 mg sodium

Daily averages for Week 1 with 1 tablespoon added margarine: **40.2 g total fat** (20%); 10.8 g saturated fat; 135 mg cholesterol; 1,819 calories; 34 g fiber; 2,668 mg sodium

WEEK 2

DAY 8

BREAKFAST
2 Corny Breakfast Cakes (5 g fat); syrup (optional); ½ grapefruit; 1 cup skim or low-fat milk (0–3 g fat); coffee or tea
Total fat: 5–8 g

MID-MORNING SNACK
1 banana
Total fat: 0

LUNCH
1 serving **Italian Tuna Salad** (6 g fat); 2 slices mixed-grain bread (2 g fat); lettuce and tomato slices; 1 ounce pretzels (1 g fat); 1 apple; beverage
Total fat: 9 g

AFTERNOON SNACK
2 cups assorted raw vegetables; ½ cup seasoned nonfat or low-fat yogurt for dip (0–1 g fat)
Total fat: 0–1 g

DINNER
1 serving pasta with **Thick and Zesty Spaghetti Sauce** (10 g fat); 1 cup zucchini; tossed salad; no- or low-cal dressing (2 tablespoons = 0–3 g fat); 1 slice Italian bread (1 g fat); ½ cup seedless grapes; 2 fig-bar cookies (2 g fat); beverage
Total fat: 13–16 g

EVENING SNACK
4 cups air-popped popcorn (2 g fat)
Total fat: 2 g

Total fat for Day 8: 29–36 g
Nutrient analysis with 1 tablespoon margarine added: **43 g total fat** (19%); 9.4 g saturated fat; 130 mg cholesterol; 1,946 calories; 40 g fiber; 3,525 mg sodium

DAY 9

BREAKFAST

1 ounce Raisin Bran or other ready-to-eat cereal (1–3 g fat); 1 cup skim or low-fat milk (0–3 g fat); 1 slice mixed-grain toast (1 g fat); 1 teaspoon jelly or jam (optional); coffee or tea

Total fat: 2–7 g

MID-MORNING SNACK

1 peach

Total fat: 0

LUNCH

Easy Bean Burritos for Two (12 g fat for 2 burritos); 1 cup assorted raw vegetables; 1 orange; beverage

Total fat: 12 g

AFTERNOON SNACK

2 fig-bar cookies (2 g fat)

Total fat: 2 g

DINNER

1 serving **Teriyaki Beef Stir-fry** (12 g fat); ½ cup brown or wild rice (1 g fat); tossed salad; no- or low-cal dressing (2 tablespoons = 0–3 g fat); 1 2-inch-diameter whole-grain roll (2 g fat); 1 cup fresh fruit salad; beverage

Total fat: 15–18 g

EVENING SNACK

1 cup berries of choice; 1 cup nonfat or low-fat yogurt (0–2 g fat)

Total fat: 0–2 g

Total fat for Day 9: 31–41 g
Nutrient analysis with 1 tablespoon margarine added: **47.5 g total fat** (23%); 13.3 g saturated fat; 118 mg cholesterol; 1,822 calories; 43 g fiber; 2,911 mg sodium

DAY 10

BREAKFAST

Toasted bagel or English muffin (1–2 g fat); 2 tablespoons blenderized cottage cheese with jam for spread; 1 cup strawberries or seasonal fruit; 1 cup skim or low-fat milk (0–3 g fat); coffee or tea

Total fat: 1–5 g

MID-MORNING SNACK
1 orange
Total fat: 0

LUNCH
1 serving **Collard Soup** (6 g fat) or 1 cup other broth-based soup
(2–3 g fat); 1 ounce breadsticks or whole-grain crackers (2–4 g fat);
1 cup assorted raw vegetables; ½ cup fresh peaches or seasonal fruit;
beverage
Total fat: 4–10 g

AFTERNOON SNACK
1 slice raisin bread (1 g fat); 1 teaspoon jelly or jam (optional)
Total fat: 1 g

DINNER
4.5 ounces **Royal Indian Salmon** (8 g fat); ½ cup steamed new
potatoes; 1 serving **Greens Casserole** (6 g fat); tossed salad; no- or
low-cal dressing (2 tablespoons = 0–3 g fat); 1 slice mixed-grain
bread (1 g fat); ½ cup **Pineapple-Orange Frozen Yogurt** (0–2 g
fat); beverage
Total fat: 15–20 g

EVENING SNACK
1 ounce pretzels (1 g fat)
Total fat: 1 g

Total fat for Day 10: 22–37
Nutrient analysis with 1 tablespoon margarine added: **45.2 g total fat**
(23%); 12.3 g saturated fat; 187 mg cholesterol; 1,742 calories; 30
g fiber; 2,395 mg sodium

DAY 11

BREAKFAST
1 ounce ready-to-eat cereal (1–3 g fat); ½ sliced banana; 1 cup skim
or low-fat milk (0–3 g fat); 1 slice mixed-grain toast (1 g fat); 1
teaspoon jelly or jam (optional); coffee or tea
Total fat: 2–7 g

MID-MORNING SNACK
1 ounce raisins
Total fat: 0

LUNCH
1 serving **Shrimpy Tomato Aspic** (1 g fat); ½ cup low-fat cottage cheese (1–3 g fat); 1 ounce breadsticks or whole-grain crackers (2–4 g fat); ½ cup seedless grapes; beverage
Total fat: 4–8 g

AFTERNOON SNACK
½ cup frozen yogurt (0–3 g fat)
Total fat: 0–3 g

DINNER
1 serving **Easy Vegetarian Chili Texas Style** (2 g fat); ½ cup brown or wild rice (1 g fat); 1 cup asparagus or other green vegetable; 1 serving **Crusty Buttermilk Cornbread** (1 g fat); 1 cup citrus fruit mixture; beverage
Total fat: 4 g

EVENING SNACK
4 cups air-popped popcorn (2 g fat)
Total fat: 2 g

Total fat for Day 11: 12–24 g
Nutrient analysis with 1 tablespoon margarine added: **33.3 g total fat** (18%); 9.6 g saturated fat; 101 mg cholesterol; 1,631 calories; 41 g fiber; 3,036 mg sodium

DAY 12

BREAKFAST
1 serving **Fruity Breakfast Rice** (1 g fat); 1 slice mixed-grain toast (1 g fat); 1 teaspoon jelly or jam (optional); 1 cup skim or low-fat milk (0–3 g fat per cup); coffee or tea
Total fat: 2–5 g

MID-MORNING SNACK
½ bagel (1 g fat)
Total fat: 1 g

LUNCH
Medium baked potato topped with ½ cup low-fat cottage cheese (1–3 g fat), diced green onions, and Cajun seasoning or salsa; assorted raw vegetables; 1 orange or fresh fruit of choice; beverage
Total fat: 1–3 g

AFTERNOON SNACK
1 pear

Total fat: 0

DINNER
1 serving **Chicken Cacciatore** (4 g fat); 1 cup pasta (1 g fat); 1 cup green beans; tossed salad; no- or low-cal dressing (2 tablespoons = 0–3 g fat); 1 slice Italian bread (1 g fat); 1 serving **Cocoa Zucchini Cake** (5 g fat); beverage

Total fat: 11–14 g

EVENING SNACK
1 slice whole-grain bread (1 g fat) with 2 teaspoons peanut butter (7 g fat)

Total fat: 8 g

Total fat for Day 12: 23–31 g
Nutrient analysis with 1 tablespoon margarine added: **36.6 g total fat** (17%); 9.0 g saturated fat; 91 mg cholesterol; 1,878 calories; 35 g fiber; 2,236 mg sodium

DAY 13

BREAKFAST
1 cup melon or other seasonal fruit; **Fruity Oat-Bran Muffin** (4 g fat); 1 cup nonfat or low-fat yogurt, or skim or low-fat milk (0–3 g fat); coffee or tea

Total fat: 4–7 g

MID-MORNING SNACK
1 tangerine or nectarine

Total fat: 0

LUNCH
2 ounces sliced lean ham in whole-grain pita with pineapple slices and lettuce leaves (3–5 g fat); 1 ounce pretzels (1 g fat); beverage

Total fat: 4–6 g

AFTERNOON SNACK
2 rice cakes or popcorn cakes (0–1 g fat); salsa (optional)

Total fat: 0–1 g

DINNER
1 serving **Dijon Swordfish** (11 g fat); 1 serving **Beets to Beat All** (2 g fat); ½ cup brown rice (1 g fat); 1 slice mixed-grain bread (1

g fat); tossed salad; no- or low-cal dressing (2 tablespoons = 0–3 g fat); **Baked Apple** (1 g fat); beverage
Total fat: 16–19 g

EVENING SNACK
1 ounce 40% Bran Flakes or other ready-to-eat cereal (1–3 g fat); 1 cup skim or low-fat milk (0–3 g fat)
Total fat: 1–6 g

Total fat for Day 13: 25–39 g
Nutrient analysis with 1 tablespoon margarine added: **45.6 g total fat** (21%); 10.9 g saturated fat; 130 mg cholesterol; 1,913 calories; 28 g fiber; 3,355 mg sodium

DAY 14

BREAKFAST
½ grapefruit; 1 serving **Scrambled Eggs with Cheese** (6 g fat); 2 slices mixed-grain toast (2 g fat); tomato slices; 1 cup skim or low-fat milk (0–3 g fat); coffee or tea
Total fat: 8–11 g

MID-MORNING SNACK
2 plums
Total fat: 0

LUNCH
1 serving **Norwegian Cottage Cheese** (6 g fat) on 2 slices toasted mixed-grain bread or bagel (2 g fat); 1 cup assorted raw vegetables; 1 apple; beverage
Total fat: 8 g

AFTERNOON SNACK
½ cup frozen yogurt (0–3 g fat)
Total fat: 0–3 g

DINNER
1 serving **Oysters Rockefeller** (5 g fat); 1 serving **Pork Scallopine in Lemon, Dill, and Fennel Sauce** (10 g fat); ½ cup green peas; 1 serving **Cauliflower with Crumb Topping** (2 g fat); tossed salad; no- or low-cal dressing (2 tablespoons = 0–3 g fat); ½ cup pineapple chunks; beverage
Total fat: 17–20 g

EVENING SNACK
4 cups air-popped popcorn (2 g fat)
Total fat: 2 g

Total fat for Day 14: 37–48 g
Nutrient analysis with 1 tablespoon margarine added: **56.3 g total fat** (25%); 15.7 g saturated fat; 359 mg cholesterol; 1,921 calories; 49 g fiber; 2,849 mg sodium

Daily averages for Week 2 as listed without added margarine: **32.5 g total fat** (16%); 9.5 g saturated fat; 159 mg cholesterol; 1,734 calories; 37 g fiber; 2,748 mg sodium

Daily averages for Week 2 with 1 tablespoon added margarine: **43.9 g total fat** (21%); 11.5 g saturated fat; 159 mg cholesterol; 1,836 calories; 37 g fiber; 2,901 mg sodium

(Note: I have totaled separately for each week the average daily intakes for the above nutrients with and without any added fat for spread and seasoning to demonstrate how well the menus fall within the guidelines on a weekly basis.)

CHAPTER 10

LOSING WEIGHT WITH THE ONE MEAL AT A TIME PROGRAM

Almost all overweight people lose a certain amount of weight just by switching to a low-fat diet. There are several reasons for this, not the least of which is that it's hard to eat as many calories when you substitute bulkier, lower-calorie carbohydrate foods for the denser, higher-calorie fatty foods you may have been eating in the past. You get filled up much faster and chances are you will end up eating around 200 fewer calories each day.

Another reason that weight loss is likely to occur when you switch to a low-fat diet has to do with the sources of energy that your body burns in its basic metabolic processes and in physical activity. Your body tends to burn both fat and carbohydrate in its fuel mixture. In a person eating the typical American high-fat diet, the fuel mixture is close to 50-50 fat and carbohydrate over a 24-hour period (after the energy in the protein foods you eat has been used up). By switching from a high-fat to a low-fat diet, your body must draw fat from its fat stores to meet the energy mixture to which it is accustomed. It can take considerable time (and considerable fat loss) before your body fine-tunes its fuel mix to match the new ratio of fat and carbohydrate in a low-fat diet.

Two other factors also aid weight loss. It takes three to five times more energy to put carbohydrate to immediate use than it does for fat (about 5 to 7 percent of the total energy content of carbohydrate versus 1.5 percent for fat). That is, the body has to work to get the energy out of food, and it must work harder on carbohydrate than on fat. Thus, when it comes to supplying fuel to keep bodily functions going, more of the carbohydrate fuel is not available, or "wasted," compared with fat.

In addition, continuous high-carbohydrate intake tends to elevate your metabolic rate, especially if you outeat your energy needs for any length of time. Again, when your metabolic rate goes up, fewer calories are available for use or storage.

Perhaps the greatest benefit of a high-carbohydrate diet is in weight mainte-nance. It's really quite hard to get fat on a high-carbohydrate/low-fat diet. That's because it takes about 25 percent of the caloric value of carbohydrate foods to fuel the metabolic processes that turn carbo-hydrate into fat for storage. It takes only about 3 percent of the calories in dietary fat to convert fat to storage. This should be intui-tively obvious to you if you compare an apple with a pat of butter. It takes a lot more work to convert apples to body fat than it does to turn butter (or any other fat) to body fat.

So between the greater caloric cost of turning carbohydrate to fat compared with dietary fat, which I've just described, and the need to eat more bulk to get as many calories out of carbohydrate foods as you get from fatty foods, which I mentioned earlier, there is a built-in protection against putting on weight when you eat a high-carbohy-drate/low-fat diet.

All of this means that if you have some weight to lose, and you have had trouble maintaining a weight loss in the past, you're going to be much better off losing weight with an approach that uses the same low-fat principles you will need to stick with for the rest of your life if you want to keep that weight off.

But overweight people tend to be in a hurry once they make up their minds to lose weight and one of the most frequent questions I'm asked is:

"SHOULD I GO ON A LOW-CALORIE DIET TO LOSE WEIGHT?"

The answer is "No! Not unless you understand what you will need to do afterwards in order to keep off whatever weight you lose. *And do it!*"

You probably know at least one person who has gone on a low-calorie diet, perhaps used one of the liquid fasting programs, and ended up regaining all of the weight that was lost—or even more weight than was lost—in the first place. That's because prolonged use, or repeated use, of a low-calorie diet can increase the body's fat-storing ability. You get fatter and fatter on less and less food the more you diet!

If you have ever gone on a reduced-calorie diet, even a moderately reduced-calorie diet, and lost and regained weight in the past, you know what I'm talking about. The dieting approach to losing weight rarely works. You go "on" a diet, but ultimately you go "off" the diet. *No approach to losing weight except the one I recommend has any chance of working.* That is, *you must learn how to eat* while you are losing weight so that, once you reach your weight goal, *you are already doing exactly what it takes to keep off all the weight you lost.* If you have any more than a few pounds to lose, you must learn how to eat a nutritious diet that can satisfy you *at several hundred calories a day less than what you have been accustomed to eating at your heavier weight.* If you don't wish to do that, then you better get several hundred calories a day more active!

Although it's normal for people who are slightly overweight to lose a few pounds, and for people who are considerably overweight to lose as much as 10 or 15 percent of their body weight, just by switching to a low-fat diet, people who have a great deal of weight to get rid of usually stop far short of their goal. So I've simply got to put it to you straight:

If you are a sedentary overweight person with more than a few pounds to lose, I'll give you 10 to 1 odds that you cannot lose it all and keep it off without getting active. It means semi-starvation or using some other uncomfortable and unhealthy strategy forever.

Think about this. The average overweight person needs about 10 or 11 calories per pound of body weight each day to maintain his or her weight. If you lose 30 pounds, your body needs 300 fewer calories each day to maintain its new lower weight. A 50-pound loss means 500 fewer calories each day. Although a low-fat diet by itself will take off and keep off considerable weight, very few people are able to eat so little each day to sustain a loss of more than 10 or 15 percent of their initial body weight. They tend to put back at least part of what they have lost.

Assuming no severe metabolic abnormality, the only way that I can assure you of losing 30, 50, or even 75 pounds if you need to, and keeping them off, *is to get active.* You've got to burn up—by physical activity—the calories your body used to use to keep its enlarged fat cells alive. I'll have more to say about this in Chapter 13, but for now let me assure you that unless you can find something physical that you like to do almost every day, you are not likely to lose all the weight you need to lose and keep it off. Part, yes. All, no.

THE VERY BEST WAY TO LOSE WEIGHT

I repeat: The very best way to lose weight and keep it off is *to learn how to eat the way you will need to eat when you finish losing the weight you want to lose!*

So my goal is to show you how to eat, once and for always, not how to diet.

To lose weight, you use exactly the same strategy that I have been describing throughout this book. That is, right from the start, you follow a low-fat diet that assures you of *weight maintenance.* To help weight loss proceed a bit faster, *you just cut the fat content to a slightly lower level.* You will use exactly the same foods, meal plans, and menus that you can use to maintain your weight—all you do to lose is cut the portion sizes of foods that contain appreciable fat and add less fat for spread or seasoning.

The strategy I'm suggesting is the one I wrote about in *The T-Factor Diet.* Our research shows that people who are moderately overweight will lose an average of one-half to two-thirds of a pound a week, and severely overweight people considerably more, without paying any attention to counting calories, if they restrict their fat intake to the following levels:

Women	20 to 40 grams of fat per day
Men	30 to 60 grams of fat per day

Stick to the lower end of the recommended range of fat intake for a somewhat quicker loss.

The fat-gram approach to weight loss teaches you where the fat is in the foods you like to eat. If you have chosen a fat-gram quota at the lower end of the recommended range, you will be able to add a bit of fat when you reach your weight goal. But you will still eat the same variety of foods that you ate while you were losing weight and you will not exceed your maintenance level. If you are a woman, you should be able to maintain whatever you lose by staying at, or slightly below, 50 grams of fat a day. A man should be able to do this at about 60 grams of fat a day. *Provided you get physically active as I describe in Chapter 13.* [1]

Do not reduce your fat intake below the lower limits that I have suggested. Remember that the first sign of too little fat in your diet is likely to be dry skin or a cracked lip. If this happens, add a little fat back to your diet. An almost sure cure consists of a salad with a dressing made with 1 or 2 teaspoons of olive oil (or your own favorite vegetable oil) each day.

When you reach your weight goal you can, if you like, determine your actual calorie needs by keeping an eating record for a week or two. Then you can determine what would be 25 percent of total calories in fat, in fat grams, by using Table 3–1 in Chapter 3. Or you might decide on some other percentage of calories in fat and adjust fat grams accordingly. In the end, like most people, you will probably prefer to forget calories and simply count fat grams, adjusting up or down slightly on an ad hoc basis. Find some fat-gram count within the recommended maintenance range that I have just suggested that works for you, and remember the basic principle of sound nutrition:

Eat a wide variety of different foods from each of the food groups, especially grains, fruits, and vegetables, and choose low-fat meats, poultry, fish, and dairy products.

A ONE MEAL AT A TIME EATING PLAN FOR WEIGHT LOSS

When you put the meals and snacks together from Chapters 5 through 8, *with little or no added fat as spread or in food preparation,* they result in daily menus that contain between 20 and 30 grams of fat. They thus become ideal for weight loss when used in this manner. If you would like specific daily meal plans, go back and use the menus we entered into our nutritional analysis in Chapter 9. Follow those

[1] Follow-up research on the T-Factor Diet indicates that women prefer to stay at 18 to 22 percent of calories from fat in their diets, which tends to average between 30 and 40 grams of fat a day.

menus, but leave off the daily 1 tablespoon of added fat and, for the most part, choose the lower-fat alternatives (for example, no-fat instead of low-fat dressing) in the meal plans.

You can, and should, work to devise your own meal plans within the fat-gram quota you set for yourself. As a general rule, if your evening meal is, for social or other reasons, the main meal of the day, I suggest you count fat grams and limit your before-dinner intake to one-half your quota. With half remaining, and with everyone following a low-fat eating plan, no special food preparation will be required and you can have a satisfying dinner.

If you follow this plan, women will be eating no more than 20 grams of fat before dinner, and saving up to 20 grams for the evening meal (and snack). Men will be eating no more than 30 grams of fat before dinner, and saving up to 30 grams for the evening meal (and snack). Control the portion sizes of foods that contain more than a few grams of fat to make sure your fat-gram totals before and at dinner do not go over these limits. Limit snacks to nonfat items or those very low in fat.

If you feel that you need specific help in designing several weeks of low-fat menus, take a look at *The T-Factor Diet.* [2] You will find many great recipes in that book, too.

"Can I cut calories in addition to using the fat-gram approach, and lose weight even faster?"

I'm often asked this question by people who have a great deal of weight to lose, or for other reasons need to lose more quickly than the one-half to two-thirds of a pound weekly average that follows a switch to a low-fat diet. I can answer with a qualified yes. You must assure yourself that you both know and can practice what it will take to maintain your loss. If you decide to speed the process, it becomes especially important that you integrate a lower-calorie diet with the recommended range of fat intake of 20 to 40 grams a day for a woman and 30 to 60 grams for a man. After losing several pounds the first week (a good part of it water), women will average 1 to 2 pounds a week by restricting themselves to 1,200 calories a day, and men will lose at about the same rate, or slightly faster, at 1,800 calories a day. *The T-Factor Diet* contains such a quick-loss plan in Chapter 5, called "The Quick Melt." It presents daily menus that help you learn where the fat is in your food as you restrict your

---

[2] Published by W. W. Norton & Company, Inc., New York, 1989, and available in paperback from Bantam Books.

calories for a quicker weight loss. You also can use the Nutrient Counter in Appendix B to count calories on your own. Your main focus, however, should be on fat grams.

Our follow-up research in the Vanderbilt Weight Management Program shows that when people combine a reduced-calorie diet with the fat-gram approach to losing weight, they do not rely on counting calories for successful future weight maintenance. They use the knowledge they have gained from counting fat grams and continue to use the low-fat foods and methods of preparation they learned while counting fat grams. Many of them tell us they keep a subconscious fat-gram count in the back of their minds each day, but *they no longer focus on, or count, calories.* As this and other research shows, the key to permanent weight management is a low-fat diet and an active life-style.

WHAT ABOUT BREAKFAST?

Although eating breakfast as part of a meal pattern that includes six or more eating episodes daily is associated with lower weight and other health benefits in the long run, a recent study reported a strange result when it comes to losing weight in the first place. On a temporary basis it seems that changing your eating habits with respect to breakfast can facilitate weight loss. Overweight people who formerly did not eat breakfast and began as part of the study, and overweight people who normally ate breakfast and stopped, lost significantly more weight than those that continued with their established habits.

Obviously a study such as this needs replication. If you presently eat breakfast and decide to alter your habits as an aid to losing weight, I still strongly advise you to learn to eat a nutritious breakfast when you switch back to a maintenance diet. And remember, if you are like most overweight people who come into the Vanderbilt program and are skipping breakfast, it's much better for losing weight to start eating breakfast as part of your weight-loss program.

A WORD OF WARNING

Although it's hard to do, it is possible to cut your *fat intake* to the weight-loss levels I recommend and still eat enough on a high-carbo-hydrate diet so that you end up not losing any more than a few pounds. It's most easily done by overeating on sweets (such as jelly beans or mints) or grains (such as bread or pretzels). You're not likely to stop your weight loss with fruits and vegetables, since they have much greater bulk due to their fiber and water content.

From our follow-up research with the T-Factor Diet, we have seen people prevent weight loss by eating a whole loaf of bread or a large bag (10 or more ounces) of pretzels daily, as snacks, over and above their basic meal plans. In some other cases, it was 6 or more ounces of nonfat candy such as jelly beans every day. In almost all such cases, this overeating was combined with a low level of activity.

Many people find that moderate physical activity every day helps regulate the tendency to lose control over one's appetite, as the people in my examples in the previous paragraph have done. Physical activity also is often a useful remedy for stress-related overeating. If you just happen to have what my mother called "a healthy appetite," and simply love good food, then you must compensate by developing an equal love for physical activity. I'll have more to say about this in Chapter 13.

HOW MUCH SHOULD YOU WEIGH?

No one can tell you as a unique individual what your ideal body weight or your ideal percentage body fat should be!

Recommended weights in weight tables are derived from statistics that predict longevity in large numbers of people. That's very important for setting insurance rates or public health goals. But the weight suggested for your age, sex, and height may be either too high or too low for your health and well-being *as a unique individual.*

Similarly, while evidence linking high levels of body fat to high serum cholesterol levels, heart disease, and certain cancers is growing, the recommended ranges for percentage body fat that you see in popular publications can be completely unsuitable for large numbers of people whose heredity predisposes them to higher body-fat levels. The recommended range of 14 to 18 percent body fat for males is not as likely to be as far off, or as unhealthy, as the often-recommended range of 18 to 22 percent for women.

I think there are three guidelines you should follow in determining what you should weigh and your percentage body fat.

First, wherever you end up by eating a nutritious low-fat diet and leading an active life is probably correct for you. That's where the interaction of your hereditary predispositions and your healthy life-style dictates that you should be healthiest and happiest. Most people will arrive at their individual "biological ideal" weight and percent-age body fat by following the One Meal at a Time program and walking briskly about 45 minutes almost every day, or its equivalent in other activity, if their work is sedentary.

Second, an existing illness or risk factor can modify the first guide-line to a certain extent. If you have high blood pressure, high serum cholesterol, diabetes, or any other illness related to weight or body fat, you might need to take more heroic measures. You might need to reduce fat below 25 percent of calories in your diet and occasion-ally engage in a more vigorous activity than walking. You may need a more complete physical conditioning program, which is always desirable even if not essential to weight management or cholesterol control. Special physical problems, such as arthritis, will require spe-cial activity programs. Obviously, when there is an existing illness or any special risk factor, the program of weight loss and physical activ-ity should be supervised by a physician.

Third, your profession or an avocation that plays an important role in your life may require that you pay special attention to your weight or body build. I hate to say this, but often other goals in life dictate that we pursue unhealthy behaviors when it comes to our weight and certain body characteristics. To become a champion marathoner, an Olympic-caliber gymnast, or a prima ballerina will almost always require that body fat be kept below the normally acceptable ranges, and that you practice your profession many hours a day, often to the point of pain.

I was once approached by a student at the university who had obtained a contract to be on the cover of a leading women's maga-zine. The job was a true "plum" for her. But at 5 feet 7 inches she was "too fat" at 120 pounds. She was told to be at a maximum of 105 pounds for the picture and asked me to supervise her weight-loss program. Although she had several months in which to lose the weight and could do it slowly, I suggested that if this assignment was crucial to her career as a model, she do it under medical supervision. I was not sure that the lower weight, and the means necessary to attain it, would be healthy for her.

My point is this: If you wish to be at some other weight or percent-age body fat than the one at which you arrive naturally by following a nutritious low-fat diet and a sensible activity program, you may need to engage in eating and exercise behaviors that can be dangerous to your health. You need to weigh the costs against the benefits. There are published cases of death among marathon runners, evidently caused by overtraining and efforts to achieve too low a body-fat percentage.

Health officials from the government and professional associations are working on new guidelines for determining ideal weight. The new guidelines will incorporate a person's body mass, waist and hip size, and medical status.[3] Such guidelines will be an improvement over the use of height and weight relationships alone. However, even these new guidelines will be derived from the use of large group averages, and may possibly not be suitable to you as a unique individual. *The most natural and best weight for you is the weight you arrive at with proper diet and physical activity. To aim for any other weight must have some other compelling reason.*

Among the first signs that you are engaging in unhealthful dietary or exercise behaviors to reach or maintain a weight that is unnatural and too low *for you* are fatigue, anxiety or depression, sleep disturbances, and chonic aches and pains. Among women, another sign of too little body fat is a disruption of the menstrual cycle.

Nevertheless, after warning against *overdoing* it, I want to reemphasize that *if you are a sedentary person,* permanent weight loss is not likely without increasing your physical activity. A low-fat diet can take you only part of the way if you have more than a few pounds to lose. Take what I have to say on how to develop an enjoyment of physical activity in Chapter 13 very seriously, and do it.

---

[3]Body mass is a measure that relates quite well to percentage body fat. It's computed by the formula "weight in kilograms divided by height in meters squared." An index greater than 27.8 for men and 27.3 for women is indicative of obesity. The reason for including waist and hip size is that a relatively greater waist-to-hip measurement is associated with obesity-related illnesses such as heart disease, stroke, and diabetes. To find your waist-to-hip ratio, measure your waist near your navel while standing in a relaxed posture (don't pull in your stomach). Measure your hips over your buttocks at the largest point. Divide the waist measurement by the hip measurement. A ratio of 0.80 or less is recommended for women, and 0.95 or less for men. Certain medical or psychological conditions may make weight loss more advisable than others, or may even advise against it. You should check with your doctor before going on a reduced-calorie diet.

CHAPTER 11

RECIPES

GUIDELINES

Before getting into my own One Meal at a Time recipes, I'd like to make explicit the three guidelines to low-fat food selection and preparation that have formed the basis for my suggestions in earlier chapters of this book. They are represented by the words **Switch**, **Avoid**, and **Modify**.

- **Switch** to lower-fat versions of the foods you like in your own recipes, as well as when you eat out. Choose the leaner cuts of beef, ham, and pork, and dairy products with the lowest fat that will still satisfy your taste buds. Check the labels of all packaged foods and when there is a choice, *switch* to the lowest-fat versions. You will discover considerable differences in fat content, especially among processed meats and snack foods. Some cereals, such as granola, also can be high in fat.
- **Avoid** certain high-fat foods and methods of preparation either most of the time or entirely. For example, you will be far ahead of the game if you never prepare or eat fried food again! *Avoid* preparing or choosing high-fat baked goods, butter and cream sauces, and rich desserts most of the time. You will find recipes for some low-fat sauces in this chapter. If you don't wish to avoid entirely—for example, skip the pie for a piece of

fruit—then *switch* to a lower-fat version of pie, cake, or cookies, such as you will find among my desserts or in other low-fat cookbooks.

- **Modify** your own favorite recipes, if they happen to be higher in fat than similar recipes that you find in this chapter. Try cutting the fat by one-third or one-half as a starter. Substitute another liquid if necessary to make up for the lower fat content. Note the fat content of my combination dishes and baked goods. You will rarely see more than 1 or 2 tablespoons of added fat in a recipe with 4 to 6 servings. You will find yogurt, evaporated skim milk, and reduced-calorie spreads used *in combination with or in place of* higher-fat items such as canned creamed soup and regular mayonnaise. If you are not experienced in low-fat food preparation, the best training you can get is to try all of my recipes until you get the hang of it.

SAM is the acronym for *Switch, Avoid, and Modify.* Think SAM when it comes to making healthful low-fat food choices and preparing lower-fat meals.

A word on kitchen utensils: You will become more expert and take greater pleasure in cooking when you have the proper utensils. At the top of the list are fine knives and cookware. Your knives must sharpen to a fine edge and hold it well for chopping vegetables and trimming meat easily. Treat yourself to Henckels or Wüsthof knives, or something of equal quality, and purchase a good stone or ceramic for sharpening. Ask for advice on cookware from the salesperson at a store that specializes in fine cookware. Many fine stores have a policy that permits you to return utensils that don't perform satisfactorily. This can be important if an expensive pot or pan warps and won't conduct the heat evenly.

A word on finding recipes mentioned within other recipes: The index to this book contains the names of every recipe in this chapter, set in **bold print,** and is the quickest way to locate the particular recipe you wish to find.

MICROWAVE COOKING

Just about all of these recipes can be adapted to microwave cooking, but I think you will prefer that meat be cooked in a regular oven. (However, as I noted in Chapter 7, you can remove more fat from hamburger if you cook it in a microwave oven.) I have good luck with all the fish and vegetable recipes in my microwave.

Microwaves vary in their power, so consult the instruction booklet that comes with yours for cooking times for recipes similar to those included in this chapter.

We do just about all our vegetables in the microwave, using 11 to 12 minutes per pound, depending on the thickness of the pieces. A medium-size baked potato takes just 6 minutes in our microwave. I never add fat during the microwave cooking of any vegetable, but I have discovered that just a few drops of olive oil, added and mixed just before serving, improve the texture and flavor of many vegetables. If you find yourself skipping them because you don't like the texture of plain steamed or microwaved vegetables, try just ¼ teaspoon of olive oil (mixed with an entire recipe for four). It will add a gram of fat per serving, but it can make all the difference between liking and disliking, and therefore eating and not eating, many vegetables.

NUTRITIONAL ANALYSES

The nutritional contents of all recipes were analyzed using the ESHA Food Processor II Nutrition and Diet Analysis System computer program. After each recipe you will find information about total fat, saturated fat, cholesterol, calories, fiber, and sodium. Cholesterol and sodium values are rounded up or down to the nearest milligram, while fiber is rounded to the nearest gram. Total fat includes all fat (saturated, polyunsaturated, and monounsaturated) in each recipe. The saturated-fat component is given for people who are particularly interested in controlling that portion of their fat intake.

A note on butter and margarine. When either butter or margarine is called for in a recipe, the recipe was tested both ways but the analysis was performed using margarine, since that is what Jamie prefers and she was in charge of doing the analyses. In addition, some of the recipes were created by participants in the Vanderbilt program, and they preferred to use margarine. As I mentioned elsewhere, I prefer the flavor of butter. However, while total fat remains the same whether you use butter or margarine, butter contains cholesterol and a higher proportion of saturated fat than does margarine. If you prefer to use butter, you must add 5 grams of saturated fat and 30 milligrams of cholesterol per tablespoon used and then divide by the number of servings to determine the additional saturated fat and cholesterol contained in each serving. In the amounts that butter would be used in place of margarine, the extra saturated fat and cholesterol in your diet should prove to be negligible. For example, in my favorite Pork Scallopine in Lemon, Dill, and Fennel Sauce, butter would add less than 1 gram of saturated fat and only 5 milligrams of cholesterol per serving. It's even less in most other recipes. Thus, I don't think you need to bother going through these calculations provided you stick to the small amounts called for in the recipes and keep within my recommendations for total fat in your diet.

HERBS AND SPICES

Table 11–1 is a guide to the use of herbs and spices that can add to your cooking and eating pleasure. If you are not already sensitive to the different tastes of various herbs and spices, I recommend that you try one at a time with some of the different foods that are suggested in the list.

One of the best ways to cut down on the use of salt is to blend it with herbs and spices. You can make your own "Herb Salt" by combining 1 part salt with 5 parts herbs, using an assortment of different herbs. For starters, try ¼ teaspoon salt with ¼ teaspoon each of basil, thyme, dill weed, celery seed, and dried parsley. Then experiment with your own combinations.

TABLE 11–1.   HERBS AND SPICES TO ACCOMPANY DIFFERENT FOODS

Allspice—Meats, fish, gravies, relishes, tomato sauce

Anise—Fruit

Basil—Green beans, onions, peas, potatoes, summer squash, tomatoes, lamb, beef, shellfish, eggs, sauces

Bay Leaves—Artichokes, beets, carrots, onions, white potatoes, tomatoes, meats, fish, soups and stews, sauces, gravies

Caraway Seed—Asparagus, beets, cabbage, carrots, cauliflower, coleslaw, onions, potatoes, sauerkraut, turnips, beef, pork, noodles, cheese dishes

Cardamom—Melon, sweet potatoes

Cayenne Pepper—Sauces, curries

Celery Seed—Cabbage, carrots, cauliflower, corn, lima beans, potatoes, tomatoes, turnips, salad dressings, beef, fish dishes, sauces, soups, stews, cheese

Chervil—Carrots, peas, salads, summer squash, tomatoes, salad dressings, poultry, fish, eggs

Chili Powder—Corn, eggplant, onions, beef, pork, chili con carne, stews, shellfish, sauces, egg dishes

Chives—Carrots, corn, sauces, salads, soups

Cinnamon—Stewed fruits, apple or pineapple dishes, sweet potatoes, winter squash, toast

Cloves—Baked beans, sweet potatoes, winter squash, pork and ham roasts

Cumin—Cabbage, rice, sauerkraut, chili con carne, ground-beef dishes, cottage or cheddar cheese

Curry Powder—Carrots, cauliflower, green beans, onions, tomatoes, pork and lamb, shellfish, fish, poultry, sauces for eggs and meats

Dill Seed—Cabbage, carrots, cauliflower, peas, potatoes, spinach, tomato dishes, turnips, salads, lamb, cheese

Dill Weed—Vegetables, salads, poultry, soups

Ginger—Applesauce, melon, baked beans, carrots, onions, sweet potatoes, poultry, summer and winter squash, beef, veal, ham, lamb, teriyaki sauce

Mace—Carrots, potatoes, spinach, summer squash, beef, veal, fruits, sauces

Marjoram—Asparagus, carrots, eggplant, greens, green beans, lima beans, peas, spinach, summer squash, lamb, pork, poultry, fish, stews, sauces

Mustard—Asparagus, broccoli, brussels sprouts, cabbage, cauliflower, green beans, onions, peas, potatoes, summer squash, meats, poultry

Mustard Seed—Salads, curries, pickles, ham, corned beef, relishes

Nutmeg—Beets, brussels sprouts, carrots, cabbage, cauliflower, greens, green beans, onions, spinach, sweet potatoes, winter squash, sauces

Oregano—Baked beans, broccoli, cabbage, cauliflower, green beans, lima beans, onions, peas, potatoes, spinach, tomatoes, turnips, beef, pork, veal, poultry, fish, pizza, chili con carne, Italian sauces, stews

Paprika—Salad dressings, shellfish, fish, gravies, eggs

Parsley Flakes—All vegetables, soups, sauces, salads, stews, potatoes, eggs

Pepper—Most vegetables, meats, salads

Poppy Seed—Salads, noodles

Rosemary—Mushrooms, peas, potatoes, spinach, tomatoes, vegetable salads, beef, lamb, pork, veal, poultry, stews, cheese, eggs

Saffron—Rice

Sage—Eggplant, onions, peas, tomato dishes, salads, pork, veal, poultry, ham, cheese

Savory—Baked beans, beets, cabbage, carrots, cauliflower, lima beans, potatoes, rice, squash, egg dishes, roasts, ground-meat dishes

Sesame Seed—Asparagus, green beans, potatoes, tomatoes, spinach

Tarragon—Asparagus, beets, cabbage, carrots, cauliflower, mushrooms, tomatoes, salads, macaroni and vegetable combinations, beef, poultry, pork

Thyme—Artichokes, beets, carrots, eggplant, green beans, mushrooms, peas, tomatoes, pork, veal, poultry, cheese and fish dishes, stuffings

Turmeric—Mustards and curries, chicken

BREAKFAST FOODS

Most of the basic breakfasts that I suggested in Chapter 5 require no preparation—they come out of boxes, bags, and bottles. However, the following selection of breakfast recipes includes some specials that are so easy to prepare you may want to include them among your regular breakfast menus. There's a sampling of hot cereals and lower-fat versions of American favorites, such as Mock Danish, Scrambled Eggs with Cheese, Egg-in-a-Muffin, and Country Sausage. And, of course, there are pancakes, French toast, and popovers. Other breakfast selections can be found under Breads and Muffins. Whole-grain flours are called for in many recipes, but it's possible to blend them with refined flour to give the results a little softer or fluffier texture.

Family-Favorite Oatmeal

3 cups hot cooked oatmeal
¼ cup light brown sugar
1 teaspoon cinnamon
1 medium-large apple, at
   room temperature, cut
   into small chunks

⅓ cup raisins
2 tablespoons walnuts or
   pecans, chopped

Stir brown sugar and cinnamon into cooked oatmeal. Add apple chunks, raisins, and chopped nuts. Serve hot.

Makes 6 servings.
Per serving: **2.9 g total fat;** 0.4 g saturated fat; 0 cholesterol; 171 calories; 4 g fiber; 7 mg sodium

Fruity Breakfast Rice

This is a delicious idea for leftover rice.

2 cups cooked brown rice, heated
1 cup plain, nonfat yogurt
1 tablespoon honey or brown sugar

1 teaspoon cinnamon
1 medium apple, chopped (or other fruit of choice)
3 tablespoons raisins

Combine rice, yogurt, honey or brown sugar, and cinnamon in a bowl. Stir in chopped apple and raisins and reheat.

Makes 4 servings.
Per serving: **1.2 g total fat;** 0.3 g saturated fat; 1 mg cholesterol; 212 calories; 4 g fiber; 50 mg sodium

Mock Danish

2 English muffins, split and toasted
1 cup low-fat cottage cheese

1 teaspoon cinnamon
1 tablespoon sugar
½ cup applesauce

1. Spread ¼ cup cottage cheese on each toasted muffin half. Combine the cinnamon and sugar; sprinkle over cottage cheese.
2. Top each "Danish" with 2 tablespoons applesauce. Place on a cookie sheet or in toaster oven and broil until bubbly.

Makes 4 servings.
Per serving: **1.7 g total fat;** 0.8 g saturated fat; 5 mg cholesterol; 147 calories; 2 g fiber; 419 mg sodium

VARIATIONS: Top with sliced peaches, banana, or apples instead of applesauce.

Egg-in-a-Muffin

This is a lower-fat adaptation of the famous fast-food breakfast sandwich.

¼ cup nonfat egg substitute
  or 1 egg, scrambled
Nonstick cooking spray
1-ounce slice Canadian
  bacon or lean ham

1 English muffin
1 slice reduced-fat cheese
Salt and pepper to taste

1. Scramble the egg substitute in a nonstick skillet sprayed with nonstick cooking spray. Heat the bacon or ham slice.
2. Meanwhile, toast the English muffin and place the slice of cheese across one half. Top with scrambled egg and Canadian bacon slice. Season with salt and pepper.

Makes 1 serving.
Per serving using egg substitute: **6.1 g total fat;** 2.7 g saturated fat; 24 mg cholesterol; 269 calories; 2 g fiber; 1,405 mg sodium
Per serving using egg: **11.1 g total fat;** 4.3 g saturated fat; 236 mg cholesterol; 309 calories; 2 g fiber; 1,356 mg sodium

Scrambled Eggs with Cheese

Jamie Pope-Cordle, our nutritionist, makes this every weekend and serves it with Canadian bacon or turkey sausage. She also says it makes a super scrambled-egg sandwich for a quick evening meal.

1 cup egg substitute (Egg
  Beaters)
2 whole eggs
2 tablespoons skim or 1%
  milk

Nonstick cooking spray
4 slices (4 ounces)
  reduced-fat cheese
Salt and pepper to taste

1. In a small bowl, beat egg substitute with whole eggs and milk. Pour into a nonstick skillet that has been sprayed with nonstick cooking spray.
2. Cook over medium heat, adding cheese in pieces to egg mixture. Using a spatula, scrape the sides of the skillet and gently fold cheese into eggs. Cook until set. Season with salt and pepper.

Makes 4 servings.
Per serving (using 1% milk): **5.8 g total fat;** 2.9 g saturated fat; 117 mg cholesterol; 101 calories; 0 fiber; 322 mg sodium

VARIATIONS: Add chopped green onion, onion, green or red pepper, diced tomatoes, or mushrooms with the cheese. Cut recipe in half to make 2 servings.

Harriette's Breakfast Popovers

1 cup all-purpose flour
½ cup whole-wheat flour
1½ cup skim or 1% milk
¾ cup nonfat egg substitute

or 4 egg whites plus 1 whole egg, beaten
½ teaspoon salt
Nonstick cooking spray

1. Combine all ingredients; beat just until smooth with electric mixer.
2. Spray muffin tins with nonstick cooking spray and heat in 450 degree oven for 3 minutes. Remove muffin tins and fill ⅔ full with batter.
3. Bake at 450 degrees for 30 minutes; reduce temperature to 300 degrees and bake an additional 10 to 15 minutes. Prick with a fork to allow steam to escape.
4. Serve hot with jelly or jam.

Makes 12 popovers.
Per popover (using 1% milk): **0.7 g total fat;** 0.2 g saturated fat; 20 mg cholesterol; 104 calories; 1 g fiber; 170 mg sodium

French Toast

This is good served with a breakfast spread, fresh fruit, applesauce, or a tablespoon or two of real maple syrup. When it comes to French toast, or pancakes for that matter, which many people are accustomed to drowning with butter, I think it's important to look for the finest alternative condiments when you cut the fat.

1 egg	Dash salt
2 egg whites	2 slices whole-grain bread
2 tablespoons skim milk	Nonstick cooking spray
¼ teaspoon cinnamon	

1. Beat the egg, egg whites, and milk with the cinnamon and salt until frothy. Dip the bread in the egg mixture, coating both sides.
2. Heat a skillet or griddle and spray with nonstick cooking spray. "Fry" the bread in the heated skillet, turning once, until golden brown on both sides.

Makes 2 servings.
Per serving: **5.0 g total fat;** 1.5 g saturated fat; 107 mg cholesterol; 200 calories; 4 g fiber; 453 mg sodium

VARIATIONS: Omit the cinnamon, and substitute ¼ teaspoon of grated lemon or orange peel. You can also use ½ cup egg substitute instead of the whole egg and add just 1 egg white.

Basic Pancakes

Make your own nutritious, homemade pancake mix. Store the dry mix in an airtight container—add the wet ingredients when you are ready to prepare the pancakes.

THE MIX

4 cups whole-wheat flour
4 cups all-purpose flour
2 cups wheat germ
1 cup nonfat dry milk
⅓ cup baking powder
1 teaspoon salt

THE PANCAKES

1½ cup dry mix
1 egg, beaten well
1¼ cup skim milk or water
1 tablespoon oil
Nonstick cooking spray

1. Combine the mix with the egg, milk, and oil. Do not overmix; the batter will be slightly lumpy.
2. Heat a Teflon pan, or other pan sprayed with nonstick cooking spray, over medium heat. Pour about ¼ cup of batter per pancake onto the heated pan. When the cakes are bubbly on top and brown on the bottom, flip and brown on the other side.

Makes 12 pancakes.
Per serving of 2 pancakes: **4.0 g total fat;** 0.6 g saturated fat; 37 mg cholesterol; 153 calories; 2 g fiber; 224 mg sodium

Corny Breakfast Cakes

Serve with warm pancake syrup or topped with fresh fruit. These are great as leftovers, too.

1¼ cups all-purpose flour
½ cup cornmeal
1 tablespoon baking
   powder
¼ teaspoon salt
1 tablespoon sugar
1 whole egg plus 1 egg
   white, beaten

1½ cups skim or 1% milk
2 tablespoons oil or melted
   margarine
1 8¾-ounce can cream-style
   corn
Nonstick cooking spray

1. Combine first five ingredients in a bowl.
2. In another bowl, whisk together the egg, milk, and oil. Stir in cream-style corn.

3. Add to flour mixture and stir just until combined—batter will be lumpy.
4. Preheat a 12-inch nonstick skillet or griddle. Spray with nonstick cooking spray and cook 2–3 cakes at a time, using approximately ¼ cup batter for each. Cook until bubbles form around the edges and each cake is lightly browned underneath, then flip and cook about 1 minute longer.

Makes 16 4-inch cakes.
Per serving of 2 cakes (using 1% milk): **4.7 g total fat;** 0.9 g saturated fat; 27 mg cholesterol; 187 calories; 1.7 g fiber; 320 mg sodium

Country Sausage

1 pound ground turkey, lean pork, beefalo, or extra-lean beef
½ cup breadcrumbs
2 cloves garlic, minced
2 tablespoons fresh parsley, finely chopped (2 teaspoons dry)
1 teaspoon thyme

1 teaspoon sage
½ teaspoon marjoram
½ teaspoon salt
Freshly ground black pepper to taste
½ to 1 teaspoon crushed hot red pepper
Nonstick cooking spray

1. Combine all ingredients and form into 8 small patties.
2. "Fry" in a Teflon pan or skillet sprayed with nonstick cooking spray until brown and crisp on both sides, about 20 minutes. Add a little water during cooking if patties begin to stick.

Makes 8 servings.
Per serving: **7.2 g total fat;** 2.0 g saturated fat; 35 mg cholesterol; 139 calories; 0 fiber; 221 mg sodium

VARIATIONS: This can be made as a loaf with extras like chopped onion and mushrooms. It can also be made with canned salmon: Add 1 large egg or 2 egg whites to two 7½-ounce cans of salmon and form into a loaf or patties. Made with salmon it's incredibly good and one of my favorite recipes.

BREADS AND MUFFINS

We have quite a sampling here. Most are mixed grain—that is, part all-purpose and part whole-wheat flour since all whole wheat can make a rather heavy bread. Sweet Honey Bread, however, is made entirely from whole wheat and it's a delightful, sweet bread for breakfast or desserts. It's one I like to nibble on, along with sipping a cup of hot coffee, brewed strong from fresh ground beans.

We include four muffin recipes, a light wheat biscuit, and corn-bread in addition to the other bread recipes. These are all designed with meals in mind. Several are well suited to breakfast and others, like the No-Knead Herb Bread and Herb-Bran Muffins, are perfect for lunch or dinner. All these good breads are low in fat and make excellent snacks in place of chips and higher-fat crackers.

Be sure to check the expiration date on the package(s) of yeast before making any of the recipes that include yeast as an ingredient.

Quick Honey-Wheat Bread

4½–5cups all-purpose flour
2 cups whole-wheat flour
2 packages *fast-acting* yeast
1½ teaspoon salt
2 cups skim or 1% milk

½ cup honey
2 tablespoons oil
½ cup water
Nonstick cooking spray

1. In a large electric mixer, combine 2 cups of the all-purpose flour, the 2 cups of whole-wheat flour, the yeast, and salt.
2. In a saucepan or in the microwave, heat the milk, honey, oil, and water until warm (110°–115°F). Add to flour mixture. Mix at low speed to blend, then beat at medium speed for 5 minutes.
3. Stir in remaining all-purpose flour. Turn out on a floured surface and knead for approximately 10 minutes. Cover and let rise in a warm place for 10 minutes.

4. Divide dough in half and shape into loaves. Coat two 4½ × 8½ × 2-inch loaf pans with nonstick cooking spray. Place dough into pans and cover with dishcloth until doubled, about 45 minutes.

5. Bake at 375 degrees for 30 to 45 minutes until browned.

Makes 2 loaves, 16 slices per loaf.
Per slice (1.7 ounces) (using 1% milk): **1.2 g total fat;** 0.1 g saturated fat; 0 cholesterol; 120 calories; 2 g fiber; 109 mg sodium

Sweet Honey Bread

This dark, whole-grain bread is a real breakfast treat or can serve as a delicious dessert bread with fresh fruit.

2½ cups whole-wheat flour
1 cup honey
1 cup skim or 1% milk
3 tablespoons oil or melted margarine

1 teaspoon baking soda
1 teaspoon salt
1 egg, beaten
Nonstick cooking spray

1. Combine all ingredients in an electric mixer bowl. Beat 2 minutes.

2. Coat a 4½ × 8½-inch loaf pan with nonstick cooking spray. Transfer bread mixture to pan and bake 1 hour or until toothpick or knife comes out clean.

Makes 20 slices.
Per slice (1.7 ounces) (using 1% milk): **2.6 g total fat;** 0.3 g saturated fat; 11 mg cholesterol; 128 calories; 2 g fiber; 159 mg sodium

Raisin-and-Cinnamon Bread

This recipe is worth the time it requires. Try making it on a rainy Saturday when there's not much else to do and you will have some super breakfast bread all week long.

1 package yeast
½ cup warm water
1¾ cups skim or 1% milk
3 tablespoons sugar
1½ teaspoons salt
½ cup margarine
4½–5 cups all-purpose flour

1½–2 cups whole-wheat flour
2 cups raisins, soaked in
    water 15–30 minutes
Nonstick cooking spray
½ cup sugar
1 tablespoon cinnamon

1. In a large bowl, dissolve yeast in water that tests warm (not hot) on wrist. Set aside.
2. Heat milk, the 3 tablespoons sugar, salt, and margarine to *lukewarm.* Add to yeast mixture.
3. Stir in flours (the smaller amount in each case) and raisins. Mix to form a stiff dough.
4. Turn out onto a floured surface and knead for 10 minutes, adding the extra flour as needed (dough should be elastic but not sticky).
5. Shape into a ball, place in a bowl that has been sprayed with nonstick cooking spray, turn dough over to coat all sides with the oil from the spray, then cover loosely with plastic wrap and let rise in warm place (on top of pilot light of a gas oven or inside an electric oven that has *not* been turned on) for 1¼ to 1½ hours (dough should look doubled in size).
6. Punch down dough (punch your fist into the middle). Gather edges into the punched-in center and turn out onto a lightly floured surface. Knead for 30 seconds, divide in half, and shape into 2 balls. Cover with a damp towel for 10 minutes.
7. Flatten each ball with a rolling pin and roll out into an 8 × 15-inch rectangle. Combine the ½ cup sugar and cinnamon and sprinkle half over each rectangle. Roll up like a jelly roll, sealing edges and seams. Place, with seam side down, in 4½ × 8½-inch loaf pans that have been sprayed with nonstick cooking spray.

Cover pans loosely with plastic wrap and let rise in warm place for 1 hour or until almost doubled in size.

8. Bake in a 375-degree oven for 30 minutes. Cover with aluminum foil and bake an additional 15 minutes. Cool on wire racks.

Makes 2 loaves, 16 slices per loaf.
Per slice (2 ounces) (using 1% milk): **3.2 g total fat;** 0.6 g saturated fat; 0 cholesterol; 161 calories; 2 g fiber; 142 mg sodium

Quick Mustard-Rye Bread

There is no better bread than this for sandwiches. Try it with lean meats or sliced turkey, or with any of my salads or spreads. Since different all-purpose flours can respond differently to the other ingredients, we needed to be approximate in the amount called for in this recipe. Just follow directions, though, and you won't go wrong.

3–4 cups all-purpose flour, divided
1½ teaspoons salt
3 packages yeast
2 cups water

¼ cup Dijon mustard
⅓ cup brown sugar
3 tablespoons margarine
2 cups rye flour
Nonstick cooking spray

1. Combine 2 cups all-purpose flour, salt, and yeast in an electric mixer bowl. Set aside.
2. In a saucepan or in the microwave, heat water, mustard, brown sugar, and margarine until warm (110°–115°F). Add to the dry ingredients and mix for 3 minutes at medium speed. Add the 2 cups rye flour and 1 to 2 cups all-purpose flour until it forms a soft dough.
3. Transfer to a floured surface and knead for 5 minutes. Shape into a ball, place in a bowl that has been sprayed with nonstick cooking spray, turn ball over to coat other side, and loosely cover with plastic wrap and then a cloth towel. Let rise 15 minutes. Punch down dough (punch your fist into the middle) and divide in half. Shape each half into a round loaf. Place on cookie

sheet that has been sprayed with nonstick cooking spray, press down lightly, cover, and let rise another 15 minutes.

4. Make diagonal cuts across each loaf and bake for 25–35 minutes at 375 degrees. Cool on a wire rack.

Makes 2 loaves, 14 slices per loaf.
Per slice (1 ounce): **1.6 g total fat;** 0.3 g saturated fat; 0 cholesterol; 100 calories; 2 g fiber; 159 mg sodium

VARIATION: Brush each loaf with beaten egg white and sprinkle with caraway or poppy seeds prior to baking.

No-Knead Herb Bread

This is the perfect accompaniment to a spaghetti, lasagna, or chili dinner.

1½ cups whole-wheat flour
¼ cup sugar
¼ teaspoon onion powder
¼ teaspoon garlic powder
1 teaspoon salt
1½ teaspoons Italian seasoning

2 packages dry yeast
1 cup water
1 cup skim or 1% milk
¼ cup oil
1 egg
2½ cups all-purpose flour
Nonstick cooking spray

1. In a large bowl combine whole-wheat flour, sugar, seasonings, and yeast.
2. Heat water, milk, and oil to lukewarm (110°–115°F) in a saucepan or in the microwave. Add to the flour mixture along with the egg. Beat 3 minutes at medium speed with an electric mixer.
3. Stir in the all-purpose flour by hand to form a stiff dough. (Add a little more if it doesn't feel stiff enough.)
4. Cover. Let rise 45–60 minutes or until doubled in size. Punch down dough (punch fist into middle) and place in a 4½ × 8½ × 2-inch loaf pan that has been sprayed with nonstick cooking spray.

5. Bake at 375 degrees for 45–50 minutes until golden brown. Cool on a wire rack.

Makes 1 large loaf, 24 slices.
Per slice (1.4 ounces) (using 1% milk): **2.8 g total fat;** 0.3 g saturated fat; 9 mg cholesterol; 109 calories; 2 g fiber; 98 mg sodium

Crusty Buttermilk Cornbread

This is good to serve with any bean, chili, or soup recipe.

1 cup all-purpose flour or ½ cup all-purpose flour and ½ cup whole-wheat flour
1 cup self-rising cornmeal (cornmeal mix)

2 teaspoons baking powder
¼ teaspoon salt
1 egg, beaten
1½ cups buttermilk
Nonstick cooking spray

1. Combine flour(s), cornmeal, baking powder, and salt. Make a well in the center of the dry mixture and add the egg. Stir in the buttermilk and mix.
2. Spray an 8 × 8 × 2-inch baking tin with nonstick cooking spray. Spread batter evenly in pan.
3. Bake 25–30 minutes in a 425-degree oven.

Makes 9 servings.
Per serving: **1.3 g total fat;** 0.5 g saturated fat; 25 mg cholesterol; 133 calories; 2 g fiber; 360 mg sodium

Light Wheat Biscuits

Living in the South makes it a must to include a biscuit variation.

1½ cups self-rising flour
½–¾ cup whole-wheat flour

⅓ cup margarine
¾ cup buttermilk

1. Combine flours. Cut in margarine with two knives or pastry blender to form coarse crumbs.
2. Stir in the buttermilk with a fork, mixing only to moisten—do not overmix.
3. Transfer dough to lightly floured surface. Knead gently for 1 minute and then roll to approximately ½ inch thickness. Cut into 10 biscuits with a biscuit cutter or moistened glass.
4. Bake on an ungreased cookie sheet for 8–10 minutes in a 500-degree oven.

Makes 10 biscuits.
Per biscuit: **6.5 g total fat;** 1.3 g saturated fat; 1 mg cholesterol; 148 calories; 1 g fiber; 328 mg sodium

Apricot Muffins

This may sound exotic and, yes, it is different. But these muffins are soft, moist, and delicious. In fact, they remind me more of little cakes than muffins.

1 cup boiling water
1½ cups (approximately ½ pound) dried apricots, cut in small pieces
2 cups all-purpose flour
1 cup whole-wheat flour
1 cup sugar
1 tablespoon baking powder

1 teaspoon baking soda
½ teaspoon salt
2 eggs, beaten, or ½ cup egg substitute
¼ cup oil or melted margarine
1 cup orange juice
Nonstick cooking spray

1. In a bowl, pour the boiling water over the dried apricot pieces. Set aside to cool.
2. In a large bowl, sift together the flours, sugar, baking powder, baking soda, and salt.
3. Stir the eggs, oil, and orange juice into the liquid apricot mixture.

4. Make a well in the center of the dry ingredients and add the liquid apricot mixture, stirring enough to moisten (do not over-mix).
5. Spray 2 12-muffin tins with nonstick cooking spray or line with muffin cups. Fill each ⅔ full with batter. Bake for 20–25 minutes in a 375-degree oven.

Makes about 24 medium muffins.
Per muffin (using 2 whole eggs): **2.9 g total fat;** 0.3 g saturated fat; 18 mg cholesterol; 138 calories; 1.6 g fiber; 126 mg sodium

Fruity Oat-Bran Muffins

1½ cups oat bran
1⅓ cups quick-cooking oats
1⅓ cups all-purpose flour or ⅔ cup all-purpose flour and ⅔ cup whole-wheat flour
¼ cup sugar
2 teaspoons baking soda
1 teaspoon salt
2 teaspoons cinnamon

2 whole eggs or 1 whole egg and 2 egg whites
5–6 ripened bananas, mashed (approximately 2 cups)
1 16-ounce can crushed pineapple, packed in juice
⅓ cup vegetable oil
¼ cup honey
1 teaspoon vanilla extract
Nonstick cooking spray

1. Combine oat bran, oats, flour(s), sugar, baking soda, salt, and cinnamon in a large bowl. Set aside.
2. In another bowl, mix remaining ingredients. Combine with dry ingredients; do not overmix.
3. Coat 2 12-muffin tins with nonstick cooking spray or line with muffin cups. Fill each ⅔ full with muffin mixture.
4. Bake at 375 degrees for 20 minutes or until browned.

Makes 24 muffins.
Per muffin (using 2 whole eggs): **4.3 g total fat;** 0.6 g saturated fat; 17 mg cholesterol; 149 calories; 2 g fiber; 164 mg sodium

VARIATION: For a carrot-apple variation, substitute 1 cup grated carrots for the banana and ½ cup finely chopped apples for the pineapple and add ½ cup applesauce to mixture.

Lemon Poppy-Seed Muffins

Normally I prefer muffins with some whole grain or bran, but once I tasted this recipe, I understood why this flavor of muffin has become so popular. This recipe has less than half the fat of the commercial varieties, and it's just as good.

2 cups all-purpose flour
¼ cup sugar
½ teaspoon salt
1 tablespoon baking powder
1 tablespoon poppy seeds
¾ cup skim or 1% milk

1 6-ounce can frozen lemonade concentrate, thawed
2 tablespoons oil
2 egg whites
Nonstick cooking spray

1. Combine flour, sugar, salt, baking powder, and poppy seeds.
2. Add milk, lemonade, oil, and egg whites. Stir until moistened; do not overmix.
3. Coat a 12-muffin tin with nonstick cooking spray or line with muffin cups. Fill each ⅔ full with muffin mixture.
4. Bake for 15–20 minutes at 400 degrees or until golden brown.

Makes 12 muffins.
Per muffin (using 1% milk): **2.9 g total fat;** 0.2 g saturated fat; 0 cholesterol; 151 calories; 1 g fiber; 189 mg sodium

Herb-Bran Muffins

When you taste this recipe I think you will see why I usually prefer muffins with some whole grains and bran in the mixture.

1 cup all-purpose flour
¼ cup whole-wheat flour
1 tablespoon baking powder
¼ teaspoon salt
2 tablespoons sugar
2 tablespoons toasted sesame seeds
¼ teaspoon dry mustard
½ teaspoon herb of your choice (suggestions: sage, dill weed, oregano, sweet basil, chives, parsley, marjoram, summer savory, rosemary, coriander, or cardamom)
1 cup 100 percent bran cereal
1 cup skim milk
1 egg
2 tablespoons melted butter or margarine
Nonstick cooking spray

1. Stir together the flours, baking powder, salt, sugar, sesame seeds, dry mustard, and herb of choice. Set aside.
2. In a large mixing bowl, combine the bran cereal and the milk. Let stand 2 minutes. Add the egg and butter or margarine, blending well. Add the flour mixture, stirring only until combined.
3. Coat a 12-muffin tin with nonstick cooking spray or line with muffin cups. Fill each ⅔ full with muffin mixture.
4. Bake at 400 degrees for 18 to 20 minutes, or until a toothpick inserted in the center of a muffin comes out clean.

Makes 12 muffins.
Per muffin: **3.5 g total fat;** 0.7 g saturated fat; 17 mg cholesterol; 110 calories; 2.5 g fiber; 204 mg sodium

APPETIZERS AND SNACKS

The appetizer or snack at our house is almost always fresh fruit. I say "almost always" because, just like everyone else, we do appreciate variety on occasion. Here are two dips, nachos, and Jamie's special Super Bowl Chicken Sticks.

Hot and Cool Dip

Try this dip with fresh vegetables or as a condiment with sandwiches.

1 cup plain nonfat yogurt	½ cup cucumber, finely chopped
2 tablespoons horseradish	¼ teaspoon dill weed

Combine all ingredients. Chill before serving.

Makes 1 ½ cups (24 tablespoons).
Per 2 tablespoons: **0 total fat;** 0 saturated fat; 0 cholesterol; 13 calories; 0 fiber; 17 mg sodium

Raita

This traditional Indian dish can be prepared in a number of different ways by substituting different vegetables. Try this with finely chopped radishes or green pepper, or any of your favorite fresh vegetables.

1½ cups plain nonfat yogurt	2 teaspoons fresh ginger, minced
1 cup cucumber, finely chopped	⅛ teaspoon curry powder
	Dash cayenne

Combine all ingredients and serve chilled as a dip or vegetable side dish.

Makes 2 ½ cups.
Per ¼ cup: **0 total fat;** 0 saturated fat; 1 mg cholesterol; 23 calories; 1 g fiber; 26 mg sodium

Oven Corn Chips

This is a low-fat alternative to regular commercial corn chips. Serve as "nachos" with canned refried beans, sliced jalapeños, and salsa.

10–12 corn tortillas
Nonstick cooking spray
Seasoning of choice: garlic powder
                        onion powder
                        chili powder
                        Cajun seasoning blend

1. Stack tortillas and using a sharp knife cut through centers to make 6 sections.
2. Arrange wedges, without overlapping, on baking sheets that have been lightly sprayed with nonstick cooking spray.
3. Lightly spray arranged wedges. Sprinkle with seasoning of choice.
4. Bake at 400 degrees for approximately 8 minutes or until lightly browned and crisp.
5. Store in airtight plastic bags *after cooling.* Serve with salsa or low-fat dip.

Makes 60–72 chips.
Per serving (10 chips): **1.4 g total fat;** 0.1 g saturated fat; 0 cholesterol; 87 calories; 3 g fiber; 1 mg sodium

Nachos

Here is a lower-fat version of the popular tortilla chips with refried beans and cheese.

1 recipe Oven Corn Chips
¾ cup commercial salsa, or Salsa Rapida (see under Sauces)
1 cup canned refried beans

⅓ cup sliced jalapeño peppers (use gloves when slicing)
½ cup sharp cheddar cheese

1. Prepare Oven Corn Chips with 10 tortillas, and prepare Salsa Rapida.
2. Arrange chips in a single layer on an ungreased baking sheet.
3. Top each chip with a small amount of refried beans and sliced jalapeños. Lightly sprinkle with grated cheese.
4. Bake at 350 degrees for about 10 minutes.

Makes 6 servings.
Per serving (10 chips): **5.5 g total fat;** 2.4 g saturated fat; 10 mg cholesterol; 206 calories; 8 g fiber; 508 mg sodium

Super Bowl Chicken Sticks

2 pounds boneless, skinless chicken breasts
¼ cup "lite" soy sauce
¼ cup apple juice
2 tablespoons brown sugar

½ teaspoon ground ginger
1 teaspoon garlic powder
1 tablespoon lemon juice
4–5 drops Tabasco

1. On a cutting board, slice chicken breasts into strips (about 30 "sticks").
2. Arrange on a rack in a foil-lined broiler pan or on a baking sheet.
3. Whisk together remaining ingredients in a small bowl. Brush mixture generously on chicken.

4. Bake for about 1 hour at 350 degrees, basting frequently, until tender and browned.

Makes 10 servings.
Per serving of 3 sticks: **3.2 total fat;** 0.9 g saturated fat; 77 mg cholesterol; 166 calories; 0 fiber; 378 mg sodium

SOUPS

Hearty soups make great meals when served with crusty bread or whole-grain crackers and a fresh fruit salad. We've included a soup stock that can be used as a base for a wide variety of stock- or broth-based soups. Soup Supreme is one of my favorite examples. It's easy to prepare, nutritious, and very satisfying.

Soup Stock

This basic stock can be used for making soups of all kinds, rice or other grains, boiled potatoes, and beans.

Accumulate the giblets of 4 to 6 chickens (or turkeys), including the necks, hearts, and gizzards, but not the livers, trim all fat, and hold in the freezer until ready for use. For beef stock, substitute a large beef bone for the giblets.

Giblets of 4 to 6 birds
8 to 10 cups water
1 large bay leaf
2 large stalks celery cut into 2-inch pieces (include leaves)
2 large carrots, cut into 2-inch pieces
1 large onion, coarsely chopped
1 teaspoon each: rosemary, thyme, basil, and tarragon (or other herbs of your choice)
½ teaspoon salt
Fresh-ground black pepper to taste

1. Place giblets in a deep soup kettle with enough water to cover (8 to 10 cups). Bring to a boil and skim as necessary. When clear, add remaining ingredients.
2. Bring to a boil once again, reduce heat, and simmer for 2 hours.
3. Separate the giblets and vegetables. Blend the vegetables in a blender or food processor and return to stock. Store in 2- or 4-cup containers in the freezer until needed.

Makes 10 to 12 cups depending upon the amount of vegetables.
Per cup (10-cup recipe): **0.3 g total fat;** 0.1 g saturated fat; 22 mg cholesterol; 20 calories; 1 g fiber; 122 mg sodium

VARIATIONS: Add other greens or wilted vegetables, but avoid vegetables from the cabbage family. They have too strong a flavor for a basic soup stock.

Soup Supreme

I call this "Soup Supreme" because, besides tasting great, it is supremely easy to make!

2 cups Soup Stock (the preceding recipe)
1 medium potato, cut lengthwise and then in 1-inch pieces
1 large carrot, cut into 1-inch pieces

1 medium onion, chopped
1 large stalk celery, chopped
Herbs of your choice (depends upon what and how much you have put in your soup stock)
Dash of cayenne (optional)

Combine all ingredients in a 4-quart saucepan and bring to a boil. Reduce heat and simmer, covered, for 1 hour.

Makes 4 cups.
Per cup: **0.3 g total fat;** 0.1 g saturated fat; 11 mg cholesterol; 80 calories; 3 g fiber; 81 mg sodium

Fresh Vegetable Soup

This recipe was contributed by a former first lady of Tennessee, Betty Dunn, wife of Governor Winfield Dunn. Betty tells us that this recipe will keep for a week in the refrigerator, but that it never stays around that long at her house!

1 tablespoon olive oil
3 cloves garlic, minced
1 large stalk celery, chopped
1 green pepper, chopped
2 carrots, sliced
3 unpeeled red potatoes, sliced
2 yellow squash, coarsely chopped
2 zucchinis, sliced
2 cups fresh tomatoes, chopped, or a 1-pound can stewed tomatoes

2 quarts chicken broth
2 tablespoons chopped celery leaves
1 teaspoon oregano
1 tablespoon basil
⅛ teaspoon cayenne pepper
Tabasco to taste
1 cup cooked spaghetti or macaroni
Parmesan cheese, grated (optional)

1. Combine all ingredients except spaghetti and Parmesan in a large soup kettle. Bring to a boil, reduce heat, and simmer covered for about 50 minutes.
2. Add the 1 cup of cooked pasta and simmer 10 minutes more. Serve sprinkled with Parmesan cheese, if desired (cheese not in analysis).

Makes 12 servings.
Per serving: **2.3 g total fat;** 0.5 g saturated fat; 1 mg cholesterol; 95 calories; 2 g fiber; 530 mg sodium

Corn Chowder

½ cup scallions, chopped
1 tablespoon water
2½ cups chicken stock
½ teaspoon dry mustard
⅛ teaspoon salt
Pinch black pepper
¼ teaspoon paprika
½ teaspoon thyme

3 cups potatoes (about 1¼
    pounds), unpeeled, cubed
2 cups skim milk
2 packages (10 ounces
    each) frozen corn kernels
¼ cup instant nonfat dry
    milk

1. Steam scallions in water, covered, until wilted. Add the stock, seasonings, and potatoes. Bring to a boil, then reduce heat and simmer until potatoes are tender, stirring occasionally.
2. Gradually add skim milk, then add corn. Heat to almost scalding and let cook 1 minute.
3. Put 2 cups of the chowder in a blender or food processor with the powdered milk. Puree. Return to pot and reheat.

Makes 8 servings.
Per serving: **0.7 g total fat;** 0.2 g saturated fat; 2 mg cholesterol; 177 calories; 5 g fiber; 295 mg sodium

Vegetable-Seafood Stew

Serve this over brown rice or in a bowl as a soup.

1 tablespoon olive oil
1 tablespoon water
2 onions, diced
2 large cloves garlic, minced
3 potatoes, diced
3 large carrots, diced
6 stalks celery, diced
½ teaspoon thyme
½ teaspoon tarragon
½ teaspoon oregano
½ teaspoon crushed dried
    red pepper (optional)

14½-ounce can whole
    tomatoes
Water as needed
½ pound bay scallops
1 pound shrimp, peeled
    and cleaned
½ pound grouper
3 zucchini squash, cut in
    ½-inch slices
8 ounces fresh mushrooms,
    sliced
Salt to taste

1. In a large kettle, combine the olive oil and the 1 tablespoon of water. Brown the onions and garlic in this mixture. Add the potatoes, carrots, celery, spices, and the canned tomatoes with their juice. Add water to cover the vegetables. Cover the pan, bring to a boil, then lower the heat and simmer until the potatoes and carrots are tender.
2. Add the scallops, shrimp, grouper, zucchini, and mushrooms. Bring to a boil again, adding more water if necessary to cover the ingredients. Then lower the heat and simmer about 10 minutes until the grouper flakes easily with a fork. Add salt to taste.

Makes 10 servings.
Per serving: **2.9 g total fat;** 0.5 g saturated fat; 87 mg cholesterol; 172 calories; 3 g fiber; 328 mg sodium

Collard Soup

I had never tasted collards until I moved to Tennessee. They are now my most preferred green vegetable (although I like all greens). They are also one of the most nutritious of all greens, being especially rich in calcium and vitamin A. This particularly delicious soup makes a complete meal when served with cornbread and fresh fruit salad.

1 pound ground turkey, cooked and drained
8 cups water (2 quarts)
3 medium potatoes, peeled and diced
⅓ cup chopped onion

2 10-ounce packages frozen chopped collards
2 16-ounce cans Great Northern beans
Salt and pepper to taste

1. Add cooked and drained ground turkey to water in a soup kettle.
2. Add potatoes and onion and bring to a boil. Reduce heat and simmer for at least 10 minutes.
3. Add frozen collards and beans. Return to a boil, reduce heat, and simmer for 1 hour. Season with salt and pepper.

Makes 10 servings.
Per serving: **6.0 g total fat;** 2.0 g saturated fat; 27 mg cholesterol; 233 calories; 7 g fiber; 156 mg sodium

VARIATION: For an extra little bit of the old-time southern flavor, add about 3 ounces of lean ham, chopped, to the recipe.

SALADS

A basic vegetable or dinner salad is whatever combination of lettuce, with or without other greens, and cut-up raw vegetables you happen to like. To make a vegetable salad an entrée for lunch or a light dinner, just add a protein source such as lean ham or turkey, or garbanzo beans. Since I like sardines and canned tuna or salmon, I frequently make a dinner salad with these foods added, rather than meat. Here are a few lower-fat versions of some popular salads.

Creative Fruit Salad

Create a different salad every time, using whatever fresh or dried fruits, spices, or nuts you have on hand. Cut the fruit up into chunks, and sprinkle with lemon juice to keep the fruit looking fresh and to add a bit of tang. For every 2 cups of fresh fruit, add 1 tablespoon of any one of the following:

Grated coconut
Chopped unsalted nuts of any kind
Raisins or chopped dates

Then add a sprinkle of any of the following spices:

Cinnamon   Ginger
Nutmeg   Anise
Allspice   Cardamom

A main-course serving is 2 cups of any combination of fresh fruits, plus the tablespoon of nuts, coconut, or raisins. The spices, of course, add little or no calories.

Per 1-cup serving: **1.5 g total fat;** 0.3 g saturated fat; 0 cholesterol; 102 calories; 4 g fiber; 4 mg sodium

Potato-Vegetable Salad

6 medium potatoes, boiled
   and cubed
3 hard-boiled eggs, diced
½ small onion, grated
2 carrots, diced
1 bell pepper, diced
2 stalks celery, sliced thin
1 cup plain low-fat yogurt

¼ cup mayonnaise
¼ teaspoon garlic powder
Fresh-ground black pepper
   to taste
1 teaspoon tarragon
1 tablespoon Dijon mustard
1 teaspoon salt

Combine all ingredients, chill, and serve.

Makes 12 servings.
Per serving: **5.2 g total fat;** 1.0 g saturated fat; 56 mg cholesterol;
132 calories; 2 g fiber; 263 mg sodium

VARIATION: Substitute reduced-calorie mayonnaise to cut fat by 50
percent.

Sweet-and-Sour Bean Salad

1 cup cooked kidney beans
1 cup cooked garbanzo
   beans
½ cup carrots, diced
1 small red onion, thinly
   sliced

¼ teaspoon salt
⅛ teaspoon pepper
½ teaspoon dry mustard
3 tablespoons vinegar
1 tablespoon honey

Combine all ingredients in a large bowl and toss gently to mix. Chill
before serving.

Makes 6 servings.
Per serving: **0.9 g total fat;** 0.1 g saturated fat; 0 cholesterol; 100
calories; 5 g fiber; 95 mg sodium

Shrimpy Tomato Aspic

1 envelope plain gelatin
⅓ cup water
1 3-ounce package lemon
  Jell-O
1 24-ounce can tomato
  juice
1 6-ounce can tomato
  paste
¼ teaspoon salt
¼ teaspoon pepper
4 teaspoons freshly
  squeezed lemon juice
¾ cup chopped celery

½ pound shrimp, cooked,
  peeled, deveined, and cut
  into pieces (frozen
  cooked shrimp that has
  been thawed may be
  substituted for the fresh
  shrimp)
Nonstick cooking spray
Lettuce leaves
16 ounces low-fat cottage
  cheese
2 teaspoons lemon herb or
  lemon pepper seasoning

1. Dissolve plain gelatin in water; set aside.
2. Dissolve lemon Jell-O according to package directions.
3. Pour tomato juice and tomato paste into a saucepan and mix
   well. Add salt and pepper and bring to a boil. Remove from heat
   and stir in prepared Jell-O and softened gelatin. Cool until par-
   tially set.
4. Stir lemon juice, chopped celery, and shrimp into gelatin mixture.
5. Pour mixture into a 6-cup circular mold that has been lightly
   sprayed with nonstick cooking spray and chill until firm.
6. Unmold on a lettuce-lined serving plate and fill center with cottage cheese mixed with lemon herb or lemon pepper seasoning.

Makes 8 servings.
Per serving (with cottage cheese): **1.1 g total fat;** 0.5 g saturated fat; 58
mg cholesterol; 142 calories; 2 g fiber; 874 mg sodium

DRESSINGS

A great many low-calorie and low-fat dressings are commercially
available as a result of the growing interest in low-fat eating. If you

don't like to create your own dressings, I suggest you try a bunch of them until you find one or more that really tempt you to eat more salad.

Dressings make or break a salad when it comes to fat content. Regular dressings contain 7 grams of fat or sometimes more per tablespoon. Since a *small* ladle of dressing contains 2 tablespoons, using two ladles means 28 grams of fat.

I prefer to make my own reduced-fat dressings, using a base with a ratio of 1 part fine olive oil, 1 part vinegar (usually red wine or white wine vinegar), and 1 part water. I then add herbs and spices, one or more, depending upon my mood at the time. I suggest you try one or a combination from the following list: basil, marjoram, parsley, oregano, rosemary, tarragon, thyme, dry mustard, a bit of honey, a little lemon or orange juice, onion powder and garlic powder (or squeeze some fresh onion or garlic), fresh-ground black or white pepper, salt, and cayenne pepper. I strongly suggest you try just one herb at a time until you get a feel for the flavor that it adds to the dressing. For example, one of my favorites includes just tarragon, a teaspoonful of lemon juice, and a bit of salt added to the base. I can't give you an exact recipe, since I never measure my ingredients for salad dressing. But the result, while never the same twice in a row, is always interesting. The above recipe will always contain about 3 grams of fat, mostly monounsaturated if you use olive oil.

Here are some specific recipes for some tasty dressings that are all lower in fat than my basic version.

Acapulco Dressing

1 cup tomato juice
¼ cup lemon juice
1½ tablespoons minced onion
1½ tablespoons minced green pepper
1 teaspoon fresh cilantro or parsley, chopped

½ teaspoon minced jalapeño (optional; use gloves when mincing)
⅛ teaspoon black pepper

Combine all ingredients. (Use a blender if you prefer a smooth texture.) Store in refrigerator.

Makes about 20 tablespoons.
Per 2 tablespoons: **0 total fat;** 0 saturated fat; 0 cholesterol; 6 calories; 0 fiber; 88 mg sodium

No-Fat Italian Dressing

¼ cup lemon juice
¼ cup cider vinegar
¼ cup unsweetened apple
  juice
½ teaspoon oregano
½ teaspoon dry mustard

½ teaspoon onion powder
 1 clove garlic, cut in half
½ teaspoon paprika
¼ teaspoon basil
⅛ teaspoon thyme
⅛ teaspoon rosemary

Combine all ingredients. Chill for an hour or two to allow herbs to blend. Remove garlic clove pieces before serving.

Makes 12 tablespoons.
Per 2 tablespoons: **0 total fat;** 0 saturated fat; 0 cholesterol; 9 calories; 0 fiber; 1 mg sodium

Honey-Mustard Salad Dressing

This is a delicious low-fat version of the popular honey-mustard dressing.

¾ cup plain nonfat
  yogurt
¼ cup reduced-calorie
  mayonnaise
¼ cup honey

2 tablespoons Dijon
  mustard
2 tablespoons prepared
  (wet) mustard
1 tablespoon cider vinegar

Combine all ingredients in a small bowl or airtight container. Cover and chill for at least 1 to 2 hours.

Makes 1 ½ cups.
Per 2 tablespoons: **1.1 g total fat;** 0.2 g saturated fat; 1 mg cholesterol; 42 calories; 0 fiber; 58 mg sodium

Sunshine Dressing

Delicious served over fresh fruit salad.

1 cup plain nonfat yogurt
½ cup orange juice
Juice of ½ lemon

⅛ teaspoon cinnamon
Dash cardamom or nutmeg

Combine all ingredients. Chill.

Makes 1 ½ cups.
Per ¼ cup: **0 total fat;** 0 saturated fat; 1 mg cholesterol; 31 calories; 0 fiber; 29 mg sodium

LUNCHES

Here are the recipes for spreads, tuna and chicken salads, easy bean burritos, and ideas for sandwiches referred to in Chapter 6 on lunch. Other lunch ideas and recipes can be found under Soups, Salads, and Pasta.

Salmon-Herb Spread

1 cup plain nonfat yogurt
1 15-ounce can salmon
   packed in water, drained
2 tablespoons green onions,
   finely chopped
1 tablespoon fresh parsley,
   minced

1 tablespoon
   reduced-calorie
   mayonnaise
¼ teaspoon dill weed
¼ teaspoon thyme
⅛ teaspoon salt

1. Put yogurt in a strainer that has been lined with a large coffee
   filter or (better) several layers of cheesecloth. Allow to drain
   over a bowl for at least 1 hour.
2. Meanwhile, combine remaining ingredients in a bowl.
3. Fold in yogurt. Store in an airtight container. Serve chilled.

Makes 1 ½ cups.
Per ¼ cup: **5.7 g total fat;** 1.3 g saturated fat; 32 mg cholesterol; 137
calories; 0 fiber; 468 mg sodium

Norwegian Cottage Cheese

1 cup low-fat cottage cheese
½ 3.75-ounce can sardines,
   drained, or 1 6½-ounce
   can minced clams,
   drained

2 tablespoons red onion,
   minced
Fresh-ground black pepper
   to taste
Pinch of cayenne pepper

Mix well with a fork and let sit for at least half an hour. Serve as
sandwich spread, dip, or on lettuce or greens for a salad.

Makes 2 servings for salad, or 4 fillings for sandwiches.
Per ½ recipe (1 salad serving): **10.9 g total fat;** 2.0 g saturated fat; 126
mg cholesterol; 263 calories; 0 fiber; 889 mg sodium

Mexican Bean Spread (or Dip)

I have searched for spreads that would compensate me for forgoing the peanut butter with which I quite frequently overindulged myself in the past. Frankly, nothing quite matches peanut butter, but this spread, with a thick consistency (although a different taste), is very satisfying as an open-faced sandwich on whole-wheat, rye, or pumpernickel bread or a bagel half. Spread with additional salsa or ketchup, or serve with sliced tomatoes. Makes an excellent dip with crackers, toast, pita, or bagel chips.

2 16-ounce cans red kidney
  beans, drained
2 tablespoons onion, minced
½ teaspoon garlic powder
1 tablespoon ketchup

1 tablespoon hot salsa
½ teaspoon salt
¼ teaspoon fresh-ground
  black pepper

Blend in food processor until beans are well mashed and the consistency is thick and smooth.

Makes about 3 ½ cups.
Per ½ cup: **0.5 g total fat;** 0.1 g saturated fat; 0 cholesterol; 114 calories; 10 g fiber; 622 mg sodium

Italian Tuna Salad

I think this is about the tastiest low-fat way to prepare an old standby. If you have the time, you can make canned tuna far more tantalizing if you soak it in a small amount of chicken bouillon for an hour before making a tuna salad. You can reduce the fat in this recipe even further by using only 1 teaspoon of mayonnaise or substituting reduced-calorie mayonnaise.

1 6½-ounce can light-meat tuna in water, drained
1 medium stalk celery, minced
1 scallion (or green onion), minced
6 small pimiento-stuffed green olives, minced
1 teaspoon capers (optional)
½ teaspoon oregano
2 teaspoons mayonnaise
2 teaspoons white wine Worcestershire sauce
Fresh-ground black pepper to taste

Blend all ingredients except capers until you reach the desired consistency. The capers may be spread on top when served as a salad on your favorite lettuce or leafy green vegetable.

Makes 2 salad servings (or enough for 4 sandwiches).
Per ½ recipe (1 salad serving): **5.9 g total fat;** 0.9 g saturated fat; 49 mg cholesterol; 160 calories; 1 g fiber; 619 mg sodium

Sweet-'n'-Savory Chicken Salad

½ cup plain nonfat yogurt
1 tablespoon lemon juice
¾ teaspoon tarragon
2 cups cooked white-meat chicken, cut in chunks
1 20-ounce can pineapple chunks, in own juice, drained
1 10½-ounce can mandarin oranges, drained
1 4-ounce can water chestnuts, drained and sliced
1 small cucumber, diced
1 scallion, finely chopped
Lettuce leaves

1. Mix the yogurt, lemon juice, and tarragon to make a dressing.
2. In a large bowl combine the remaining ingredients except the lettuce leaves. Pour the dressing over the chicken mixture and toss lightly. Serve on lettuce leaves.

Makes 6 cups.
Per 1 cup: **2.3 g total fat;** 0.6 g saturated fat; 40 mg cholesterol; 196 calories; 3 g fiber; 58 mg sodium

Easy Bean Burritos for Two

4 large flour tortillas,
  preferably whole wheat
1 15-ounce can refried
  beans
2 cups lettuce, shredded
1 cup tomatoes, chopped
¼ cup onion, chopped
2 tablespoons jalapeño

peppers, chopped
(optional; use gloves
when chopping)
¼ cup shredded sharp
  cheddar cheese
½ cup plain nonfat yogurt
½ cup salsa or taco sauce

1. Warm tortillas (microwave if available) and heat refried beans.
2. Spread each tortilla with ¼ can of refried beans. Top with vegetables and shredded cheese. Add a dollop of plain nonfat yogurt.
   Serve with salsa or taco sauce.

Makes 2 servings of 2 burritos each.
Per burrito: **6.2 g total fat;** 2.7 g saturated fat; 9 mg cholesterol; 248
calories; 8 g fiber; 696 mg sodium

Sandwich Ideas

Combine your favorite sandwiches with a cup of broth-based soup,
cut-up fresh vegetables, fresh fruit, pretzels in place of chips, and
beverage.

1. Sliced turkey breast (2 ounces) with 2 pieces whole-grain bread,
¼ cup cranberry sauce, and alfalfa sprouts.

Per sandwich:
4.4 g **total fat;** 1.3 g saturated fat; 39 mg cholesterol; 336 calories; 6
g fiber; 417 mg sodium

2. Sliced lean ham (2 ounces) in whole-grain pita with 2 pineapple
slices and lettuce leaves.

Per sandwich:
3.9 g total fat; 1.0 g saturated fat; 27 mg cholesterol; 317 calories; 4 g fiber; 1,152 mg sodium

3. Canned refried beans (½ cup) or Mexican Bean Spread recipe (above) on a bagel with red onion and tomato slices.

Per sandwich:
2.5 g total fat; 0.7 g saturated fat; 0 cholesterol; 332 calories; 13 g fiber; 839 mg sodium

4. Leftover meat loaf or ground-turkey loaf (2½ ounces) on a whole-grain sandwich roll with lettuce leaves, mustard or ketchup if desired.

Per sandwich:
15.6 g total fat; 6.1 g saturated fat; 84 mg cholesterol; 363 calories; 3 g fiber; 500 mg sodium

5. Open-faced: 1 large slice pumpernickel or rye bread spread with Dijon mustard and topped with ¼ cup drained sauerkraut and sliced tomatoes. Then top with a 1-ounce slice cheddar cheese and broil.

Per sandwich:
10.9 g total fat; 6.2 g saturated fat; 30 mg cholesterol; 215 calories; 4 g fiber; 811 mg sodium

6. Sliced lean roast beef (2 ounces) in a whole-grain pita with 2 tablespoons plain nonfat yogurt, chopped onion, sliced cucumbers, and thinly sliced green or red peppers.

Per sandwich:
6.5 g total fat; 2.1 g saturated fat; 55 mg cholesterol; 321 calories; 3 g fiber; 391 mg sodium

BEEF

Always start with the leanest cuts of beef and trim visible fat. If you cook beef with fat on it, melted fat will spread between the lean muscle fibers as the meat cooks. Compared with meat trimmed before cooking, meat trimmed after will contain about twice the amount of fat.

Lean cuts are eye of round for roasts and stews; flank, tenderloin, and round steak (London broil) for steaks; and extra-lean hamburger (at least 90 percent lean) for ground meat. The names of the different cuts of beef vary from one section of the country to the next, and sometimes among supermarkets. Ask your butcher to help you pick the leanest cuts, and if you don't like to trim meat yourself, ask the butcher to do it for you. Talk to the manager of the meat section and encourage him or her to label the leanest cuts or to put the fat content clearly on the packages.

The lean cuts of beef for steak, except for tenderloin, tend to be tougher than the fatty cuts. They need marinating for at least a few hours before cooking. Soy sauce, Worcestershire, vinegar, and wine make good tenderizing agents. Use them alone or in combination for different flavors. Punch holes in the meat with the tines of a fork to allow the marinade to sink in more completely.

You can design a healthful low-fat diet with beef as a main-meal dish once a week (or twice a week if you don't use pork once a week as well). But you will end up with less fat, especially saturated fat, in your diet if you replace some of your meat dishes with fish or meatless main courses. I would normally avoid hamburger in restaurants or fast-food establishments, where it is usually much higher in fat (less than 80 percent lean) than the ground meat you can purchase in the supermarket yourself. Sliced lean roast beef for sandwiches, should you enjoy these for lunch occasionally, is much preferable to hamburger. Beware of the added mayonnaise dressings used in many restaurants for beef or hamburger sandwiches: They can add 12 to 20 grams of fat. Use mustard and ketchup instead.

Beef Stroganoff

¾ pound round steak,
boneless, trimmed of fat
8 ounces fresh mushrooms,
sliced
1 large onion, sliced
1 cup beef stock
1 tablespoon ketchup

¼ teaspoon black pepper
2½ tablespoons whole-wheat
flour
½ cup skim milk
½ cup plain nonfat yogurt
2 tablespoons sherry
2 cups cooked noodles

1. Julienne steak across the grain.
2. Heat a nonstick skillet over medium heat and brown the beef, mushrooms, and onion.
3. Stir in the stock, ketchup, and pepper. Cover and simmer until the beef is cooked through and tender, about 45 minutes.
4. In a small bowl, mix together the flour and milk until well blended. Stir in the yogurt and sherry and pour into the beef mixture. Cook over low heat, stirring constantly, until thickened. Serve over cooked noodles.

Makes 4 servings.
Per serving: 7.5 g **total fat;** 2.5 g saturated fat; 85 mg cholesterol; 329 calories; 4 g fiber; 333 mg sodium

Simple Beef Marinade

I have made this and other marinades with and without a bit of oil. The meat tastes fine either way, but the oil seems to enhance both tenderness and flavor. I think it's worth the extra few fat calories, especially if you use olive oil.

For each pound of steak or other beef, combine:

¼ cup chopped green
   onions
2 cloves garlic, minced
2 tablespoons soy sauce

1 tablespoon red wine
1 tablespoon water
1 teaspoon olive oil

Marinate cuts of beef such as flank steak or round steak (London broil) for at least 4 hours (preferably overnight) in the refrigerator. Use marinade for basting while broiling or grilling.

Entire marinade: **5 g total fat;** 0.6 g saturated fat; 0 cholesterol; 108 calories; 0 fiber; 1,657 mg sodium (marinade adds less than 1 gram of fat per serving; with low-sodium soy sauces the whole marinade contains 952 mg sodium)

VARIATION: Mince a 1-inch piece of fresh ginger (peeled) and add to the marinade for an Oriental flavor.

Mexican Meat Loaf

This is a very tasty, medium-spicy meat loaf that's quick and easy to prepare. Be sure to drain the fat as directed.

1½ pounds extra-lean ground
   beef, ground round, or
   ground turkey
1 8-ounce can tomato sauce
1 cup packaged cornbread
   stuffing mix
1 medium onion, chopped

2 cloves garlic, minced (or
   ½ teaspoon garlic
   powder)
1 4-ounce can green chiles,
   diced
1 egg
1 tablespoon chili powder

1. In a large bowl, mix meat, ½ can of tomato sauce, and all other ingredients.
2. Place in a shallow baking dish and cook at 375 degrees for 1 hour.

3. Drain the fat into a heat-resistant dish or bowl.
4. Spread the remaining tomato sauce over the meat loaf and bake for another 5 minutes. Allow to stand for 5 minutes before slicing.

Makes 8 servings.
Per serving (using extra-lean ground beef): **13.2 g total fat; 5.5 g** saturated fat; 84 mg cholesterol; 229 calories; 1 g fiber; 225 mg sodium

Teriyaki Beef Stir-fry

3 tablespoons teriyaki sauce
4 teaspoons vegetable oil, divided
2 teaspoons cornstarch
1 pound top round of beef, cut in thin strips

2 red, green, or yellow bell peppers, cut into ¾-inch cubes
6 green onions, cut into 2-inch slices

1. Combine teriyaki sauce, 2 teaspoons oil, and cornstarch in a medium to large bowl.
2. Add the beef strips and marinate in refrigerator for at least 45 minutes.
3. In a wok or skillet, stir-fry bell peppers and onions in 2 teaspoons oil for about 3 minutes. Remove from pan.
4. Stir-fry beef (half at a time) for 3 minutes.
5. Return vegetables to pan and cook until hot. Serve with rice and steamed broccoli.

Makes 4 servings.
Per serving (without rice and broccoli): **11.5 g total fat; 2.8 g** saturated fat; 70 mg cholesterol; 230 calories; 1 g fiber; 231 mg sodium

Fajitas

¼ cup lime juice
2 tablespoons white wine, tequila, or water
1 tablespoon olive oil
2 cloves garlic, minced
2 tablespoons jalapeño peppers, chopped (use gloves when chopping)
¼ teaspoon salt
¼ teaspoon black pepper
1 pound beef flank steak (well trimmed) or

boneless, skinless chicken breasts
1 15-ounce can refried beans
8 large flour tortillas, preferably whole wheat
2 cups lettuce, shredded
1 cup fresh tomatoes, chopped
1 cup commercial salsa or Salsa Rapida (see recipe)
1 cup plain nonfat yogurt

1. Whisk together lime juice, wine, oil, garlic, jalapeño peppers, salt, and pepper in the bottom of a shallow dish. Add steak or chicken; cover and refrigerate, turning occasionally, for at least 8 hours, or overnight.
2. Remove steak or chicken from marinade (reserve marinade) and grill or broil until done (do not overcook).
3. Heat beans and warm tortillas according to package directions. Slice meat into thin strips and place on a warm platter.
4. Wrap the meat, beans, shredded lettuce, and tomatoes in tortillas. Serve with salsa and yogurt.

Makes 4 servings.
Per serving of 2 fajitas using beef: **17.5 g total fat;** 4.4 g saturated fat; 72 mg cholesterol; 602 calories; 13 g fiber; 1,340 mg sodium
Per serving of 2 fajitas using chicken: **14.2 g total fat;** 2.9 g saturated fat; 86 mg cholesterol; 13 g fiber; 1,360 mg sodium

PORK

Pork can truly be the "other white meat." Breeders have created lean strains of animals during the last 20 years and pork today is much leaner and lower in cholesterol than in the past.

Tenderloin is the leanest cut you can buy. A regular loin roast can be either fat or lean, depending both on the breeding and diet of the animal and on how well it's trimmed. If you buy the loin cut, ask the butcher about the fat content, and ask to have it trimmed. He or she will probably do a better, neater job than you can do. A lean loin can be as low as 10 percent fat—that is, about 3 grams of fat per ounce. Today's lean *tenderloin* contains only about 1 gram of fat per ounce.

Pork chops and ribs are normally loaded with fat. The closest thing to a relatively lean chop is the butterfly cut, but you must trim the fat closely. Remember that any fat left on the meat will melt during cooking and permeate the lean tissue, doubling the fat content in the finished product.

Roast Pork Tenderloin

Pork tenderloin makes a roast to remember. Two pounds of raw meat will reduce in cooking and yield about six 4-ounce servings.

½ teaspoon thyme
½ teaspoon marjoram
½ teaspoon sage
½ teaspoon garlic powder
½ teaspoon onion powder
½ teaspoon ground ginger

Fresh-ground black pepper
   to taste
2 tablespoons soy sauce
1 tablespoon
   Worcestershire sauce
2 pounds pork tenderloin

1. Place all dry ingredients in a small bowl.
2. Add soy sauce and Worcestershire sauce and mix well.
3. Spread mixture evenly over meat and allow to marinate for an hour or two in the refrigerator.
4. Roast at 350 degrees until internal temperature reaches 170 degrees Fahrenheit (about 45 minutes).
5. To serve, slice in ¼-inch pieces and arrange on a platter with rice or vegetables.

Makes 6 servings.
Per 4-ounce serving of meat alone: **5.6 g total fat;** 2.0 g saturated fat; 105 mg cholesterol; 193 calories; 0 fiber; 77 mg sodium

VARIATIONS:
1. If you wish, you can add 1 teaspoon olive oil to the marinade. The oil helps the marinade stick to the meat and since some of the marinade cooks away during roasting, and some sticks to the pan, you will add only a couple of grams of fat to the entire roast.
2. Company version: Use 4 cloves of minced garlic, 3 chopped green onions, and a 1-inch piece of ginger, minced, in place of the dry ingredients.
3. When you are in a hurry for a roast, one of my friends who is a master chef recommended that you forget everything else and just rub the meat with 2 tablespoons of Dijon mustard and 2 cloves of garlic, minced, before roasting.

Pork Scallopine in Lemon, Dill, and Fennel Sauce

This scallopine of pork is a favorite dish at our house. It requires a bit of preparation time, but if you serve it to company, they will talk about it forever. The inspiration came from a chef at the Johnstown, Pennsylvania, Holiday Inn, where against the advice of my travel agent I had elected to stay instead of going on to Pittsburgh during a media tour. This recipe was my reward. While the original version was higher in fat, I knew the moment I tasted it that I had never had pork with a more congenial assortment of flavors.

Nonstick cooking spray
4 green onions, minced
3 cloves garlic, minced
1 tablespoon olive oil
2 pounds pork tenderloin, cut in ¼-inch slices
1 tablespoon margarine or butter
1 tablespoon fresh lemon juice

2 ounces white wine
1 teaspoon fennel seed, ground with mortar and pestle
1 teaspoon dill weed
Fresh-ground black pepper and salt to taste
Lemon wedges

1. In a large frying pan that has been sprayed with nonstick cooking spray, sauté the onions and garlic in olive oil over medium heat until translucent. Do not allow pan to become so hot that onions and garlic stick or brown.
2. Add slices of pork evenly to the pan, and sauté over medium heat about 2–3 minutes per side (until redness disappears). Keep moving the pork so that it doesn't stick. If you cannot cook all the pork at once, remove the pieces when they are done and keep in a warm oven. After all of the pork is done, transfer to an ovenproof dish and keep in a warm oven.
3. To make the sauce, melt the butter or margarine in the frying pan over medium heat, then add the lemon juice and white wine. Add the ground fennel, dill weed, salt, and pepper and heat for about 2 minutes.
4. Return the pork to the pan and mix with the sauce over medium heat for a minute or two. Serve immediately with a slotted spoon. Pour remaining sauce into a small serving cup for use as desired. Serve with lemon wedges.

Makes 6 servings.
Per serving: **9.7 g total fat;** 2.7 g saturated fat; 105 mg cholesterol, 237 calories; 0 fiber; 145 mg sodium

POULTRY

When it comes to choosing a low-fat, low-cholesterol meat, there's good reason that chicken and turkey are good "diet" standbys. They contain only about 1 gram of fat per ounce of white meat, of which just 0.3 gram is saturated. The dark meat has 2 grams of fat per ounce, but that is less than most other meats. The extra fat in the dark meat makes it more appealing to many people. If you don't care much for white meat, and have been avoiding chicken for this reason, you won't be making a bad choice if you eat the dark!

There's absolutely no reason to ever tire of poultry—that's because the meat is so delicate, it can take on many different and interesting flavors from sauces and seasonings. I think these recipes will stimulate your taste for poultry and give you some ideas for creating your own variations. We include some traditional favorites (barbecued, oven-fried) plus casseroles using chicken or turkey.

Because poultry (and fish) can play such an important part in a healthful low-fat diet, I hope you will try all my recipes. There is considerable variety in this collection, and the different styles will give you ideas for creating your own recipes.

Remember, you can substitute ground turkey for ground beef in meat loaf and spaghetti sauce, but be sure you are selecting *lean* ground turkey. Many butchers and processors add all the fat they can sneak into ground turkey, and it ends up containing 15 percent or more fat (5 to 6 grams per ounce), whereas the white meat is less than 5 percent fat (only 1 gram per ounce).

Barbecued Chicken

You can use my Barbecue Sauce (see recipe) or a store-bought variety. Look for one without added fat.

3½ pounds chicken pieces, skin removed
  1 cup barbecue sauce

1. Skin the chicken pieces. Place the pieces "skin" side down in a large, shallow baking pan. (You may wish to line the pan with foil for easy cleaning.)
2. Baste the chicken pieces liberally with barbecue sauce, and place in the oven.
3. Bake at 350 degrees for 20 minutes, basting halfway through. Then turn the chicken pieces over and bake another 25 minutes, or until chicken is tender, basting occasionally.

Makes 6 servings (approximately 4 ounces each).
Per serving (using commercial barbecue sauce): **6.1 g total fat;** 1.5 g saturated fat; 96 mg cholesterol; 223 calories; 0 fiber; 427 mg sodium

Crispy Chicken

1 frying chicken, about 3
pounds, skinned and cut in
pieces
1 cup crushed cornflakes
¼ teaspoon paprika

⅛ teaspoon garlic powder
⅛ teaspoon onion powder
⅛ teaspoon black pepper
1 cup skim milk

1. Remove all skin and fat from the chicken. Rinse and dry the chicken thoroughly.
2. In a medium bowl mix together the cornflake crumbs and seasonings.
3. Dip the chicken pieces in the milk, shake to remove excess liquid, and roll in the cornflake crumbs. Place the chicken in a shallow nonstick baking pan, making sure the pieces don't touch each other. Let stand for a minute so the crumbs will stick.
4. Bake for 25 minutes in a 400-degree oven, turn, and bake 20 minutes longer or until chicken tests done.

Makes 6 servings.
Per serving: **7.5 g total fat;** 2.1 g saturated fat; 89 mg cholesterol; 221 calories; 0 fiber; 154 mg sodium

Tender Chicken-in-a-Pot

This one-dish meal is very low in fat. The layer of onions and celery on top of the skinned chicken helps keep it moist.

8 small new potatoes, cut in
half
4 carrots, cut in 2-inch
chunks
4 chicken breasts, skinned
⅛ teaspoon garlic powder
1 teaspoon curry powder
½ teaspoon ground mustard

1 teaspoon tarragon
½ teaspoon dried crushed
red pepper
2 tablespoons lemon juice
½ cup wine
4 stalks celery, sliced thin
4 onions, sliced thin

1. Combine potatoes and carrots in a casserole dish. Place chicken breasts on top.
2. Combine spices, lemon juice, and wine and pour over chicken. Top chicken with celery and onions.
3. Cover and bake at 350 degrees for 1 hour.

Makes 4 servings.
Per serving: **3.5 total fat**; 1.0 g saturated fat; 73 mg cholesterol; 408 calories; 7 g fiber; 136 mg sodium

VARIATION: You can turn this into a delicious chicken stew by adding about 2–3 cups of stock or bouillon (enough to cover everything in the pot). Add about half an hour to the cooking time. The meat is done when it separates easily from the bone (if you use bone-in chicken breasts) or when it is no longer pink and is tender. You may thicken the stock before serving by blending in 1 tablespoon of flour or a small amount of cornstarch.

Chicken-and-Spinach Mostaccioli Casserole

10 ounces uncooked mostaccioli (tubular pasta or other pasta)
1 10-ounce package frozen chopped spinach, thawed and drained
Nonstick cooking spray
2 teaspoons vegetable oil
1 large onion, chopped
4 garlic cloves, minced
1 pound boned, skinned chicken breasts, cut into 1-inch pieces
1 28-ounce can whole tomatoes, undrained, coarsely chopped
3 tablespoons tomato paste
1¼ teaspoon dried basil
¾ teaspoon oregano
¼ teaspoon crushed hot red pepper
½ cup grated Parmesan

1. Cook mostaccioli or other pasta according to package directions. Drain. Place spinach on paper towels; squeeze until barely moist.

2. Coat large nonstick skillet with cooking spray; add oil and place over medium heat until hot.
3. Add onion and garlic and sauté until tender.
4. Add chicken and cook until it loses its pink color, stirring constantly.
5. Stir in tomatoes, tomato paste, basil, oregano, and crushed pepper. Bring to a boil and then reduce heat. Simmer 5 minutes, uncovered, stirring occasionally.
6. Combine pasta, spinach, chicken mixture, and ¼ cup cheese in a bowl; stir well. Spoon into a 13 × 9 × 2-inch baking dish coated with nonstick cooking spray. Sprinkle remaining ¼ cup cheese over top.
7. Bake at 350 degrees for 20 minutes.

Makes 8 servings.
Per serving: **4 g total fat;** 1.4 g saturated fat; 37 mg cholesterol; 272 calories; 4 g fiber; 228 mg sodium

Turkey or Chicken Divan

Jamie adapted this favorite Sunday dinner recipe for the Harper family in Madison, Tennessee. When Suzanne Harper first served this lower-fat version to her family, they couldn't tell the difference. Suzanne's original Turkey Divan, which contained far more mayonnaise, creamed soup, and cheese, totaled 47 grams of fat per serving. The Harpers now regularly enjoy this recipe at only 10 grams of fat per serving. The reduction in fat was achieved by:

• Substituting evaporated skim milk for 1 can of creamed soup
• Substituting reduced-calorie mayonnaise and nonfat yogurt for part of the regular mayonnaise
• Using less of a sharp cheddar in place of a larger amount of mild cheddar cheese

These three ideas for reducing fat in casserole recipes should be part of your own repertoire.

2 10-ounce packages frozen broccoli or 2 bunches fresh broccoli, cut in pieces
2 to 3 cups cooked white meat of turkey or chicken, skinless and boneless
Nonstick cooking spray
2 tablespoons flour
1 teaspoon chicken bouillon or 1 bouillon cube

1 12-ounce can evaporated skim milk
1 10½-ounce can cream of chicken soup
¼ cup reduced-fat mayonnaise
1 cup plain nonfat yogurt
½ teaspoon curry powder
½ cup sharp cheddar cheese, grated
½ cup plain breadcrumbs

1. Layer broccoli and turkey (or chicken) in a 13 × 9 × 2-inch casserole that has been lightly sprayed with nonstick cooking spray.
2. In a bowl, combine the flour and bouillon and add a small amount of the evaporated skim milk, stirring to form a paste. Gradually add the remaining milk, cream soup, reduced-fat mayonnaise, yogurt, and curry powder, mixing well. Pour over the broccoli and turkey.
3. Top with the grated cheese and then the breadcrumbs.
4. Bake at 350 degrees for 25 to 30 minutes.

Makes 6 servings.
Per serving: **10.3 g total fat;** 3.9 g saturated fat; 51 mg cholesterol; 293 calories; 3 g fiber; 792 mg sodium

Chicken Cacciatore

1 small onion, chopped
1 clove garlic, minced (or ½ teaspoon garlic powder)
⅓ cup water
1 14½-ounce can whole tomatoes, chopped
1 6-ounce can tomato paste

1 teaspoon oregano
Salt and fresh-ground black pepper to taste
4 chicken breasts, skinless and boneless
4 cups hot cooked spaghetti or rice

1. In a skillet over medium heat, cook onion and garlic with water, covered, for 5 minutes or until onion is tender.
2. Stir in the tomatoes, tomato paste, and seasonings. Reduce heat, cover and simmer for 10–15 minutes.
3. Add the chicken and cook, covered, for 30 minutes. Uncover and cook another 15 minutes.
4. Serve over spaghetti or rice.

Makes 4 servings.
Per serving with 1 cup spaghetti: **4.6 g total fat;** 1.1 g saturated fat; 73 mg cholesterol; 402 calories; 5.4 fiber; 394 mg sodium

Meal-in-a-Pepper

4 large green peppers
Water
Dash salt
Nonstick cooking spray
1 pound ground turkey
½ cup finely chopped onion
1 16-ounce can tomatoes, chopped, undrained
½ cup long-grain rice

½ cup water
¼ teaspoon salt
¼ teaspoon pepper
1½ tablespoons Worcestershire sauce
½ teaspoon dried oregano, crushed
¾ cup part-skim mozzarella, grated

1. Halve peppers lengthwise, removing membranes, seeds, and stems. Cook peppers in boiling water for 3 minutes; drain and sprinkle insides of peppers with a small amount of salt.
2. Spray a skillet with nonstick cooking spray. Cook turkey and onion until onion is tender. Drain well.
3. Stir in tomatoes (undrained), uncooked rice, ½ cup water, salt, pepper, Worcestershire sauce, and oregano, bring to a boil, then reduce heat to simmer.
4. Cover and simmer for 20 minutes, or until rice is tender. Stir in half of the cheese and fill pepper halves with the rice-meat-cheese mixture.
5. Place stuffed peppers in an ovenproof baking dish and bake for

15 to 20 minutes at 375 degrees. Remove from oven and immediately sprinkle with remaining cheese.

Makes 8 servings.
Per serving: **8.9 g total fat;** 3.0 g saturated fat; 40 mg cholesterol;
208 calories; 2 g fiber; 294 mg sodium

FISH

I've explained one of the health reasons for increasing your consumption of fish in Chapter 2: the presence of omega-3 fatty acids,
which are especially high in the cold-water varieties. But fish does
not have to be taken as a "prescription." Prepared correctly, it's
really good. Here are some important rules:

* *Do not overcook fish.* Follow the cooking times closely.
* Keep interest high by using different methods of cooking: Broil, steam,
  bake, grill, and poach.
* Experiment with different herbs, spices, and sauces.

Fish is mild in flavor and best when fresh. If you buy in quantity for
freezing, make sure fish is wrapped especially for the freezer or it
will suffer "freezer burn." This is also true of meat. Ask the meat or
fish manager to double-wrap and heat-seal the package at the time of
purchase.

I've recommended you eat fish at least once a week, better twice.
If you don't particularly enjoy fish, be sure to try my recipes and see
if you can cultivate more of a taste for this healthful food. This chapter contains only my most favorite recipes, including one my daugh-
ter Terri created many years ago and which has appeared elsewhere—Royal Indian Salmon. This recipe is outstanding and has
been adopted by many restaurants around the country. The very first
one I present, Fish Fillets in Lemon-Tarragon Sauce, is a basic, convenient method of preparation for almost all fillets and steaks. It's a
must for your repertoire.

Fish Fillets in
Lemon-Tarragon Sauce

To get the full flavor of the tarragon, let it soak in the lemon juice for at least 15 minutes while you assemble the other ingredients for your dinner. While the recipe calls for fillets, it's equally good with swordfish and just about any other fish steak except tuna, which I think has too strong a flavor for this somewhat delicate sauce.

1 tablespoon lemon juice	½ teaspoon onion powder
½ teaspoon tarragon	¼ teaspoon salt
1 tablespoon olive oil	Fresh-ground black pepper to
1 tablespoon dry white	taste
table wine (optional)	1½ pounds fish fillets
½ teaspoon garlic powder	

1. Combine the lemon juice and tarragon in a small bowl, mix well, and set aside.
2. Pour the oil and (optional) wine into a foil-lined broiling pan.
3. Sprinkle the dry ingredients all around the pan.
4. Add the lemon and tarragon mixture to the pan.
5. Swish the fish fillets around the pan until they are well coated on both sides.
6. Broil about 6 minutes to a side (less or more depending upon thickness, but do not overcook).

Makes 4 servings, 4.5 ounces cooked weight.
Per serving: **5.4 g total fat;** 0.9 g saturated fat; 82 mg cholesterol; 188 calories; 0 fiber; 271 mg sodium

With swordfish steaks: **10.2 g total fat;** 2.3 g saturated fat; 66 mg cholesterol; 239 calories; 0 fiber; 287 mg sodium

Oven-Fried Catfish

Only like fish if it's fried? Well, this is a low-fat alternative that any fried-fish lover will appreciate.

2 tablespoons skim or 1% milk
1 whole egg or 2 egg whites
½ cup yellow cornmeal
¼ teaspoon paprika
¼ teaspoon salt
¼ teaspoon onion or garlic powder
1 pound catfish fillets (or other white fish)
Nonstick cooking spray
½ teaspoon olive oil

1. In a shallow bowl, beat the milk and egg together. In another shallow bowl, combine the cornmeal and dry ingredients.
2. Dip each fish fillet in the egg mixture and then coat thoroughly in the cornmeal.
3. Spray a shallow baking dish with nonstick cooking spray and then add the olive oil, turning the dish to coat. Place the fish in a single layer in the baking dish.
4. Bake in a 500-degree oven for about 12 minutes or until fish flakes easily with a fork.

Makes 4 servings.
Per serving using whole egg and 1% milk: **7.2 g total fat;** 1.6 g saturated fat; 119 mg cholesterol; 213 calories; 2 g fiber; 229 mg sodium
Per serving using egg whites and 1% milk: **6.0 g total fat;** 1.2 g saturated fat; 66 mg cholesterol; 203 calories; 2 g fiber; 242 mg sodium

Dijon Swordfish

This marinade is also delicious with chicken.

2 tablespoons Dijon
mustard
½ cup white wine
¼ cup lemon juice
¼ cup olive oil
1 clove garlic, minced

¾ cup fresh basil, shredded
(or 2 tablespoons dried)
6 swordfish steaks, 1 inch
thick (about 6 ounces
each)

1. In a bowl, combine the mustard, wine, lemon juice, and olive oil
   with a wire whisk. Add the garlic and basil.
2. Arrange the swordfish in a shallow baking dish.
3. Pour the marinade over the fish, turning to coat both sides.
   Refrigerate for 1 hour, turning once.
4. Place steaks on broiling rack and broil 7 inches from heat for 5
   to 6 minutes on each side.

Makes 6 servings.
Per serving: **11.4 g total fat;** 2.4 g saturated fat; 64 mg cholesterol;
262 calories; 0 fiber; 214 mg sodium

Royal Indian Salmon

This recipe is one of our all-time favorites, delicately flavored and
very easy to prepare.

4 salmon steaks, 1 inch thick
(about 6 ounces each)
¼ cup chicken or vegetable
bouillon
2 tablespoons lemon juice
½ teaspoon fennel seeds,
crushed

¼ teaspoon cumin
¼ teaspoon ground
coriander
Dash of salt and
fresh-ground black
pepper

1. Place the steaks in a shallow pan. Combine the bouillon and lemon juice and pour over the steaks. Add the seasonings. Marinate, covered, in the refrigerator for at least 2 hours, turning the steaks occasionally.
2. To cook, place the steaks on a foil-covered broiling pan. Spoon 2 teaspoons of the marinade on top of each steak. Place under the broiler on low broil for 8 to 10 minutes, or until slightly brown on the edges. Turn steaks over, spoon on the remaining marinade, and broil for an additional 8 to 10 minutes.

Makes 4 servings.
Per serving: **8.2 g total fat;** 1.3 g saturated fat; 70 mg cholesterol; 185 calories; 0 fiber; 105 mg sodium

VARIATION: If you like your salmon with a teriyaki sauce, as I sometimes do, replace half the bouillon with 1 tablespoon of soy sauce and replace the fennel with either ¼ teaspoon of powdered ginger or ½ inch of fresh ginger, peeled and minced. It's terrific.

Easy Italian Fish Fillets

This dish is good served over cooked pasta, bulgur wheat, or rice.

2 onions, chopped
1 6-ounce can V8 juice
1 8-ounce can tomato sauce
1 tablespoon whole-wheat
   flour

½ teaspoon basil
1 pound scrod fillets,
   or other white firm
   fish

1. Sauté the onions in the V8 juice until tender.
2. Stir in the remaining ingredients except for the fish and heat through.
3. Place the fish in another saucepan and pour the sauce on top. Cover and cook on medium heat for about 10 to 15 minutes, until fish loses its translucency and flakes easily with a fork.

Makes 4 servings.
Per serving (using sole): **1.6 g total fat;** 0.4 g saturated fat; 54 mg cholesterol; 150 calories; 2 g fiber; 591 mg sodium

Oysters Rockefeller

3 tablespoons dry
  breadcrumbs
2 teaspoons olive oil
1 tablespoon grated onion
Tarragon, fresh-ground
  black pepper, and Tabasco
  sauce to taste

1 10-ounce package
  chopped frozen spinach,
  thawed and drained
6 ounces raw or canned
  oysters (not smoked)
2 tablespoons grated
  part-skim mozzarella
1 tablespoon Parmesan

1. Combine the breadcrumbs, oil, onion, and seasonings. Toss together with the spinach.
2. Broil the oysters, if using raw, for 5 to 7 minutes. Drain liquid if using canned.
3. Top oysters with spinach mixture and broil 3 to 4 minutes. Sprinkle with the cheeses and broil just until melted.

Makes 4 servings.
Per serving: **4.6 g total fat;** 1.3 g saturated fat; 27 mg cholesterol; 103 calories; 2 g fiber; 183 mg sodium

Halibut with
Ginger-and-Shallot Sauce

1 tablespoon margarine or
  butter
1½ pounds halibut steaks, cut
  into 4 pieces
2 tablespoons flour (all
  purpose or whole
  wheat)

½ cup fish or chicken stock,
  or clam juice
2 shallots, finely chopped
¼ cup white wine
¼ cup 1% milk
2 teaspoons fresh
  gingerroot, julienned

1. Melt the margarine in a skillet on medium-low heat. Dredge the fish in the flour to coat. Lightly brown the fish on both sides in the melted margarine, then cover and let steam for 5 minutes, or until fish flakes easily with a fork. Remove the fish to a platter and cover.
2. To prepare the sauce, add 2 tablespoons of the stock or juice to the pan, then add the shallots, cover, and sauté for 3 minutes. Add the remaining stock and wine and boil uncovered until the liquid is reduced by half, about 8 to 10 minutes.
3. Reduce the heat and stir in the milk and gingerroot. Simmer 1 minute.
4. Pour the sauce through a strainer over the fish, and serve.

Makes 4 servings.
Per serving: **6.9 g total fat;** 1.2 g saturated fat; 56 mg cholesterol; 244 calories; 1 g fiber; 199 mg sodium

PASTA

National food consumption surveys show we are beginning to catch on. Not only is pasta good for you, it can taste good, too, without having to be soaked in a high-fat sauce.

Pastas can be made from a variety of sources, including wheat, soy, rice, corn, buckwheat, or even beans and seaweed. Pasta comes in an assortment of different shapes, from thin to thick and from shells to corkscrews. In this country we are used to durum-wheat semolina (made into the typical white spaghetti) or egg noodles, but I think you will have fun trying different varieties. There also are interesting colors, including black (squid ink), brown (whole wheat), green (spinach), and red (tomato, usually). Using a variety of sources, shapes, and colors, together with the different sauces, you can create countless fascinating dishes.

Pasta normally contains very little fat and no eggs or cholesterol, while egg noodles contain a bit more fat and about 50 milligrams of cholesterol per serving. For your basic everyday dish, I suggest using a mixture of regular (white) and whole-wheat (brown) spaghetti.

Here are some sauces for your favorite varieties of pasta, some luncheon pasta salads, and a special entrée—cannelloni.

Red Clam Sauce

Here is a challenge: I think this is the greatest red clam sauce there is, but if you can come up with a better—or even an equal—send it to me (care of the publisher) and I will arrange with you for permission to publish it. You can make this sauce without the oil—just sauté the ingredients in Step 1 below in the water. Then the sauce is almost fat free (the clams have a small amount of fat). However, the olive oil adds to the flavor and consistency and, with just 4 grams of fat for a whole cup of sauce, I think it's well worth it.

2 cups chopped onions
1 large green pepper, chopped
8 cloves garlic, minced
12 ounces mushrooms, sliced
2 tablespoons olive oil
2 tablespoons water
4 6½-ounce cans minced clams, with liquid

1 teaspoon dried basil
2 dried red peppers (hot) or ½ teaspoon crushed hot red pepper
¼ teaspoon fresh-ground black pepper
1 15-ounce can tomato sauce
1 6-ounce can tomato paste

1. In a 4-quart covered saucepan, sauté onions, green pepper, garlic, and mushrooms in olive oil and water over medium-low heat until onions are translucent.
2. Add remaining ingredients and simmer, covered, over low heat for 45 minutes.

Makes about 10 cups.
Per 1 cup: 4 g **total fat;** 0.5 g saturated fat; 26 mg cholesterol; 139 calories; 3 g fiber; 389 mg sodium

Thick and Zesty Spaghetti Sauce

Nonstick cooking spray
1 tablespoon olive oil
3–4 medium onions, sliced
4 cloves garlic, minced
1 green pepper, chopped
10 ounces mushrooms, sliced
Water as needed
1 pound ground turkey
1 28-ounce can tomato
  sauce

1 6-ounce can tomato paste
1 10-ounce can tomato
  puree
1 teaspoon salt
½ teaspoon fresh-ground
  black pepper
½ teaspoon crushed red
  pepper (cayenne)
1 teaspoon basil

1. Spray the bottom of a deep saucepan with nonstick cooking spray, add the olive oil, then add the onions, garlic, green pepper, and mushrooms. Sauté covered over medium heat until vegetables are tender, adding a tablespoon or two of water if necessary to prevent vegetables from sticking.
2. Meanwhile, in a skillet, cook the ground turkey until browned. Drain liquid. Add to cooked vegetables. Stir in tomato sauce, tomato paste, tomato puree, and the seasonings.
3. Simmer covered for 1 to 2 hours. Serve over your favorite pasta.

Makes 8 servings.
Per serving with 1 cup pasta: **10.1 g total fat;** 2.3 g saturated fat; 34 mg cholesterol; 419 calories; 7 g fiber; 1,087 mg sodium

Summer Pasta Salad

A colorful, tasty, and easy pasta salad that makes use of those vegetables in the hydrator! Can be served as a main course for lunch or as a side dish.

8 ounces tri-colored pasta (green, red, white)
2 cups assorted raw vegetables, chopped (try all
   or some of the following to make 2 cups:
   green or red pepper, summer squash, onions,
   tomatoes, cauliflower, broccoli, carrots)
1 cup oil-free commercial Italian dressing

1. Cook and drain pasta according to package directions.
2. Add chopped vegetables and dressing. Toss well.
3. Chill before serving.

Makes 6 servings.
Per serving: **2.3 g total fat;** 0.3 g saturated fat; 2 mg cholesterol; 172 calories; 3 g fiber; 320 mg sodium

Easy Pasta Toss

This is a dish for which the ingredients can always be kept on hand, and it can be served hot or cold. It is a great idea for brown-bag lunches.

1 medium onion, chopped
1–2 cloves garlic, minced
Nonstick cooking spray
3 cups beef or chicken stock
   or broth or 3 cups water
   and 3 bouillon cubes
1 8-ounce can sliced
   mushrooms with liquid
1 12-ounce box of pasta (try
   a garden trio)

1 19-ounce can garbanzo
   beans
½ cup parsley (optional)
1–2 cups cooked vegetables
   (leftovers are great!)
Salt and fresh-ground black
   pepper to taste

1. Sauté onion and garlic in a medium-large pot sprayed with non-stick cooking spray. Add a tablespoon or two of water or of the broth if onion and garlic begin to stick.
2. Add the stock or the water and bouillon cubes and bring to a

boil. Add the mushrooms with liquid and the pasta. Cover and simmer for 20–25 minutes or until pasta is tender.

3. Add the garbanzo beans, parsley (optional), and cooked vegetables (broccoli, carrots, summer squash, green peas, whatever!). Season with salt and pepper. Toss and serve hot or chilled.

Makes 8 cups.
Per 1 cup: **3 g total fat;** 0.4 g saturated fat; 0 cholesterol; 295 calories; 7 g fiber; 421 mg sodium

Shrimp-Feta-Pasta Salad

Although I have cut way back on my consumption of cheese of all kinds, I remain a fan of feta. Nothing quite compares with feta cheese in a Greek salad, or this pasta salad. When it's used in moderation, as it is in this salad, it makes for a real treat.

½ pound cooked, deveined shrimp
⅔ cup crumbled feta cheese (3 ounces)
2 large fresh tomatoes (chopped)
1 large cucumber, peeled and chopped
½ cup low-fat or no-fat commercial Italian dressing

2 tablespoons fresh-squeezed lemon juice
1½ teaspoons oregano
½ teaspoon fresh-ground black pepper
3 cups cooked and cooled pasta

1. Mix shrimp, feta cheese, tomatoes, cucumber, dressing, lemon juice, and seasonings.
2. Toss with prepared pasta.
3. Chill.

Makes 8 servings.
Per serving: **5 g total fat;** 2.6 g saturated fat; 87 mg cholesterol; 211 calories; 2 g fiber; 405 mg sodium

Cannelloni

This recipe takes a bit of extra time, which I think you will find well worthwhile. It's another illustration of how to use cheese in moderation to produce a very tasty dish that remains relatively low in fat.

SAUCE
- 1 clove garlic, crushed
- 1 tablespoon olive oil
- 3 tablespoons water
- ¼ cup flour
- 1½ teaspoons instant chicken bouillon
- ⅛ teaspoon white pepper
- 2 cups evaporated skim milk
- ¼ cup grated farmer or sapsago cheese

OTHER INGREDIENTS
- 6 cannelloni (or manicotti) shells
- Nonstick cooking spray

FILLING
- 3 tablespoons sliced green onions
- 2 tablespoons water
- 1 10-ounce package frozen, chopped spinach, thawed and well drained
- 1 cup finely chopped cooked chicken
- ¼ cup grated farmer or sapsago cheese
- 1 egg, beaten
- 2 tablespoons skim milk
- ¾ teaspoon liquid Italian seasoning
- ¼ teaspoon pepper

1. To make the sauce, sauté the garlic in the olive oil and water in a medium saucepan over moderate heat.
2. Stir in the flour, bouillon, and pepper.
3. Remove from heat and gradually stir in the milk.
4. Return to heat and bring to a boil, stirring constantly. Boil and stir for 1 minute.
5. Reduce heat to low. Stir in the cheese until melted. Set aside.
6. Parboil the pasta shells according to package directions. Rinse and drain.
7. While shells are cooking, make the filling: Sauté the onions in water in a nonstick skillet just until tender.
8. Combine remaining ingredients in a bowl, add onion, and mix well.
9. Fill shells with mixture and arrange in a shallow 2-quart casserole dish that has been sprayed with nonstick cooking spray.

10. Spoon sauce over filled cannelloni.
11. Bake for 20 minutes at 350 degrees, then broil for 5 minutes or until sauce is bubbly and golden. Serve immediately.

Makes 4 servings of 1 ½ shells with sauce.
Per serving: **10.1 g total fat;** 3.2 g saturated fat; 95 mg cholesterol; 468 calories; 4 g fiber; 889 mg sodium

MEATLESS MAIN COURSES

I think you should begin to make it a practice to include at least one meatless main course, if not an entire meatless day, in your meal plans each week. It's even better when you do two. Bean dishes, pastas, pizza, and vegetable casseroles can make this easy and tasty. These dishes will contain little or no cholesterol (depending upon your use of dairy products) and usually less fat than meat courses. Remember that wherever people eat more plant foods and less saturated fat, there is less heart disease and cancer.

Some people worry about getting enough protein when they cut back on their meat intake. They have heard that plant protein is "incomplete." That is, since protein is made up of 22 different amino acids, and requires that enough of the eight essential amino acids be available for the body to use the rest, they worry that they will fail to obtain the "complete" protein that's available in animal products, but missing in plant foods.

This fear is groundless for two reasons. First, although plant foods may be low in one or another of the essential amino acids, the large portions that we can eat on a low-fat diet make plenty of protein available even when we eat wheat, legumes, or rice all by themselves. Second, and even more important, we tend to combine plant foods that make up for the deficiency in one or the another, or to add a small amount of dairy product, which makes the dish "complete"—for example, beans and rice, seeds in our bread, or a bit of cheese with pasta and pizza. Even a small amount of a meat or dairy product will complete the protein available in grains and vegetables, as in a stir-fry.

I have published a recipe for spinach lasagna in the past, but as it is such a favorite among people in the Vanderbilt program (it is one of the most frequently recorded dishes in their food diaries) I repeat it here because I think it will become one of your favorites, too. The bean, pizza, and chili recipes are all new creations and among my best.

Champ Beans

2 cups assorted dried beans (e.g., pinto, black, kidney, garbanzo)
6 cups soup stock (or 6 cups water and 6 teaspoons instant bouillon)
2 bay leaves
1 teaspoon each sage, thyme, rosemary, and savory

4 dried red peppers (hot)
1 cup chopped onions
1 green pepper, chopped
2 large cloves garlic, minced
2 large carrots, sliced in ½-inch chunks
4 stalks celery, sliced in ½-inch chunks
Salt and fresh-ground black pepper to taste

1. Rinse beans and then place in a large bowl with stock, bay leaves, sage, thyme, rosemary, and savory. Cover and refrigerate overnight.
2. Place entire mixture in a large pot and add hot peppers and the remaining ingredients. Bring to a boil, then reduce heat and simmer for at least 3 hours, stirring occasionally to prevent sticking to the bottom of the pot. The longer they cook, the better they get! (The garbanzos remain crunchy while the other beans will get soft.) Serve plain, with rice, or over a baked potato.

Makes 8 servings.
Per serving (without rice or potato): **0.9 g total fat;** 0.2 g saturated fat; 0 cholesterol; 205 calories; 8 g fiber; 605 mg sodium

Baby Vegetarian Pizzas

This is the first pizza sauce I ever made, and it remains my best! I sometimes use whole-wheat English muffins, but I must admit it tastes more "original" with the regular-flour variety. The muffins do not need toasting in advance.

½ cup minced onions
2 large cloves garlic, minced (or ½ teaspoon garlic powder)
1 tablespoon olive oil
1 cup chopped mushrooms
1 15-ounce can tomato sauce
1 tablespoon grated Parmesan

½ teaspoon each oregano and sage
1 teaspoon basil
Dash of cayenne pepper
Fresh-ground black pepper to taste
6 English muffins, split
1 cup grated part-skim mozzarella (4 ounces)
¼ cup chopped olives

1. In a saucepan sauté onions and garlic in oil until tender.
2. Add remaining ingredients except muffins, mozzarella, and olives. Stir well and simmer, covered, for 10 minutes.
3. Place muffins cut side up on a baking sheet. Sprinkle half of the mozzarella cheese over the muffins and then spread 2 tablespoons of the sauce over the cheese.
4. Sprinkle the olives and the remaining cheese over the sauce.
5. Bake in a 450-degree oven for 5 minutes, or until the cheese melts.

Note: The sauce can also be made in a microwave oven. Cook the onions on high heat, covered, for about 3 minutes and simmer the sauce on 75 percent power for 8 to 10 minutes. Leave the sauce uncovered in the microwave, so that it thickens. Prepare the pizzas in the oven as directed above.

Makes 12 baby pizzas.
Per pizza: **3.7 g total fat;** 1.4 g saturated fat; 5 mg cholesterol; 124 calories; 2 g fiber; 475 mg sodium

Easy Vegetarian Chili Texas Style

This is a recipe for folks who don't want to bother cooking dried beans from scratch. I was surprised at how good it was when I first made it since I normally prefer to use a variety of dried beans and cook them all day long. This recipe does require about an hour's simmering, or the flavor will not develop fully.

1 cup chopped onions (2 medium-size onions)
4 cloves garlic, minced
2 cups vegetable stock (or use vegetable bouillon)
1 15-ounce can whole tomatoes, cut up, with juice
1 6-ounce can tomato paste
3 tablespoons chili powder
1 teaspoon vinegar (cider or red wine)

1 teaspoon ground cumin
½ teaspoon ground coriander
½ teaspoon oregano
¼ teaspoon fresh-ground black pepper
3 whole dried red peppers (hot)
2 16-ounce cans red or kidney beans, drained

1. In a 4-quart saucepan, simmer the onions and garlic in 3 tablespoons of the stock until translucent.
2. Add all remaining ingredients except the beans and simmer for 45 minutes.
3. Add beans and simmer another 15 minutes.

Makes about 8 cups.
Per cup: **1.7 g total fat;** 0.3 g saturated fat; 0 cholesterol; 170 calories; 12 g fiber; 875 mg sodium

Spinach Lasagna

½ pound lasagna noodles,
preferably whole wheat
1 medium onion, chopped
2 cloves garlic, minced
1 tablespoon olive oil
Water as needed
1 pound "lite" or part-skim
ricotta cheese or low-fat
cottage cheese
¼ cup grated Parmesan
1½ pounds fresh spinach,
chopped and packed
(about 2 cups) or 1

10-ounce package frozen
chopped spinach, thawed
and drained
2 egg whites, beaten
¼ teaspoon fresh-ground
black pepper
2 to 3 tablespoons fresh
parsley, chopped
Nonstick cooking spray
6 cups tomato or meatless
spaghetti sauce
6 ounces part-skim
mozzarella, grated

1. Cook the lasagna noodles according to package directions.
2. While the noodles are cooking, sauté the onion and garlic in the olive oil, adding a tablespoon or two of water as needed to keep from sticking.
3. Combine the ricotta, Parmesan, spinach, egg whites, black pepper, parsley, and sautéed onion and garlic, mixing well.
4. Spray a 9 × 13 × 2-inch casserole dish with nonstick cooking spray. Spread ¼ of the tomato or spaghetti sauce over the bottom and then arrange a layer of noodles, top with ⅓ of the ricotta-spinach mixture, sprinkle with ⅓ of the mozzarella, and top with tomato sauce. Repeat layers twice more, ending with sauce.
5. Cover pan with aluminum foil, crimping edges tightly. Bake at 350 degrees for 40 minutes; remove foil and bake 10–15 minutes more.

Makes 12 servings.
Per serving: **7.5 g total fat;** 3.9 g saturated fat; 21 mg cholesterol; 222 calories; 3 g fiber; 903 mg sodium

250 One Meal at a Time

VEGETABLE SIDE DISHES

If you will only trust yourself to try them, you may find that just
about all vegetables taste great steamed or microwaved, with very
little if any fat or seasoning added. Taste them first after cooking, and
add salt and pepper at the table if desired. Adding a small amount of
salt at the table normally results in a lower intake than attempting to
bring the dish to full flavor while cooking.

When I do want to add flavor during cooking, I use just a bit of salt
with other seasonings. Salt helps bring out the flavor of many vegetables and grains and other herbs and spices, *but you don't need to add
very much during cooking.* You can achieve excellent results with vegetables and grains, with little or no fat, by using a variety of herbs and
spices. If you have been cooking with fatty ham hocks, frankfurters,
or sausage, replace these with lean ham, bones, bouillon, or broth.

For example, cook rice in broth instead of water and fat. Add any
one or more of other ingredients to the broth, including onion, bell
peppers, or mixed vegetables. Give the dish a little edge with one or
two dried (hot) red peppers. If you like a butter flavor, try one of the
butter-flavored sprinkles, such as Molly McButter, Butter Buds, or
McCormick's.

Whenever possible, leave edible skins on the vegetables. They
contain much of the fiber and many other nutrients. Green and yellow vegetables are good to excellent sources of vitamin A, and the
same goes for calcium in greens. Collards, for example, are almost as
good a source of calcium as milk—and contain no fat!

The recipes below illustrate several different ways to prepare
vegetables that can be adapted to other vegetables with a little imagination. Read them through and you will see what I mean.

Cauliflower with Crumb Topping

2 cups water
1 large head cauliflower, cut
  into small flowerettes
1/4 cup green onions, finely
  chopped
2 cloves garlic, chopped
1/2 teaspoon salt

1/4 teaspoon fresh-ground
  black pepper
2 tablespoons
  reduced-calorie
  margarine, melted
1 cup breadcrumbs

1. In a saucepan, bring 2 cups water to a boil. Add cauliflower, cover, and cook until tender, about 10 minutes. Drain well. Transfer to a 9 × 13 × 2-inch casserole dish and spread evenly.
2. In a bowl, combine green onions, seasonings, and melted margarine. Toss gently with the breadcrumbs.
3. Sprinkle over the cauliflower and bake in a 425-degree oven for 10 minutes. Turn on the broiler and broil about 7 inches from the heat for 4–5 minutes or until lightly browned.

Makes 6 servings.
Per serving: **2 g total fat;** 0.5 g saturated fat; 1 mg cholesterol; 112 calories; 5 g fiber; 345 mg sodium

VARIATIONS: Try the above approach with other crunchy vegetables such as broccoli, celery, and summer squash, but be sure not to overcook the vegetables before putting in the oven.

Greens Casserole

This delicious vegetable casserole can be made with a combination of spinach and broccoli or any other greens you choose. I am especially fond of kale or turnip greens mixed about half and half with any more mildly flavored greens.

2 eggs or 1 whole egg and 2 egg whites
6 tablespoons whole-wheat flour
½ teaspoon each thyme, sage, marjoram, crushed red peppers (peppers optional, but highly recommended)
2 10-ounce packages frozen chopped greens, thawed
¼ teaspoon garlic powder
1 cup low-fat cottage cheese
1½ cups grated extra-sharp cheddar cheese
Nonstick cooking spray
3 tablespoons stuffing mix or seasoned breadcrumbs

1. Combine the eggs, flour, and spices in a bowl and mix until smooth.
2. Add all ingredients except the stuffing mixture or breadcrumbs and mix well.
3. Transfer to a 1½-quart casserole dish that has been sprayed with nonstick cooking spray.
4. Sprinkle stuffing mixture or breadcrumbs over the top of the greens-and-cheese mixture.
5. Bake at 325 degrees for 45 minutes.

Makes 10 servings.
Per serving (using 2 whole eggs): **6.0 g total fat;** 3.4 g saturated fat; 51 mg cholesterol; 115 calories; 2 g fiber; 212 mg sodium

Steamed Oriental Vegetable Medley

6–8 green onions, sliced
1 medium red pepper, chopped
4 stalks celery, sliced
1 teaspoon minced gingerroot
¼ cup soy sauce
1 cup water chestnuts, sliced
1 cup mushrooms, sliced
1 bunch broccoli, cut into spears

1. In a saucepan, sauté the onions, pepper, celery, and gingerroot in the soy sauce until onions are tender.
2. Add the remaining vegetables. Cover and steam for 6–8 minutes.

Makes 6 servings.
Per serving: **0.4 g total fat;** 0.1 g saturated fat; 0 cholesterol; 54 calories; 4 g fiber; 735 mg sodium

VARIATIONS: This is another recipe that's suitable for any variety of crunchy vegetables.

Glazed Orange-Spice Carrots

2½ cups carrots, thinly sliced
Water
½ cup orange juice
1½ teaspoon cornstarch
⅛ teaspoon powdered ginger
⅛ teaspoon nutmeg
Fresh cilantro or parsley sprigs (optional)

1. Steam carrots over water until just tender.
2. Meanwhile, combine orange juice, cornstarch, ginger, and nutmeg in a saucepan. Heat over medium heat until sauce begins to thicken. Stir in carrots and heat through. Serve garnished with cilantro or parsley sprigs if desired.

Makes 4 servings.
Per serving: **0 total fat;** 0 saturated fat; 0 cholesterol; 48 calories; 2 g fiber; 24 mg sodium

Summer Squash with Lemon-Dill Sauce

1 tablespoon olive oil
2 tablespoons water
½ cup onion, finely chopped
3–4 yellow summer squash,
   cut into 3-inch by ½-inch
   strips
½ teaspoon salt

½ teaspoon paprika
1 teaspoon dried dill (or 2
   tablespoons fresh dill,
   chopped)
1 tablespoon lemon juice
½ cup plain nonfat yogurt
Fresh parsley (optional)

1. Heat oil and water in a saucepan, add onion, and sauté/steam until tender, about 5 minutes.
2. Add squash, seasonings, and lemon juice. Cover and simmer for 10 minutes. Remove cover and continue cooking over medium heat until squash is tender.
3. Immediately before serving, transfer to a serving dish and stir in the yogurt. Garnish with fresh chopped parsley if desired.

Makes 6 servings.
Per serving: **2.6 g total fat;** 0.4 g saturated fat; 0 cholesterol; 55 calories; 2 g fiber; 194 mg sodium

VARIATIONS: Use zucchini or any other summer squash, alone or in combination with yellow squash.

Beets to Beat All

With a recipe like this I think you will begin to include beets for variety a little more often in your diet.

1 1-pound can julienned
  beets (reserve ½ cup of
  the liquid)
1½ teaspoons cornstarch
1 teaspoon grated orange
  peel

1 tablespoon orange juice
½ teaspoon honey
½ tablespoon margarine or
  butter
Fresh-ground black pepper
  to taste

1. Drain beets and reserve ½ cup of the liquid.
2. Combine the ½ cup beet juice with the cornstarch and cook
   until it starts to clear and thicken.
3. Add the other ingredients except the beets to the juice-corn-
   starch mixture and stir until smooth.
4. Place drained beets in a small casserole dish and pour mixture
   over it.
5. Heat in oven or microwave until hot and bubbly.

Makes 4 servings.
Per serving: **2.0 g total fat;** 0.4 g saturated fat; 0 cholesterol; 58
calories; 2.0 g fiber; 321 mg sodium

Rice Pilaf

1 cup brown rice, uncooked
2 stalks celery, chopped
1 medium onion, chopped
2 tablespoons
  reduced-calorie margarine
1 4-ounce can small
  mushrooms, whole

1 10¾-ounce can beef
  consommé
¼ teaspoon fresh-ground
  black pepper
1¼ cups water

Combine all ingredients in a 1½-quart casserole dish. Cook, covered, at 350 degrees for 1 hour.

Makes 6 servings.
Per serving: **2.8 g total fat;** 0.6 g saturated fat; 0 cholesterol; 147
calories; 2.2 g fiber; 819 mg sodium

SAUCES

Garlic Soy Sauce

This is a good sauce for broiling seafood, poultry, and meats.

1 garlic clove, crushed
1 tablespoon sherry
1 tablespoon lemon juice

1 tablespoon honey
2 tablespoons soy sauce

Combine all ingredients in a small bowl.

Makes about 5 tablespoons.
Per 1 tablespoon: **0 total fat;** 0 saturated fat; 0 cholesterol; 22 calories;
0 fiber; 412 mg sodium

Salsa Rapida

This is a quick Mexican-style hot sauce.

2 tomatoes, peeled and
  chopped (about 1½ cups)
½ cup onion, finely chopped
1 clove garlic, crushed
½ teaspoon crushed dried
  hot red pepper
3 sprigs fresh parsley

½ teaspoon ground dried
  coriander
½ teaspoon salt
Pinch of marjoram and
  cloves
Fresh-ground black pepper
  to taste

Mix the chopped vegetables, then add the seasonings and mix. Refrigerate for at least 2 hours before serving. Serve with meat, burritos, and tacos.

Makes about 2 cups.
Per tablespoon: **0 total fat;** 0 saturated fat; 0 cholesterol; 3 calories;
0.2 g fiber; 34 mg sodium

Roux

This roux can be used to thicken soups, sauces, or just about any
cooked item that needs thickening. It is also the basis for gravies.
Although you can use it for making a white sauce when you are in a
hurry, my recipe for Light Béchamel, which follows, contains other
ingredients that I think are necessary for a good white sauce.

1 tablespoon vegetable oil or margarine
2 tablespoons flour (all purpose or whole wheat
   or combination)

Heat the oil in a skillet over medium heat. Slowly add the flour,
stirring constantly. Cook until golden brown, stirring constantly. Stir
into the main recipe.

TO MAKE GRAVY: Add to the above 1 cup of stock, and stir over
medium-low to medium heat until thickened. Season your gravy
with a dash of salt and fresh-ground black pepper if desired; add a
few pinches of rosemary, sage, marjoram, or thyme for flavoring.

Makes about 1 cup of gravy.
Per ¼ cup: **3.4 g total fat;** 0.2 g **saturated fat;** 0 cholesterol; 44
calories; 0 fiber; 63 mg sodium

Light Béchamel (White Sauce)

This is an excellent sauce for vegetables. One recipe can be used in
place of the tomato paste and tomato sauce in my recipe for Red

Clam Sauce, and you will end up with a great white clam sauce! I would definitely use a vegetable seasoning (optional below) when making the clam sauce.

¼ cup chicken or vegetable stock
¼ cup flour or 2 tablespoons cornstarch
2 cups skim milk
½ cup nonfat dry milk

1 bay leaf
½ teaspoon thyme
½ teaspoon white pepper
1 teaspoon vegetable seasoning (optional)

1. Heat stock in a saucepan over moderate heat.
2. Gradually add the flour or cornstarch and blend with a wire whisk or wooden spoon.
3. Simmer on very low heat until heated through but not browned.
4. Remove from heat and add remaining ingredients.
5. Return to heat and simmer, stirring occasionally, until thickened.

Makes 2 ½ cups.
Per ¼ cup (using flour): **0 total fat;** 0 saturated fat; 1 mg cholesterol; 42 calories; 0 fiber; 63 mg sodium (without vegetable seasoning; however, a salt-free seasoning such as Mrs. Dash will add no sodium)

Barbecue Sauce

1 12-ounce can tomato paste
⅓ cup dry red wine (or water)
1 ½ cups water (or stock)
1 tablespoon vinegar (red wine or cider)
2 teaspoons lemon juice
½ cup finely chopped onion
½ cup finely chopped bell pepper
1 tablespoon Worcestershire sauce

1 tablespoon brown sugar
1 tablespoon honey
1 teaspoon garlic powder
1 tablespoon chili powder
1 tablespoon dry mustard
Cayenne pepper to taste
2 teaspoons dry basil (or 2 tablespoons fresh, minced)
¼ teaspoon celery seed
½ teaspoon salt (optional)

1. Combine all ingredients except basil and celery seed (and salt, if you are using any) in a large saucepan; bring to a low boil, then reduce heat and simmer 20 minutes.
2. Add the basil and celery seed (and optional salt if desired) and simmer for another 5 minutes.

Makes about 1 quart.
Per tablespoon (without salt and using water in place of stock): **0 total fat;** 0 saturated fat; 0 mg cholesterol; 7 calories; 0 fiber; 5 mg sodium

Cocoa Fudge Sauce

Do you remember that wonderful chocolate sauce that hardens when poured over your ice cream, or when you dip a cone? Here is a fantastic recipe that Harriette created that will delight children of all ages. But you must make it with cocoa! If you use the unsweetened baker's chocolate it will contain two to three times more fat. I think this recipe is just a little bit better with butter so I insisted on analyzing it that way! But you can use margarine if you prefer (it's about 0.75 gram less saturated fat per serving and has no cholesterol). Serve it over frozen yogurt.

6 tablespoons cocoa powder	1 cup sugar
3½ teaspoons butter or margarine	2 tablespoons white corn syrup
⅓ cup boiling water	1 teaspoon vanilla

1. Put cocoa and butter in saucepan; pour the boiling water over them and stir well. (The boiling water will melt the butter.)
2. Add sugar and corn syrup to the mixture and stir just once or twice to blend. Then increase heat to the point where the mixture boils readily but not furiously. DO NOT STIR. Cook for 8 minutes without any additional mixing.
3. Remove from heat and allow to cool for 10 minutes.
4. Add vanilla, stir lightly, and serve immediately. Store leftover sauce in refrigerator. Reheat in a double boiler over boiling water.

Makes 1 cup.
Per 2 tablespoons (using butter): **2.4 g total fat;** 1.5 g saturated fat; 4.5 mg cholesterol; 136 calories; 1.2 g fiber; 18 mg sodium

DESSERTS

This section includes a sampling of many different kinds of desserts, just to prove that nothing need be sacrificed when you reduce the fat in your diet. There's a frozen dessert, a pudding, a pie, a cake, baked fruit desserts, cookies, and candy.

The first step in making desserts lower in fat is using ingredients lower in fat. The second is reducing the added fat by ⅓ to ½ whenever feasible. Replace the fat with another liquid (for example, milk, juice, applesauce, or yogurt).

You need never sacrifice a tasty dessert just because you are following a low-fat diet. There are many commercially prepared low-fat desserts for everyday use. Here are some examples:

- Angel food cake, served with fruit sauce or chocolate fudge sauce
- Frozen yogurt, or the new no-fat ice creams
- Lower-fat cookies, such as fig bars, gingersnaps, and graham crackers

Fresh fruit should be a frequent first choice.

Remember that some of our breads and muffins also make satisfying and delicious meal endings.

Pineapple-Orange Frozen Yogurt

1½ cups plain low-fat yogurt
½ cup orange juice
½ 8-ounce can crushed
  pineapple

2 tablespoons sugar
2 teaspoons vanilla

Combine all ingredients, and make in an ice cream maker according to manufacturer's instructions. Serve immediately.

Makes 4 servings.
Per serving: **0.2 g total fat;** 0.1 g saturated fat; 2 mg cholesterol; 103 calories; 0 fiber; 66 mg sodium

Southern-Style Banana Pudding

1 7-ounce package vanilla or banana cream pudding mix (regular or instant)
3 cups skim or 1% milk
32 vanilla wafers
3–4 bananas, sliced

3 egg whites, at room temperature
1/8 teaspoon cream of tartar
1/2 teaspoon vanilla
1/4 cup sugar

1. Prepare pudding with milk according to package directions.
2. In the bottom of an 8 × 8-inch baking dish, arrange half of the vanilla wafers. Top with a generous layer of sliced bananas and then half of the pudding. Repeat with a layer of remaining vanilla wafers, bananas, and pudding.
3. Beat egg whites, cream of tartar, and vanilla at highest speed of electric mixer until the mix forms soft peaks. Gradually add sugar, beating until stiff peaks form. Spread meringue evenly over pudding mixture, sealing to edge of dish.
4. Bake at 350 degrees for about 10 minutes or until golden brown.

Makes 8 servings.
Per serving (using 1% milk): **3.2 g total fat;** 0.9 g saturated fat; 12 mg cholesterol; 256 calories; 1 g fiber; 129 mg sodium

Pumpkin Pie

CRUST
1½ cups graham-cracker
    crumbs
2 tablespoons honey
1 tablespoon oil or melted
    margarine

TOPPING
1 cup vanilla nonfat or
    low-fat yogurt

FILLING
2 cups cooked pumpkin,
    mashed, or 1 16-ounce
    can pumpkin
⅓ cup brown sugar
¼ cup granulated sugar
1 12-ounce can evaporated
    skim milk
1 carton (1 cup) Egg
    Beaters (or 2 whole eggs
    plus 3 large egg whites)
1 teaspoon cinnamon
½ teaspoon ginger
¼ teaspoon nutmeg or
    allspice
⅛ teaspoon cloves

1. Combine graham-cracker crumbs, honey, and oil. Mix well. Press into a 9-inch pie pan. Set aside.
2. In a large bowl, combine all filling ingredients and beat until smooth.
3. Pour into pie crust and bake in a 350-degree oven for approximately 50 minutes or until knife inserted into center comes out clean. Cool and serve with a dollop of yogurt.

Makes 8 slices.
Per slice using the eggs and egg whites, without the topping: **4.8 g total fat;** 1.1 g saturated fat; 28 mg cholesterol; 249 calories; 2 g fiber; 227 mg sodium
Per slice using the eggs and egg whites, with low-fat yogurt as topping: **5.2 g total fat;** 1.3 g saturated fat; 30 mg cholesterol; 273 calories; 2 g fiber; 246 mg sodium

Fruit Crisp

4 cups fruit, sliced or
chopped (try Rome or
Granny Smith apples,
peaches, blueberries, or
blackberries)
¼ cup sugar
2 teaspoons lemon juice
½ teaspoon cinnamon
(optional—best for apple
crisp)

¾ cup quick-cooking oats,
uncooked
¼ cup all-purpose flour
¼ cup firmly packed brown
sugar
2 tablespoons margarine
1 egg white

1. Combine fruit, sugar, lemon juice, and cinnamon in an 8 × 8 ×
   2-inch baking dish. Toss well.
2. In a bowl, combine oats, flour, and brown sugar. With a pastry
   blender or two knives cut in margarine and egg white until
   mixture resembles coarse crumbs. Sprinkle evenly over fruit
   mixture.
3. Bake at 350 degrees for about 40 minutes. Serve warm with
   frozen yogurt or ice milk if desired.

Makes 6 servings.
Per serving (without yogurt or ice milk): **3.7 total fat;** 0.7 g saturated fat;
0 cholesterol; 173 calories; 3 g fiber; 73 mg sodium

Baked Apples

4 apples, cored
½ cup raisins
2 tablespoons brown sugar

1 teaspoon cinnamon
½ cup apple juice (or
water)

1. Place apples in a shallow baking dish.
2. Combine the raisins, brown sugar, and cinnamon. Spoon into
   centers of the apples. Pour apple juice over apples.

3. Bake at 350 degrees for 45 minutes or until apples are tender, basting occasionally. Serve warm with frozen yogurt or ice milk if desired.

Makes 4 servings.
Per serving (using apple juice and without yogurt or ice milk): **0.6 g total fat;** 0.1 saturated fat; 0 cholesterol; 175 calories; 5 g fiber; 7 mg sodium

Cocoa Zucchini Cake

This cake is moist and lightly sweet, with a satisfying, rich texture.

1¼ cups granulated sugar
½ cup vegetable oil
1 teaspoon vanilla extract
1 egg
2 egg whites
½ cup skim or 1% milk
1 teaspoon baking soda
1½ cups all-purpose flour

1 cup whole-wheat flour
¼ cup cocoa powder
½ teaspoon cinnamon
½ teaspoon salt
2 cups grated zucchini, unpeeled (about 1½ squashes)
Nonstick cooking spray

1. Combine first 6 ingredients in a large bowl.
2. In another bowl, sift together the baking soda, flours, cocoa, cinnamon, and salt. Add alternately with the zucchini to the first mixture.
3. Bake at 350 degrees for 1 hour in a Bundt pan that has been sprayed with nonstick cooking spray, or for 45 minutes in a 9 × 13 × 2-inch baking pan. Let stand 5–10 minutes before removing from pan.

Makes 24 servings.
Per serving (using 1% milk): **5.1 g total fat;** 0.5 saturated fat; 9 mg cholesterol; 137 calories; 1 g fiber; 90 mg sodium

Gingerbread Cookies

⅓ cup margarine
½ cup sugar
½ cup molasses
2¼ cups all-purpose flour
1 egg

1 teaspoon cinnamon
1 teaspoon dry ground
   ginger
½ teaspoon ground cloves
1 teaspoon baking soda

1. In a mixing bowl, cream margarine with an electric mixer. Add the sugar, molasses, 1 cup of the flour, egg, seasonings, and baking soda. Beat until well blended. Blend in remaining flour.
2. Shape into 1-inch balls. Bake 2 inches apart on ungreased cookie sheets at 375 degrees for about 8 minutes. Cool on a wire rack.

Makes 48 cookies.
Per cookie: **1.4 g total fat;** 0.3 g saturated fat; 4 mg cholesterol; 48 calories; 0 fiber; 36 mg sodium

VARIATION: To make gingerbread people, chill dough for at least 3 hours. Divide, and on a floured surface roll to ½ inch thickness. Cut into desired shapes with a cookie cutter. Bake 6–7 minutes at 375 degrees.

Candied Orange or Grapefruit Peel

I've included this recipe because it's like the one my grandmother used to make when I was a child, and I loved it. I could hardly stand waiting those two days for the fruit to dry. The fruit peel is a good source of fiber.

Don't be put off by the amount of sugar in this recipe. When it's made up, a 1-ounce serving contains only 55 calories, including the calories in the peel. By comparison, a 1-ounce serving of jelly beans contains 100 calories, *and all the calories are derived from sugar.* This is obviously a preferred way to go when you want a piece of candy!

2 large grapefruits with
thick peel or 6 oranges
Cold water
1 teaspoon salt

1 cup granulated sugar
½ cup light corn syrup
1 cup water
Sugar for coating

1. Cut peel from grapefruits or oranges into 4 lengthwise sections. If white membrane is thick, remove some of it; otherwise leave intact.
2. Cover peel with cold water and the 1 teaspoon salt; bring to a boil. Boil 10 minutes (5 minutes if using orange peel) and drain. Repeat three more times, omitting salt after first procedure.
3. With kitchen scissors, cut peel into ½-inch strips.
4. In a 3-quart saucepan, combine the sugar, corn syrup, and the 1 cup water. Stir over low heat until sugar dissolves.
5. Add peel and boil gently, uncovered, for about 40 minutes or until most of the syrup is absorbed. Drain in strainer or colander.
6. Lightly roll peel a few pieces at a time in granulated sugar.
7. Arrange in a single layer on wax paper and let dry for 2 days. Store in an airtight container.

Makes 1–1 ½ pounds candy.
Per 1-ounce serving: **0 total fat;** 0 saturated fat; 0 cholesterol; 55 calories; 1 g fiber; 22 mg sodium

CHAPTER 12

THE ONE MEAL AT A TIME PROGRAM FOR CHILDREN AND ADOLESCENTS[1]

The silent example—that's about the strongest weapon we have at our disposal when it comes to steering our children toward a healthful life-style. We also can help initiate a preference for healthful foods and the enjoyment of physical activity early in life by making it a family affair.

Our schools can play a role, too, of course. I believe that nutrition and physical education courses should have a place in the standard curriculum simply because sound nutrition and physical activity are so important to our personal health and national well-being, economically as well as physically. However, I'm not sure we should blame our schools for failing to promote nutrition and physical activity when so many of us don't take responsibility for promoting healthy eating and exercise in our own homes.

Many of us are not doing a very good job of helping our children toward a healthful diet and active life. The main reason is that we haven't been doing a very good job with ourselves. We don't pro-

[1]Much of the material for this chapter was furnished by Ms. Jamie Pope-Cordle, M.S., R.D., director of nutrition, Vanderbilt Weight Management Program.

vide those potent silent examples and a proper home environment. I think you will find it quite easy to make the One Meal at a Time nutrition changes for the whole family. It will take a little more planning, and perhaps even greater commitment, to make being active a family project.

I have some specific suggestions that can help you meet the needs of both children and adolescents. First, I want to review some startling facts about the health of our youth and the causal factors. I hope this review will help you to understand the environmental and motivational factors that provide the unhealthy influences.

DID YOU KNOW THAT...

- 77 percent of young men have detectable coronary artery lesions by the age of 22; 15 percent have blockage of 50 percent or more?
- 40 percent of children under 8 years of age already show at least one risk factor for heart disease?
- The average consumption of calories from fat among children is almost exactly the same as that of adults (38 percent or more)?
- Food commercials comprise 55 percent of the advertising on Saturday morning television? (Very little of it for fruit!)
- There is a significant relationship between requests by children and purchases by parents of foods advertised or shown on television?
- There is no relationship between television content and requests for sports items or an interest in physical activity?
- The more time spent in front of the TV, the more children are likely to eat?
- Fewer than 1 in 10 parents do any physical activities with their children on a regular basis?
- Only about 1 in 3 children have regularly scheduled physical education classes available to them in their schools?
- Almost 70 percent of American children and adolescents *cannot* pass a basic fitness test that *is passed* by over 90 percent of children in European countries?
- Obesity among children is at an all-time high; that it increased by 39 percent in a recent 10-year period, with superobesity increasing by 64 percent?
- Children average about 25 hours of television watching each week? (It's more time than they spend in school on a yearly basis, and next to sleeping, it's the most frequent activity.)

- Prevalence of obesity increases by 2 percent for each hour of television viewing?
- There is a direct relationship between watching TV and children's serum cholesterol levels—the more they watch, the higher the serum cholesterol?

HELPING YOUR CHILDREN TO A HEALTHFUL LIFE-STYLE

Your own behavior when you adopt the One Meal at a Time program will be the strongest influence in the family environment and in your children's lives. You don't have to do anything special with pre-adolescents. Adolescents are another story.

I'll focus first on creating a healthful eating environment for children in general and then add some suggestions for the overweight child.

REQUIREMENTS IN CHILDREN'S DIETS

Except for more calcium, iron, and calories per pound of body weight, nutritional recommendations for children over the age of 2 are very much like those for adults. More calories per pound of body weight are needed to meet the growth demands and the tendency to be more active than adults.

Like the average adult, children and adolescents are consuming far too much fat, especially saturated fat. The guidelines for reducing fat consumption that I spelled out in Chapters 2 and 3 apply to children. However, while I suggested that the average adult aim for 25 percent of calories in fat, I don't think we need aim quite so low with healthy children because of their need for more energy. The consensus among health organizations is to aim for 30 percent of calories or less after the age of 2. (More fat may be needed for growth and neural development up to that age.)

The key health consideration for children as well as adults is to keep saturated fat at or below 10 percent of calories. This is accomplished by using low-fat dairy products and lean meats and poultry.

The need for vitamins and minerals as well as adequate protein, carbohydrate, and fat for growth and energy needs can be met by following these daily guidelines for children after the age of 2:

- 4 servings of low-fat milk products
- 2 *or more* servings of lean meat, fish, or poultry
- 4 *or more* servings of vegetables and fruits, including one citrus fruit and a green or yellow vegetable
- 4 *or more* servings of breads and cereals (whole-grain or mixed-grain preferred)

Obviously, servings for a 4-year-old will be smaller than those for a 17-year-old, but, in general, when we use the word "serving" we mean a standard cafeteria-size portion. Just use discretion when you have children of different sizes and ages.

"More" is an important word in these recommendations, especially in the grains and fruit-and-vegetable categories. Children between the ages of 4 and 10 will require between 1,700 and 2,100 calories a day, and adolescents between 11 and 17 will generally require 2,100 to 2,800 calories a day. The actual amount will depend on increasing age, height and weight, and level of physical activity. As children's energy needs increase for any of these reasons, focus on that word "more" in the fruit-and-vegetable and bread-and-cereal groups of foods.

Translating 30 percent of calories as fat to grams of fat, within these overall calorie guidelines, children between 4 and 10 would have a fat quota of between 57 and 70 grams, and adolescents between 11 and 17 of between 70 and 93 grams, *but please consider these figures as "theoretical."*

We don't believe in having children get into the counting frame of mind.

Counting encourages an obsessional attitude toward food, and is likely to encourage on-again, off-again dieting behavior should a child become concerned about weight. This is exactly what we don't want. Our goal for children is the same as for you—to help them learn how to eat, not diet, and how to do it as a matter of course, without thinking twice about it.

You help your child to a healthful attitude toward food by constructing a healthful eating environment that permits your children to eat until their appetite is satisfied whenever they are hungry. Your children's diets will fall within the fat guidelines without conscious concern when the eating environment is a healthful one.

There are two possible restrictions on this freedom to eat whenever hungry. First, a regular pattern of eating is better than an irregular one. Second, whatever pattern fits a child's needs should blend with the family schedule. Not everyone needs to eat at the same time, but we tend to eat a more healthful diet when whoever is in charge of meals can plan around a fairly dependable schedule for the family as a whole.

Children will not choose a healthful diet spontaneously any more than adults do if high-fat "designer" foods are freely available alongside the healthier choices.

As I mentioned in Chapter 1, food scientists work hard to design foods that blend flavors the human animal likes best. Fat and sweeteners or salt are usually important basic ingredients. Food processors take that knowledge and produce foods that are more attractive for most human beings than anything found growing naturally on trees and bushes. Apples and grapes are not likely to be first choices for our children any more than they are for ourselves when cookies, cakes, and candies are within an arm's reach at all times.

Be aware that food processors try to play it both ways. That is, they know what sells by taste and texture, but they also know that there is a growing concern about the impact of too much fat on our health. So you will see banners such as "No cholesterol" on potato chips and "Made with real fruit" on cereals. When you see such claims, read the labels carefully. "No cholesterol" does not mean a low-fat product, and "real fruit" may tempt you to think "low fat" or "low sugar" when fat or sugar may really be primary ingredients. Unless the new labeling rules and laws now being discussed by the Food and Drug Administration, the Department of Agriculture, and Congress prevent the use of health-related statements ingeniously designed to be misinterpreted by the general public, we are likely to see more statements of this kind on many products, including those aimed at children.

DESIGNING A PROPER FOOD ENVIRONMENT: "EVERYDAY FOODS" AND "OCCASIONAL FOODS"

To design a proper food environment for the entire family, it's good, once again, to think in terms of "everyday" foods and "occasional" foods. This will help put all foods in their proper place, since we believe everything—including cakes, candy, ice cream, and so on—

can have an "occasional" place in a healthful low-fat diet for everyone in the family.

Everyday foods include everything I have been talking about in Chapters 5 through 8 as the core of the One Meal at a Time program. Assuming everyone is in good health, there is no reason to make special foods for anyone in the family over the age of 2. However, since children have smaller stomachs than adults, they are much more likely to need to eat more often, and that means snacks. Take a look at Table 12-1 (page 275) for some snack ideas that make it possible to have healthful, everyday choices available whenever a child is hungry.

What about peanut butter, and those "quick-energy" candy bars (there we go with the advertising again) aimed at children as snacks? As long as a child is of normal weight and doesn't eat half a jar at a time, peanut butter in moderation is a fine food for growing children. Overweight children might consider substituting apple butter. As for fatty candies (chocolate bars can contain over 50 percent of their calories in fat), it's better to substitute no-fat sweets such as hard candies, jelly beans, gum drops, and so on most of the time. However, be sure sugary foods are not present in the mouth for very long, since they do encourage cavities. Fresh fruit and dried fruit are preferable to candy, most of the time. Although they, too, contain sugar, they also contain vitamins and minerals not present in candy.

Homemade sweets using cereals such as Rice Krispies are preferable to commercial fatty candies. Rice Krispies squares contain almost no fat, and provide vitamins and minerals generally lacking in candy, cake, and cookies. The same will be true of muffins made from cereal products. Adding raisins, dates, or other dried fruit turns muffins into a healthful sweet treat, and they should be included as a choice within the everyday food group.

Do not keep occasional foods on hand at all times—they will become everyday foods if you do. Control the eating environment by making high-fat treats available only on the occasions when they can fit into your family's otherwise low-fat diet. Consider going out for them, rather than bringing them into the house. A trip to the ice cream parlor, for example, is often more fun for the family than going to the freezer. Besides, everyone is likely to eat a little less than if they were at home and could go back for seconds.

Here are some additional suggestions, together with a few comments, for dealing with the home environment, school, fast-food establishments, and exercise:

- Find out what is to be offered at school if your child purchases lunches there and obtain advice on the lower-fat food choices.
- Pack a healthful lunch if the choices at school are limited or disliked by your child.

    Did you know that some school systems have given up providing lower-fat foods and using lower-fat methods of preparation because the children rejected them? The attitude of those school systems was "Why fight city hall? We'll give them what they want."

- If your child eats at any fast-food establishments, check them out—get nutritional information on the foods they serve, and counsel your child on the best choices. Go with your child and taste-test the lower-fat items. Occasional high-fat burgers and so on are no problem as long as they don't become an everyday affair.
- If they will not be otherwise available, children should carry appropriate snack foods when they have to be away from the house at snack times. (See Table 12–1 for suggestions.)
- The One Meal at a Time program will help the adults of your family cultivate a positive, healthful attitude toward foods and eating. Make this enjoyment of good, healthful food an important part of family life.
- Set a good example for your children in the foods you choose and the amounts you consume—both at home and away.
- Try new foods, be adventurous, but don't force these new foods on your children. Let them serve themselves a small portion. Young children are especially sensitive to strong tastes or extremes in temperature or texture, but taste buds change, so don't cast a refused food from the family dinner table forever.
- Do not force children to finish everything on their plates when their appetites are satisfied with less.
- Establish dependable mealtimes. This helps regulate your child's appetite and lends some structure to the day. This can be very important for an overweight child.
- Small children have relatively high energy needs, so, since their stomachs cannot hold a lot of food at one time, make healthful low-fat snacks available throughout the day. Snacks do not have to be scheduled like meals, but they should not interfere with meals.
- Don't forbid "junk food," but don't keep it around the house all the time. If you feel that all your child will eat is junk food, think about who is buying it!

With respect to exercise:

- Provide a safe environment for your child to run and play.
- Don't carry a child who can walk.
- Make your daily routine and your child's more active by walking more and driving less.

- Ration television time if you need to. Have your child list TV programs in order of preference, if you have to make some choices. But watching TV should not replace physical activity in your child's life.
- Encourage your children to play outdoors in all seasons. Make sure they have appropriate attire for these seasons, or they will be limited in movement or will be uncomfortable, which may lead them to dislike physical activity.
- Share enjoyable, physical activities with your children. Plan family walks, hikes, bike rides, and active outings.
- Encourage children to engage in active play with other children.
- Plan active family vacations, reinforcing that exercise is fun and worth pursuing.
- Give an older child responsibility for exercising the family pet.

I make some other suggestions for encouraging physical activity that really can apply to all in the section below where I give advice to parents of overweight children.

FOOD AS A REWARD AND PACIFIER?

You probably already know that it's not a good idea to give your children cookies and sweets just to stuff their mouths and keep them quiet when they've been making nuisances of themselves. But we can't escape it: Good food is a celebration, and eating tends to reduce tension. Although it is rather easy to find other means of reducing tension that are better than eating, we will, in spite of ourselves, sometimes want to use food as a reward. In contrast with many of my colleagues, I think there are times and places where it is truly appropriate to do so.

Let's deal first with *inappropriate* use of food as a reward.

High-fat foods should not be used as a reward for eating other, healthful foods—for example, "You can't have any ice cream until you eat your spinach." This only makes spinach less attractive in its own right and ice cream more tantalizing. It also tends to attach feelings of guilt to the eating of ice cream, and can sow the seeds for future eating problems.

High-fat foods should not be used to quiet children while you're doing things like shopping in the grocery store. It illustrates that one way to keep Mom or Dad in line or embarrass them in such situations is to make a fuss, and get a cookie in return.

Appropriate uses of food as reward are in connection with successes in life that are *not* food oriented. Making it to another birthday or anniversary, for example! Promotions, awards, festivals, holidays, and other celebrations feature good food, and the food is an appropriate part of the "rewards" that go with those occasions. That trip to the ice cream parlor as a family affair is a reward for liking one another so much, taking the time to be with each other, and for family solidarity. Of course, these uses can become inappropriate should they become everyday, rather than occasional, affairs. But such uses encourage a positive attitude toward food and illustrate for your children the occasional appropriate use of food in association with other rewarding experiences.

SMART SNACKING FOR YOUR KIDS

Because 60 to 80 percent of calories in many snack foods are in the form of fat, it is a good idea to encourage healthful snack foods as early in life as possible. Table 12–1 contains some of our suggestions.

TABLE 12–1. SMART SNACKING FOR KIDS

Milk and Dairy Products	Low-fat or nonfat yogurt mixed with fruit; low-fat cottage cheese or part-skim ricotta; other cheeses in moderate amounts; ice milk; low-fat frozen yogurt; hot cocoa made with low-fat milk; sherbet; pudding made with low-fat milk
Vegetables	Fresh, crisp, cut-up raw vegetables with yogurt-based seasoned dip; offer a variety of colors, shapes, and sizes of vegetables—keep in water in refrigerator for easy availability
Fruit	Fresh or dried fruit; frozen fruits (bananas and grapes) make a chilly summertime treat; try mixing fruit with nonfat or low-fat yogurt; mix fruit with gelatin (Jell-O)
Breads and Cereals	Dry cereals; bagels; pretzels; popcorn; pita bread with vegetables or lean meats or cheese; whole-grain breads or rolls spread with low-fat cottage or ricotta cheese and jam; graham crackers; Rice Krispie squares; whole-grain crackers; flour tortillas; breadsticks; muffins; raisin bread
Beverages	Water; fruit juices; low-fat or skim milk (add chocolate syrup for a treat); seltzer or club soda; hot cocoa

SOME SPECIAL WORDS OF ADVICE FOR PARENTS OF OVERWEIGHT CHILDREN

Unless your child is severely overweight, don't put your child "on a diet" or make a project of losing weight per se. Going on a diet means going off a diet and it encourages that yo-yo syndrome you've no doubt heard about.

Every suggestion offered earlier in this chapter to promote good health and an active life-style will enable an overweight child to lose weight quite naturally and grow into the height-and-weight ratio that's appropriate for that child. It's automatic with a low-fat diet that's embraced by the entire family and an increase in physical activity—also embraced by the entire family if it's to be successful.

I suspect you are already aware of the feelings of embarrassment and rejection that go along with being an overweight child. For this reason, your child needs lots of love and support rather than nagging and criticism. Being overweight doesn't make you a lousy person and the more you can do to develop self-esteem in children who are beginning to dislike themselves, the better. Cultivating your child's abilities in many areas can help develop self-esteem and perhaps reduce the drives that may be leading to inappropriate eating.

Most of all, for any lasting solution to a weight problem, you need to cultivate physical skills. Start with the basics. There is no way, for example, that anyone can become proficient in most sports unless they can throw and catch a ball. (I was appalled when I discovered that over half the women in one of my weight management groups could not do this! How could I expect them to get interested in learning to play tennis and to develop the skill they would need to enjoy the game before they could do this normally simple activity?)

To get your child interested in moving, enter into the activity yourself. Play hide-and-seek, different versions of tag, and Frisbee golf and football; practice throwing basketballs through the hoop even if you will never play the game yourself; go on hikes; and learn the interesting sport of orienteering. Check with your local YMCA or other health facility about the kinds of physical activities they offer that families can do together. To find out more about such sports and games, take the time to visit your library or bookstore and look through the books on physical activity and games.

If your child is severely obese, weight reduction should be supervised by your pediatrician or by someone experienced in helping overweight children who either is recommended by your doctor or will work with your doctor. If indicated, check into local childhood or adolescent obesity treatment programs. Often area hospitals will offer programs specializing in pediatric obesity. A team of health professionals including a registered dietitian, physician, exercise physiologist, and/or psychologist can work with parents and children about sensible diet and exercise as well as behavior change. You can write the Center for Adolescent Obesity for a listing of centers across the country utilizing this team approach (send self-addressed, stamped envelope to Center for Adolescent Obesity, University of California, Box 0900 FCM, San Francisco, CA 94143).

CHAPTER 13

PHYSICAL ACTIVITY: STEPS TO PARNASSUS[1]

With all that's been said and written, you are a rare person indeed if you haven't already heard about the health benefits of physical activity. But you're not so rare if you haven't heeded all the advice to which you've been subjected and continue to lead a sedentary life. In fact, you're in the majority!

Just in case you're unaware of the latest findings on the effects of physical activity on one's physical, psychological, and emotional well-being, I will list them a little later in this chapter. They are impressive, so I will discuss what it takes to obtain them.

But, frankly, I don't blame you if you are becoming secretly annoyed with all the preaching and the lack of true help and understanding about developing an active life-style that you receive from many health professionals. As a former fat psychologist, hypertensive and with a heart condition, I know quite well that lecturing and

[1]Mount Parnassus, according to Greek legend, was sacred to Apollo, the god of music, poetry, prophecy, and medicine, and to the Muses. Apollo exemplified youth, health, and beauty. I have subtitled this chapter "Steps to Parnassus" in the hope that you will find added youth, health, and beauty in your own life through physical activity.

preaching don't do much good. The statistics bear me out: From 50 to 90 percent of people who begin an exercise program, including those who enroll in cardiac rehabilitation programs following a heart attack, will quit within the year.

Why?

Unfortunately, many of my professional colleagues are fond of analyzing the reasons in terms of "excuses." This approach leads you to feel as though being inactive is some kind of sin for which you ought to feel guilty and need absolution. What you really need, however, is an understanding of the forces, in yourself and in the environment, that lead you either to the couch or to the open road. To put it in a more general way, what motivates those of us who can't bear to go a day without finding time to walk or run around, compared with those who, given the choice, prefer to settle into a comfortable chair, nibbling on a tasty snack, sipping a drink, and watching TV? What incentives are there that make it worthwhile to be an active rather than a sedentary person?

I think I can speak both personally and professionally on these issues. I've been both places myself, and I have tried, with only partial success, to motivate thousands of overweight persons to develop an active life-style. So here's my analysis, and I sincerely hope it will be helpful to you. I know the difference in myself, from the days when it was an effort to walk a block and climb a flight of stairs to being able to run 5 or 10 miles over mountain trails with less effort than it used to take to go for that walk. I know the difference it has made in the lives of many of the participants in the Vanderbilt program who discovered "the secret."

SOME BASIC PRINCIPLES OF MOTIVATION

Except for those situations in which most of us would risk life and limb to protect those we love and the principles by which we live, we humans are like animals that operate between a carrot and a stick. I don't mean this in a demeaning way, however. Unlike the animals we usually picture between a carrot and a stick, we humans can control our own incentives and I will try to show you how.

When it comes to being active, there's no one out there with a stick to goad us on. We live in a culture where a level of physical activity that would be best for our health is simply not required of us. It wasn't always like this, of course. If we had lived in the middle of the last century, without cars and electricity in our homes, it would have taken about 7 or 8 miles of walking every day (or its energy equivalent in other work) just to get the job of living done. Put another way, we had to expend 400 to 500 more calories each day moving about—tending fields, gardens, and livestock, climbing stairs, washing clothes, chopping wood, carrying coal, and so on—to stay alive in the last century. If we could put that level of activity back in our lives, combined with present advances in preventive public health medicine, vaccines, antibiotics, and our far better food supply, we would add many healthy years to our lives.

So without sticks behind us, we must look ahead for carrots if we're going to get active and stay that way. How can you discover a payoff that will outweigh the cost of whatever you must change in your life if you are to get active?

THE PAYOFFS

PHYSIOLOGICAL BENEFITS

There are a tremendous number of physiological benefits to being an active person. Here's an up-to-date list that might contribute to your initial motivation. Compared with sedentary people, active people tend to have:

- Lower LDL cholesterol levels (that's the "bad" cholesterol)
- Higher HDL cholesterol levels (that's the "good" cholesterol)
- Lower triglyceride levels
- Enhanced insulin sensitivity
- Improved glucose tolerance
- Lower blood pressure
- Less illness and death from heart disease

And there is growing evidence that being active offers some protection against cancers of the colon and digestive tract in both men and women, and against breast and other cancers of the reproductive system in women.

When it comes to obesity, there is no question about it. Active people have much better success at managing their weight compared with sedentary people. Since obesity is associated with diabetes and gallbladder disease, and is another predisposing factor for the illnesses and other risk factors I've already listed, being active is a kind of double insurance policy for a healthier, longer life.

Active people also maintain muscular strength, better balance, stronger bones, and greater cardiovascular endurance as they grow older, compared with inactive people. In other words, active people are *biologically* younger, by as much as 20 or 30 years, when they reach the age of 60 or 70 compared with inactive people of that same chronological age.

Finally, active people, in laboratory experiments, tend to have less dangerous physiological reactions to mental stress compared with sedentary people, including less elevation and quicker recovery in blood pressure, heart rate, and epinephrine secretion.

Physical activity is so important to our physical well-being that many epidemiologists feel its lack is our greatest national health hazard. Fully 58 percent of all adults don't even get 1 hour's worth of physical activity *in an entire week.* Think of it: A majority of Americans are not up and about on their feet an average of 8½ minutes in an entire day. We move just enough to get us from one reclining or sitting position to another.

From a public health standpoint, lack of physical activity as a risk factor for heart disease is probably far ahead of any other risk factor because it affects so many people—that is, 58 percent. By comparison, only about 31 percent of the population are affected by high serum cholesterol, 25 percent smoke, 22 percent are obese, and 17 percent have high blood pressure. In other words, lack of physical activity is present in from two to three times more people than any other risk factor for heart disease. Experts estimate that about 30 to 40 percent of deaths from heart attacks—that's 200,000 a year—could be prevented if people exercised.

Later in this chapter I'll show you how to develop an activity program that will maximize the likelihood that you will achieve all the physical benefits I've been talking about. But as important as they are, I don't think your knowledge of them or any lecturing on the health statistics to which I've just subjected you will be enough to ensure that you become an active person. I think the key, for most people, is to be found in psychological, social, and emotional factors, not physical.

PSYCHOLOGICAL AND EMOTIONAL BENEFITS

There are basically two, possibly three, conditions under which physical activity becomes an established part of one's life.

The first, and most reliable, is when you find something that contributes to your self-concept and builds your self-esteem. If being active becomes an integral part of the way you think about the kind of person you are, then it will be with you for life. It really has very little to do with the possible physical health benefits. When people who are asked to describe themselves and their interests include statements like "I'm a runner" or "I'm a tennis player," they are implying that there is something about the skill, strength, or another aspect of the activity that is an essential part of the way they think about themselves. Without it, they would be different people, less satisfied with themselves.

The second condition is governed by the pleasure principle. If you find something that gives you tremendous physical pleasure and a feeling of well-being, you are likely to stick with it even though it contributes little to your self-esteem. If you discover that brisk walking, swimming, or some other similar activity provides an antidote to stress, anxiety, or depression, you may be able to sustain your motivation to be active in the face of other daily responsibilities.

The third condition has to do with your work or an important avocation. Many people find that taking time to be alone, walking or gently jogging, is their most creative time. Philosophers, scientists, and writers are frequently walkers, alternately enjoying their changing surroundings and letting their minds ruminate about their work. More and more business people are discovering that taking time to be alone, but being physically active during that time, helps them to be more creative and better problem solvers. They also find that an early-morning walk is a good time for planning and makes them more alert and effective at the start of the workday.

Let's deal now in detail with what it takes to make sure you experience the physiological, psychological, and emotional benefits of physical activity I've been talking about.

THE PHYSIOLOGICAL BENEFITS OF A LIFETIME FITNESS PROGRAM

Physical activity can have several measurable physiological benefits that become evident within a matter of weeks. However, it takes slightly different kinds and amounts of activity to help make sure you obtain all of them, including an increase in cardiovascular endurance, an elevation in HDL level, and a significant impact on your weight. The less tangible benefits, such as protection against heart disease and cancer and the potential for a longer life, may have yet other requirements.

But it need not be confusing. I'll go over the essentials for each aspect of health and fitness, *and then put it all together in a single, simple program.*

CARDIOVASCULAR ENDURANCE

For an increase in cardiovascular endurance, you need to exercise in your "target heart range," sometimes called the "training range," three or four times a week for 20 to 30 minutes each time. The training range is between 60 and 85 percent of your maximum heart rate. Your maximum heart rate is approximately 220 minus your age. Table 13–1 will make it easy for you to determine your appropriate level.

When you first begin an exercise program it's good to begin slowly and stay at the lower end of your range. For significant improvement, you will need to work toward the higher end. If you're over 35, overweight, or have any medical condition and plan to do anything more than walking at the lower end of your training range, you should check with your physician before starting. Naturally, if

TABLE 13–1. MAXIMUM HEART RATES AND TRAINING RANGES

Age	Maximum Heart Rate (beats per minute)	60% Level (beats per minute)	85% Level (beats per minute)
20	200	120	170
25	195	117	166
30	190	114	162
35	185	111	157
40	180	108	153
45	175	105	149
50	170	102	145
55	165	99	140
60	160	96	136
65	155	93	132
70	150	90	128

any symptoms such as shortness of breath, nausea or dizziness, or chest pains develop during walking even at low levels of intensity, you should check with your doctor. The same is true for other muscular aches and pains that don't lessen in 24 to 48 hours.

Cardiovascular endurance is measured best by an exercise stress test, which can be arranged by your physician or performed at most YMCAs. This test can determine your actual maximum heart rate and training rate, which do vary quite a bit from person to person. But you can get a pretty good idea of your improvement in several ways. First, you will note that your increase in heart rate during any given physical activity decreases over time. If you are overweight and out of shape, and walk at a pace of a mile in 20 minutes, it might go up to 138 beats a minute when you start a walking program. Within 8 to 12 weeks and after losing a few pounds you may find that at the same pace it is beating only 114 times a minute. Some very fit persons show hardly any elevation at all, compared to their resting rate, when they walk at this pace. An improvement of this kind means that you are capable of more physical exertion without feeling strain or fatigue, and that your energy level is likely to be higher.

Most people show at least a small decline in resting heart rate as they get fit, but not all people do. So don't be alarmed if you note no decrease at rest. The important thing is how hard your heart must work to maintain your body during physical exertion. The less the better!

The most convenient way to take your pulse is to place the first three fingers of one hand lightly on the other arm along the radial artery, which runs along the inside edge of the arm leading to your thumb. Count the beats for 10 seconds and multiply by 6.

As fitness increases, you will find it easier to get out of a chair, to climb stairs, and to do other things such as carry packages. Upper-body strength will, however, depend on whether you do anything to increase *muscular* strength and endurance. I'll talk about that in a moment. But as a result of increased cardiovascular endurance and the loss of some weight if needed, you will, quite spontaneously and without conscious awareness, probably find yourself moving about more.

RAISING OR MAINTAINING HDL LEVEL

While active people have higher HDL levels than inactive people, what it takes for any individual to raise his or her HDL level is unclear. Not all individuals can obtain an increase in HDL level with exercise. However, a majority of people appear to be able to maintain all or almost all of the HDL component while they are reducing total cholesterol and the dangerous LDL component (via diet, weight loss, and possibly drugs) by adding exercise to the treatment. Should there be a slight decline in HDL, exercise almost always assures that the LDL component drops far more dramatically than the HDL component, leading to a lower and healthier ratio of total cholesterol to HDL cholesterol.

For example, if your total cholesterol is 250 mg/dl and your HDL is 40 mg/dl, the total/HDL ratio is 6.25, which is rather high. If your total level is reduced to 200 mg/dl, but you maintain the 40 mg/dl HDL, the ratio, while not ideal, is a healthier 5.0. (See also Chapter 2.)

Some experts feel that walking 30 to 45 minutes at 3 to 4 miles per hour six or seven times a week is sufficient. While men are likely to see a greater effect than women, one recent study in England showed a significant elevation in HDL in previously sedentary women who followed a vigorous walking program for one year. However, another recent study showed that the exercise does need to be quite vigorous: Only participants who exercised at 75 percent of maximum heart rate obtained any significant elevation in HDL. Exercising at a lower intensity was not effective, although it did result in an increase in cardiovascular endurance.

WEIGHT MANAGEMENT

Weight management requires that you come as close as possible to the level of activity that was required of us in the last century (and it needs to be combined with eating a low-fat diet). We are talking about at least 45 minutes a day, six or seven times a week. In fact, making up for the missing 400 to 500 calories of *daily* energy expenditure in our present lives takes the equivalent of an hour's walk at a 4-mile-an-hour pace, or 40 to 50 minutes of jogging at a gentle pace, or an hour of vigorous singles tennis every day. But don't fret, yet! I think I can show you how to make this a joy, not a burden.

Certain forms of physical activity are more effective for weight management than others. The key is to maximize the burning of fat rather than carbohydrate in the fuel that powers the activity.

Moderate, low-intensity activity burns more fat in the fuel mixture than does high-intensity activity. For example, at the extremes, a

100-yard dash burns stored carbohydrate (glucose) almost entirely, while walking at a comfortable pace can burn about 60 percent or more in fat. The longer you go, the more fat you burn. Over time, the body switches fuel tanks, starting out with carbohydrate primarily and then gradually switching to stored fat.

In addition, the fitter you get the more fat you burn at any level of activity. That is, as you see your heart rate decreasing during exercise (or quite simply, as the exercise begins to feel easier to you), you can be confident that you are burning relatively more fat than carbohydrate. By eating a low-fat diet, you can be sure that the fat is withdrawn from your fat cells. So you see, there are some built-in assurances for weight management that are self-sustaining as you start to become active, get fit, and then maintain your low-fat diet and activity program.

THE MATTER OF LONGEVITY AND THE OTHER HEALTH BENEFITS

Walking about 30 to 45 minutes at 3 to 4 miles per hour six or seven times a week (or its energy equivalent) can result in many benefits in addition to the ones I've discussed above. These include lower triglyceride levels, better insulin and glucose control, and a reduction in blood pressure. With respect to disease and longevity, one large study over a period of eight years showed that this level of activity is associated with a reduction in the cardiovascular death rate of 70 percent, and *from all causes* of death of about 50 percent. Another study indicated that when energy expenditure hit about 2,000 calories a week there was a significant increase in longevity. Just about everything that kept people on their feet and moving about was of value, including walking, stair climbing, gardening, and so on.

How can we put these different pieces of information together into a single set of recommendations for a health-enhancing activity program that also takes your personal needs and preferences into consideration? Can the same recommendations meet our psychological, emotional, and social needs?

THE ONE MEAL AT A TIME
ACTIVITY PROGRAM

Let's start with the basic facts, put as simply as possible:
We need to find some way to move around, mostly moderately but sometimes

briskly, for at least a half-hour and up to 1 hour, six or seven times a week.
(Yes, there's a day off if you're tired!)

It really doesn't matter a great deal what you do from the physiological standpoint, *as long as it happens almost every day, is mostly moderate, but is occasionally brisk.*

The usual kinds of aerobic (or continuous steady-state) exercises that you have read about are equally good—walking, swimming, bicycling, cross-country skiing, aerobic dancing, and gentle jogging (but only if you are at or near normal weight and in good condition). So are the anaerobic, start/stop exercises such as singles tennis, volleyball, badminton, and so on—*but only if you get good enough to play quite vigorously and are in motion most of the time.* Unless you play these games with a skill equal to local tournament caliber, you are not likely to move around enough.

But you are not limited to these usually recommended activities. Gardening, raking leaves, house painting, mopping your own floor—all qualify! If you sit for a living, just getting out of your chair for five minutes on the hour and moving around the hallways or corridors of your home or office building, perhaps going up and down a flight of stairs, will add up to 40 minutes of health-giving activity every day. It can do wonders.

For example, one of my colleagues told me about a patient in his weight-loss program who worked in a ten-story hospital. Whenever he needed to go from one spot in his building to another, which he had to do several times a day, he made it a point to climb first to the top of the building and then descend to the floor where he needed to go. He engaged in no other extra physical activity outside of his stair climbing, but he became the most active person, in terms of energy expended per week, in the entire weight-loss program. He lost a great deal of weight and increased his cardiovascular endurance significantly.

THE FIRST RULE OF PHYSICAL ACTIVITY

Whatever you decide to do, the first rule is: *Never hurt yourself.* This means starting slowly. Using walking as an example, build up to 30, 45, and perhaps 60 minutes a day by starting first with 15 minutes at a time. Hold to 15 minutes per session for a full week and stay at the lower range of intensity. Next week gradually increase to 30 minutes. Then to 45. Go longer before you go faster! Then go faster in short spurts and see how it feels. The more you make a game of it, the better you will like it.

If you have never been active before, I strongly suggest you join a facility such as the YMCA. Although there are many good private, for-profit health clubs, it is hard to know their quality until you have committed yourself. So I recommend the YMCAs above all others because they employ professionals who have met certain educational and training requirements. They also are less motivated by the need to generate a profit. An exercise test at the Y will establish the guidelines for a personalized fitness program, and retesting will demonstrate your progress. You will find an assortment of supervised activities and, most likely, good companionship. Once you've started, made some advances in fitness, and found what you like to do, you will be in a better position to decide whether to stick with an exercise facility or go off on your own.

Which brings me finally to the psychological and social aspects that may be crucial to the success of any exercise program.

THE PSYCHOLOGICAL AND SOCIAL BENEFITS OF A LIFETIME FITNESS PROGRAM

When people are asked what interferes with their efforts to become active, the list usually includes lack of time, inconvenience or other barriers implying too much effort, responsibilities to family and others to which they must give a higher priority, and physical limitations (an existing illness such as arthritis).

While we need to deal with these immediate obstacles, I don't think these reasons get at the root of the problem. Going back to my basic analysis of motivation, we do the things we must do to stay alive from day to day, and with any time left over we do the things we like to do—the things that feel good. We need to recognize that physical activity may not feel good until you get fit. Some people may never reach the stage where they feel good moving vigorously. If that's the case, there has to be a payoff that's worth the effort.

If I can find a way to help you make being fit, perhaps skilled in some sport, central to your self-concept and self-esteem, we'll have the problem solved. Your entire perspective in life will change.

Being active will go down first on your daily calendar, and you will find plenty of time during the rest of the day for your work and other responsibilities, I assure you. Contributions to your self-concept and self-esteem can happen in several ways, and it's more likely to happen with certain activities than with others.

SOCIAL SPORTS THAT REQUIRE SKILL

If you decide to pursue some activity that requires skill, you need to put the time, effort, and perhaps money into it to make sure you get good enough to enjoy that activity. This is especially true of activities like tennis. Without skill you cannot enjoy the game. Being skilled has to have some meaning for you, as an expression of one of your talents. Some aspect of the game must offer you a challenge you feel you can meet.

You will need to find a group of people who enjoy the same activity, and who will become your companions, partners, or opponents. Besides enjoying your companions, you must find a level of competition where you win some, lose some, but come out in general about 50-50. Except for the professionals, where it can be worth millions in addition to championships, winning all the time can become boring, and losing all the time is depressing.

To become good enough to enjoy tennis or any other racquet sport, you must play several times a week, in addition to your coaching sessions. Since individual tennis lessons are becoming so expensive, many coaches arrange for group lessons with two or three students at a time. Drills and doubles for an hour with a coach will give you a good workout. Group lessons also provide a good way to meet other players at your level and will help you build a circle of friends who like the game as well as you do. Many tennis clubs employ professional coaches who give lessons to non-members as well as members. The clubs may offer other exercise classes and complete workout facilities which you can use if you decide to join.

I think you will be much more likely to stick with a social sport, provided you develop the skill and circle of friends that are required to make it rewarding, than if you choose another kind of physical activity that does not offer enough of a challenge or opportunity for personal fulfillment. There are many challenging and fulfilling aspects to racquet sports, including psychological, physical, and social, that are not found in other activities. While aerobic dancing, for example, can be great fun at first, people drop in and out of dancing classes because they don't offer the many aspects for self-expression that you can get from a sport that's both friendly and competitive, and which offers continual room for improvement. Other sports, such as volleyball and softball, require many people, and there is a greater likelihood of injury in the former and considerably less moving about in the latter.

THE SOLO ACTIVITIES: WALKING, SWIMMING, BICYCLING, JOGGING

You get to know others through social activities. You get to know yourself in solo activities. You also get to appreciate yourself and your time alone, but it may not happen overnight.

If you prefer to do any of the activities that can be done alone in the company of other people, you have to be sure they are as committed as you are, and will not miss appointments. In my experience, people who depend on others as companions for walking, jogging, etc., are likely to skip their activity when their companions disappoint them. That's why I think you should try to cultivate these activities as solo rather than as social occasions.

Many people who are not committed walkers or joggers remark that the activity seems too boring to them. My response is that only boring people are bored by such activities. Just give yourself a chance. In time, with a little discipline, you will discover that you are a very interesting person indeed, and have the very best conversations of all with yourself. Trust me. Here's how to find out. I'll use walking as my example, although the same principles apply to other solo activities.

First of all, you have to go for that walk almost every day and work up to at least 45 minutes at a time. As I mentioned previously, you have to move briskly a few times each week so that walking begins to feel easy to you. It also takes about 20 to 30 minutes to get really relaxed and into the mental swing of things, so you need another 15 to 25 minutes to fully enjoy it.

I don't know what to predict as the special benefits on the psychological and emotional levels for any particular individual who discovers the joys of walking. You have to do it to find out because, after a while, walking becomes addictive and as necessary to you as brushing your teeth. You will not be able to begin or finish the day without it.

For me, one of the great benefits of walking or jogging (I do both) is that no one knows where I am! I can meditate in motion, plan various activities, prepare or rehearse lectures, or outline whatever articles or book I'm writing. In your own case, you may find that walking or jogging can reduce the tension you experience in your other daily activities. It may, in one way or another, become associated with interesting changes in your life and the development of interests and talents you didn't know you had. It was so in my own case.

I took up jogging after a tennis injury made it difficult for me to play at my accustomed level and I needed to take some time off. I was 50 years old at the time. As I was jogging in the park near my home one day I began mentally to outline some short magazine articles on diet and exercise. Within two years I had published my first book. I'm now 62 years old and this is my seventh book. I'm still walking and jogging, even though I'm back to playing tennis. Some days it's really hard to make a choice!

OVERCOMING IMMEDIATE OBSTACLES

Finding time, dealing with possible inconvenience, and balancing your need to be active with other responsibilities may take ingenuity and negotiation. Sometimes you may need to manage all of these obstacles simultaneously.

Believe me, everybody can find 45 minutes to do exactly what they want to do every day except in the most extreme, life-or-death circumstances. Your first job, then, is to make a commitment to using these 45 minutes for physical activity—not for TV, the newspaper, shooting the bull, or any other sedentary activity that is not essential to your life.

To help people in the Vanderbilt program develop an active life, I have them keep a daily log, writing down everything they do every day, by the half-hour, for at least a week. It's a wonderful first step toward good management of time for work as well as recreation. Do it yourself. You will discover where the gaps are in your days. Should you find no gaps, you will discover which activities, now felt as personal responsibilities, are actually negotiable. Let me give you an illustration.

One schoolteacher with three small children was certain there was no time in her day for physical activity. She was up at 5:30 A.M. to get herself and her children ready for school, including brown-bag lunches, and then after school she had classes to prepare, children to ferry around, meals to prepare, and a home to care for. She felt that her husband was doing his share and that there was no room for any special help on his part until we discussed what he did in the morning as she was getting herself and her children ready for school. Well, nothing, except fend for himself.

I suggested she ask her husband to get the kids ready for school while she went for an early-morning walk. She couldn't believe I'd make such a suggestion. He couldn't possibly do it—it would be chaos. And indeed it was for about three days. Within two weeks, however, her children and her husband were getting to know each other better than they ever had before and were enjoying themselves immensely. At first, she found it difficult to accept that her children came to prefer that Dad, rather than Mom, get them off to school. But she had found the time to be active.

If you can't go outside your front door to take a walk, and must travel to a park or exercise facility, it is certainly less convenient. If your working schedule and other responsibilities require tight scheduling, you may have to carry your exercise clothes and other equipment with you. You may have to negotiate with family and friends for a block of time either on the way to work or on the way home. Look over your schedules jointly and see if you can't collaborate on finding an equal block of time for each person for their preferred activity. You make it possible for them to do what they want, and they make it possible for you to do what you want—in this case, be active. You may be amazed at how well this approach works. I have never seen it fail in families that love and care for each other's welfare.

If you must travel to a place for exercise and can't stand to "do nothing" for 15 or 30 minutes while you travel, you can play educational tapes in your car or on a portable cassette player. You can also do this, or play music, while walking or jogging, but I find this distracting and not nearly as valuable as having the time to think without distraction.

As for riding indoor cycles, rowing, or using a ski machine, I agree with most people: They're truly distasteful! But I found a way to make 30 minutes on a stationary cycle work for me following a knee injury during a tennis match that kept me from playing tennis or running for a few weeks. (The injury was the price I payed for trying to get ready for a tournament by playing for three hours in two tough singles matches in one day. You don't need to do this, and I think I've learned my lesson, too!) I saved up and made all my telephone calls while riding the bike, which my doctor had recommended as part of the rehabilitation for my knee. You may find that watching TV or getting a special bookstand for reading can make stationary peddling an acceptable activity. I've seen advertisements for special bookstands for stationary bikes, but a music stand placed near the handlebars works too.

THE COMPLETE FITNESS PROGRAM

I have focused on the aerobic components of an activity program since they are most closely associated with the prevention of heart disease, high blood pressure, obesity, and obesity-related illnesses such as diabetes and gallstones. A complete fitness program also includes strength training and flexibility exercises.

If you buy a set of free weights (dumbbells) at a sporting goods store you will find a set of instructions for their use. I suggest 3-pound weights for women, and 5- or 6-pound weights for men, as starters. Just a few minutes a week will tone your upper body and you will find it easier to carry packages, move furniture, and accomplish other tasks that take a bit of strength. You also will be less likely to hurt yourself doing these jobs.

You can maintain flexibility (and prevent injury while performing other activities) by doing a few stretches every morning, and repeating them just before any other activity that requires muscular exertion. Swing your upper body from side to side, rotating at the hips, to loosen up the lower-back area. Stretch the muscles at the front and back of your legs before brisk walking, jogging, or playing at racquet sports. You can do this by placing one leg at a time on a chair or table and leaning forward slowly and gently, aiming for your toes with your fingertips, but only going as far as feels comfortable. Then stand with your feet at shoulder width about three feet from a wall and lean forward. Do a few slow forward bends with knees slightly flexed. I highly recommend Richard Hittleman's *Yoga: 28 Day Exercise Plan,* published by Bantam, as a do-it-yourself introduction to a stretching program that will keep you supple and prevent injury.

As long as your major activity is no more vigorous than walking, you can skip the preliminary stretches and still prevent injury by starting slowly—no faster than a 3-mile-per-hour pace—for the first five minutes. Go more slowly if you are overweight. Then after you are loosened and warmed up, you can pick up the pace and go as briskly as you can without hurting yourself. If you work out within your training range, be sure to finish your walk by slowing down for the last five minutes, or until your heart rate drops below 100 beats per minute. This will prevent dizziness, which can result from temporary pooling of your blood supply in your legs after vigorous activity. It also will help prevent muscle cramps. Stiffness and cramping can also be arrested by stretching after vigorous exercise.

You will find some other recommendations for reading material in the fitness area in Appendix A. However, no book can guide you as well as a professional, in person. Once again, if you have no background in the fitness area, I suggest you join a YMCA when you begin an exercise program, or find some other reputable health club.

A WORD ON EQUIPMENT

The right equipment can help you avoid discomfort and injury, and make physical activity more enjoyable. Proper shoes are probably your most important piece of equipment. You also need proper clothes for all seasons. In fact, change of season is often given as the reason people stop being active. Until you have gone through all the seasons and solved whatever problems they bring, physical activity will not be reliably established as a permanent part of your life. Wear several light layers of clothing, rather than fewer heavy ones, in cold weather. They will insulate you better, and you can peel off layers as you warm up, if necessary. The most common clothing error early in a beginning fitness program is overdressing.

If you decide to pursue a racquet sport, your coach will be your best guide to equipment until you are accomplished and have a feel for what works for you. Some sporting goods stores have demonstration racquets that you can borrow before purchasing the model you come to prefer.

When it comes to walking shoes and other equipment, find a store that will let you try things out first by allowing you to go for a walk around the block, ride different bicycles in the parking lot, and so on. Stores that sell both jogging and walking shoes and cater to athletes usually permit some kind of "test run," if not outdoors in good weather then in your own home, around the house, for a day or two.

A FINAL THOUGHT

Next to throwing away your cigarettes if you are a smoker, following the One Meal at a Time low-fat diet is the most important thing you, as an individual, can do for your health. Next to being the very best you can be at the work you love, getting physically fit is probably the most important thing you can do to build self-confidence and self-esteem. Unless you discover this for yourself, I doubt the potential health benefits will keep you permanently motivated.

You must start your activity program with the intention of working at it all year round. You must approach your program as though it were a course in the development of your hidden potential and an important aspect of your character. Commit yourself for a year, and then do it. The value of physical activity is another of those things that you can only know by doing.

CHAPTER 14

EPILOGUE

You do not have direct control over your blood pressure, cholesterol level, insulin level, or even your weight, for that matter. All you can control directly is your behavior. I've been concerned with two of the most important behaviors that can have an effect on the physiological factors that determine whether you can expect to live a happier, healthier, longer life. The first behavior is what you choose to eat; the second is your level of physical activity.

I'd like to leave you with three thoughts—they are really directives—that can guarantee you will reach your objective. In my mind, they are the three most important points I've tried to make in this book. The first has to do with making sure you are successful in switching to a low-fat diet; the second has to do with making sure you develop an active life; and the third has to do with the winning attitude.

First, people who are successful in implementing a low-fat diet control their eating environment. They take my advice to customize their home eating environments so that only good, healthful foods are normally available. They put the idea of "everyday" foods into practice, and make sure that they always have on hand a large variety that will satisfy everyone in the family. They bring "occasional" foods in for treats in amounts that are calculated to fit into their overall low-fat eating plan. But they never let "occasional" foods become "everyday" foods.

Second, if nothing about the demands of everyday living requires that they move about at a healthful level of physical activity, successful people understand that they must take charge of their daily schedules and give physical activity *top* priority. I'm very serious about this. If staying alive on a day-to-day basis does not require you to move around at a healthful level of activity, then you must make the demand of yourself—that is, if you want the added assurance an active life can give you of a healthier, longer life.

Physical activity must go down first on your daily calendar. No one else can put it there but you. And believe me, unless it goes down first and has top priority in your own value scheme, it's not going to happen. Then, once started, you must keep at it, because the effects take time to make themselves known. If you choose a solo activity such as walking or jogging, and do it alone even if it can be done with other people, within a year you will get to know and like yourself better than ever before. If you choose a social activity, you will find, as I have in the sport of tennis, friendships that can grow and last a lifetime.

Third and finally, do the very best you can in following my advice on the first two points, but don't demand perfection of yourself. If you do, you are almost certain to fall short; and if you tend to berate yourself for failure, you may give up altogether to avoid the unpleasantness.

To put this thought in a more general context, the people I know who are both happiest and most successful in everything they do keep on developing their knowledge and skills in their work, and keep on learning and doing new things in other areas of their lives. But they don't try to be perfect and they are not overly competitive; they don't try to outdo everyone they interact with in every aspect of their lives.

I think you should apply this advice to the changes you are about to make, or have already started to make, in your diet and your level of physical activity. If you miss the goal you set for yourself today, get right back on track tomorrow. With this attitude, you *will* get better and better. But, as I said, don't demand perfection. Besides, I hope I've made it clear that perfection isn't necessary.

I sincerely hope the things I've said in this book will be helpful to you and that you will experience the happiness that goes with a healthier, longer life.

APPENDIX A

SCIENTIFIC
ADDENDUM[1]

The major research prior to 1989 that forms the scientific foundation for the One Meal at a Time program is reviewed in great depth in the National Research Council (NRC) report *Diet and Health.* I have relied on Helen A. Guthrie's text, *Introductory Nutrition,* for basic information in the nutrition area, and I can highly recommend this readable text for basic background in lipid metabolism and a discussion of *trans* fatty acids. The NRC's *Recommended Dietary Allowances* (1989) was consulted for the latest recommendations on vitamin and mineral requirements and for recent research on the various nutrients.

My main purposes in writing this addendum are to add a note on certain relationships between total fat and saturated fat, to present a few of the points I mentioned in Chapter 2 in greater detail, and to touch on some of the key studies published since the 1989 NRC report *Diet and Health.*

---

[1]Articles noted in this addendum are listed in the References that follow. Additional related scientific articles appear in the Bibliography. The Recommended Readings section includes practical guides in the nutrition and fitness areas.

SOME ADDITIONAL INFORMATION
RELATING TO TOTAL FAT AND
SATURATED FAT

There are three important relationships between total fat, saturated fat, and the fatty acid composition of different fats and oils that I would like to clarify.

1. I have suggested that a person aim for 25 percent of total calories as fat, with less than 10 percent of total calories from saturated fat.
2. Fats and oils are a combination of saturated, monounsaturated, and polyunsaturated fats. I illustrated this with two graphs in Chapter 2. Roughly speaking, on the average:

   • About 60 percent of the *total fat* content of butterfat is saturated.
   • About 40 percent of the *total fat* content in beef is saturated.
   • About 35 percent of the *total fat* content in pork is saturated.
   • About 30 percent of the *total fat* content in chicken is saturated.
   • Between 20 and 25 percent of the *total fat* content in fish is saturated.

   Generally, the fish that contain somewhat more fat (such as salmon) have a lower proportion of the total as saturated. And compared with meat, even fatty fish contain no more total fat than the leaner cuts.
3. Research shows that heart disease is very rare in populations that consume less than 10 percent of *total calories in saturated fat.* On the facing page are the approximate figures for percentage of total calories as saturated fat in certain dairy products, the fatty and lean cuts of beef and pork, poultry with and without skin, and fish.

   You can see from this list that lean pork, poultry without skin, and fish all have only 10 percent or less of total calories as saturated fat. Among the lean meats, only lean beef is as high as 15 percent of total calories as saturated fat. Low-fat frozen yogurt (and regular low-fat yogurt) has only 10 percent of total calories as saturated fat, and low-fat milk has 15 percent (skim milk has only a trace of fat).

   In the context of an entire day's meals and snacks, which include fruit, vegetables, and grains, it is quite easy to fall at or below 10 percent of calories in saturated fat. This was my goal in providing you with the One Meal at a Time guidelines and meal plans. If you do not exceed 25 percent of total calories as fat (of

Food	Percentage of Total Calories as Saturated Fat
Butter	60%
Milk	
Whole	30%
Low-fat (1%)	15%
Frozen Dairy Products	
Premium ice cream	40%
Regular ice cream	30%
Low-fat frozen yogurt	10%
Beef	
Fatty cuts	30%
Lean cuts	15%
Pork	
Fatty cuts	25%
Lean cuts	10%
Poultry	
With skin	15%
Without skin	Less than 10%
Fish	
Fattier varieties	Less than 10%
Leaner varieties	Less than 5%

any kind) and make low-fat choices in the dairy and meat groups of foods, you are likely to end up with about 5 to 7 percent of total calories in saturated fat (as is the case with the follow-up on participants from the Vanderbilt program, which I reported in Chapter 4).

RECENT RESEARCH ON THE RELATIONSHIP OF OTHER COMPONENTS OF SERUM CHOLESTEROL THAT MAY AFFECT CARDIOVASCULAR DISEASE

At the present time, total serum cholesterol, the low-density lipoprotein (LDL) component, the high-density lipoprotein (HDL) component, and the ratio of total cholesterol to HDL have the greatest clinical significance in the prediction and treatment of atherosclerotic cardiovascular disease. However, recent research suggests that there may be some subtle characteristics of the lipoprotein molecules that are more important than the amount of LDL or HDL in your

total cholesterol level. Because of the new findings, there are a growing number of experts who believe that there are two major factors,
acting in association with your cholesterol, that determine whether
you are likely to develop atherosclerosis. I'd like to discuss these
factors in case they assume increasing importance in the future.

The first factor has to do with the *receptors* on your body cells,
through which the cholesterol enters and performs its useful work
making the membranes of your body cells, the bile acids, and the
hormones. The second has to do with certain characteristics of the
protein part of the circulating lipoproteins themselves. Some of the
proteins act like *keys,* locking onto the receptors and facilitating the
entrance of cholesterol into the cells.

The protein that acts like a key and facilitates the entrance of
cholesterol carried by LDL into cells throughout the body is called
apolipoprotein B. This label is frequently shortened to *apo B.* Up to
and through this point, cholesterol and apo B in LDL are doing
good, necessary work. However, if the production of cholesterol
and apo B by your liver exceeds the ability of the receptors on your
body cells to extract the cholesterol in LDL, and the cholesterol
cannot be picked up fast enough by the liver and removed from the
bloodstream, it circulates at high levels. *Apparently apo B has an af-
finity for the walls of your arteries, and it may be this protein that carries a
major responsibility for the plaque buildup in atherosclerosis.*

Other apolipoproteins, apo E and apo A, appear to be associated
with the removal of excess cholesterol by the liver. Apo A is part of
the HDL molecule, and may help carry cholesterol back to the liver.
It's now commonly believed that apo A has the ability to pick up and
remove some cholesterol from the plaque that forms on arterial
walls.

Apo E is associated with a form of lipoprotein called *very low-density
lipoprotein* (VLDL). VLDL molecules are large and contain a large
amount of triglycerides, as well as cholesterol and protein. VLDL is
produced in the liver and brings triglycerides to be used as energy to
your body cells. As soon as the triglycerides are removed from the
VLDL, apo E goes to work on the remnants, removing many of them
and their cholesterol from the bloodstream. However, other remnants of VLDL are converted to LDL, from which the cholesterol is
extracted by tissue and glands. Apo E appears to have an important
regulatory function: By removing VLDL remnants and their cholesterol from the bloodstream, LDL production can be reduced and

kept within healthier bounds. Cooper (1988) provides an excellent, considerably expanded introductory discussion of the processes I have outlined in these paragraphs; Ginsberg (1990) provides a summary of lipoprotein physiology, apolipoprotein functions, and their relationship to atherosclerosis.

Scientists have identified many different varieties of apolipoproteins associated with each form of lipoprotein that circulates in the bloodstream, and research is growing by leaps and bounds in this area. Studies have shown atherogenic properties to different varieties of LDL and to VLDL (Stein and Stein, 1990) and that circulating immune complexes containing cholesterol and apo B (that is, lipoproteins that have become attached to certain immune system cells) induce the accumulation of lipid in arterial tissue (Tertov et al., 1990).

Recently, a number of studies have suggested that a particular form of low-density lipoprotein, called lipoprotein (a) or "Lp(a)" because it carries an additional protein labeled "apo (a)" attached to apo B, is a particularly dangerous variety. Production in the human body takes place in the liver and is genetically determined. Individuals can vary by 1,000-fold in the amount found in the bloodstream.

Lp(a) is an antigen—that is, it acts like a toxin in the human body and is attacked by the immune system. The resulting particles are strongly attracted to any streaks on the walls of the coronary arteries. In addition, the particles increase the coagulability of the blood at those sites by interfering with the production of a substance, plasminogen, that keeps the blood fluid. Thus this lipoprotein is a double threat: It leads to both narrowing of the arteries and increased likelihood of clotting (Albers et al., 1989; Davidoff et al., 1989; Hegele, 1989; Mezdour et al., 1990; Sandkamp et al., 1990; Stein and Stein, 1990; Tertov et al., 1990; Utermann, 1989; Wong et al., 1990). At this point there is no simple dietetic or medicinal treatment that can lower substantially serum Lp(a), although Wong et al. (1990) have developed a test that can be used in mass screenings to measure its level.

Lp(a) and LDL cholesterol are under different metabolic control. That is, they fluctuate independently. This may help explain why some individuals, with normal LDL levels but high Lp(a) levels, develop atherosclerosis and end up with heart disease.

Although there are many different physiological factors that can predispose a person to hyperlipidemia and atherosclerosis, except

for severe genetic abnormalities (for example, familial hypercholes-
terolemia) *the development of hyperlipidemia, atherosclerosis, and ultimately coronary heart disease is a complex interaction of genetic and dietary
factors* (Nestel, 1989). The genetic predispositions can vary from
mild to extreme and from few to many, but fortunately, as Nestel
also points out in reviewing current strategies for atherosclerosis and
lowering cholesterol, there are dietary actions that can be placed in
opposition to each.[2]

RECENT RESEARCH ON DIETARY FACTORS PREDISPOSING TO ATHEROSCLEROSIS AND HEART DISEASE

Research strengthening the relationship between dietary factors and
heart disease has continued to accumulate in the two years since the
publication in 1989 of the NRC report *Diet and Health*. I will note
here just a few of the most interesting studies and comprehensive
reviews. Others appear in the bibliography.

In a review of the literature, Stone (1990) concludes:

1. Saturated fat plays a key role in the determination of serum cholesterol and coronary heart disease.
2. There appears to be a link between dietary cholesterol and the
   prediction of heart disease *that is independent of serum cholesterol.*
3. Chief factors in the diet that raise cholesterol and LDL are dietary
   cholesterol, saturated fat, and excess calories leading to obesity.
4. The level of circulating lipids after meals may prove to be another
   risk factor.

In one of the clearest studies implicating a high-cholesterol diet in
heart disease, *independent of its impact on serum cholesterol,* Shekelle and
Stamler (1989) followed a group of men for 25 years and showed
that after adjusting for the effects of age, intake of other lipids, and
serum cholesterol, those eating a high-cholesterol diet were about
50 percent more likely to die of heart disease than those eating a

[2]Of course, other life-style variables such as smoking and lack of exercise also play a
significant role and often compound the damage done by poor diet. However, my
focus in this appendix is on diet primarily.

low-cholesterol diet. They conclude that lowering the intake of dietary cholesterol is advisable in everyone, regardless of serum cholesterol level.

As to one possible mechanism whereby cholesterol can have its impact, Schwenke and Carew (1989) demonstrated in a study with rabbits that were not genetically prone to heart disease that a high-cholesterol diet led to increased incorporation of LDL in certain areas of arterial walls that are susceptible to lesions. They concluded that increased concentration of LDL in the arterial wall may be a first step in the development of the fatty streaks that become the focal points for increased lipid deposition and atherosclerosis. This suggests that a high-cholesterol diet may be a factor in causing the damage to the walls of your arteries that leads to the accumulation of lipid deposits. These deposits in turn lead to a narrowing of the opening in the arteries, which cuts the flow of blood and ultimately results in heart disease. Blankenhorn and Kramsch (1989) also note that a high-cholesterol diet induces scarring of the artery walls in primates, *and that the damage is reversible when the diets are withdrawn.*

Fatty acids, in addition to cholesterol, may have an impact on the cellular membranes in the arterial walls that predisposes arterial tissue to the atherosclerotic process. Stam et al. (1989) point out that the fatty acid composition of our diets is, in fact, reflected in cellular membranes to such an extent that from the membranes themselves you can determine the kind of fat a person eats. It may be that a high saturated-fat diet creates a tissue that is particularly susceptible to those lipid particles that cause scarring and plaque deposition.

Too much total fat, too much saturated fat, and too much dietary cholesterol are implicated in a number of other ways in heart disease.

Blankenhorn et al. (1990) demonstrated, in participants in the Cholesterol Lowering Atherosclerosis Study, that an increased risk of new lesions in coronary arteries was associated with total fat (including polyunsaturated fat). Subjects in whom new lesions did not develop reduced total fat and saturated fat, and replaced lost fat calories with calories from carbohydrate and protein. *They did not increase their intake of polyunsaturated fat.* The authors conclude that when total fat and saturated fat are reduced, protein and carbohydrate are preferred sources of energy, rather than monounsaturated or polyunsaturated fat.

Both total fat and saturated fat have an impact on risk factors for heart disease that is independent of their effect on serum cholesterol. One of the important independent risk factors is the ease with which blood can clot within your arteries.

Miller et al. (1989) compared the fat intake from 170 men over five days and found that total fat was significantly correlated with coagulant activity (Factor VIIc), which is a strong predictor of coronary heart disease. The difference between those men with the highest fat intake and those with the lowest was similar to the difference found in men with and without heart disease. They concluded that a high-fat diet has consequences for both blood coagulability and coronary thrombosis.

Marckmann et al. (1990) actually manipulated the fat content in the diets of 11 healthy adults and found that a low-fat diet, even if the proportion of saturated fat was still rather high, could reduce both serum triglycerides and the likelihood of clotting. However, only a low-fat diet that was also low in saturated fat decreased the serum cholesterol level. They concluded, nevertheless, that low-fat diets reduce the risk of heart disease, even if they don't reduce serum cholesterol, by eliminating abnormally high coagulant activity and reducing the likelihood of blood clots within the arteries.

In addition to the points I've just made, Nordoy and Goodnight (1990), in a general report on the effects of dietary lipids and thrombosis, note that dietary saturated fat may increase the likelihood of clots in your veins as well as in your arteries. They also note that omega-3 fatty acids as well as other polyunsaturated fatty acids may reduce the likelihood of clotting.

Trevisan et al. (1990b) looked at the dietary habits of several thousand Italians and found that foods high in cholesterol and saturated fat (high-fat dairy products, eggs, and fatty meats) increased three risk factors for atherosclerosis: systolic blood pressure, serum glucose, and serum cholesterol. In another study with a similar population, the same authors (1990a) examined the intake of different specific fats and found that increased consumption of butter was associated with higher blood pressure, serum cholesterol, and glucose in men (but only glucose in women). They also found that in both sexes, increased consumption of olive oil and vegetable oil was associated with decreases in serum cholesterol, glucose levels, and systolic blood pressure.

Looking at the increase in total serum cholesterol and the fall in HDL that took place in a group of men between the ages of 19 and

29 over a 10-year period, Berns et al. (1989) found that increase in obesity among the subjects was a powerful determinant of the unhealthy changes that had taken place.[3] This finding simply reflects the fact that fatter people in general have unhealthier lipid profiles. Fortunately, as I noted in the main text, losing weight by eating a low-fat diet can usually correct the situation.

THE ISSUE OF *TRANS* FATTY ACIDS

In Chapter 2, I touched on the reason for hydrogenation and on its effect on the chemical formation of the fatty acids in oils that contain primarily polyunsaturated fatty acids. That is, in order to get a desirable texture and increase shelf life, polyunsaturated fats—such as soybean, cottonseed, and corn oils—are hydrogenated to make margarine or vegetable shortening for baked goods. Hydrogenation adds hydrogen atoms to the chain of carbon atoms, stiffening the product and helping to protect it from spoilage. The process increases the saturation of the fat, often back to the point where it is about as saturated as chicken or pork fat.

Hydrogenation produces a strange transformation in the structure of the fat. That is, in naturally occurring polyunsaturated fats, at most points where a double bond occurs the single hydrogen atoms line up adjacent to each other on the same side of the two double-bonded carbon atoms. However, when a fat is artificially hydrogenated, some of the double bonds in the chain do a flip-flop. The hydrogen atoms are now lined up on opposite sides of the two adjacent carbon atoms, rather than in a straight line on the same side. Besides folding over in this way, the chain gets kinky, and shortens. The fatty acids that result are said to have a *trans* configuration, rather than the more common *cis,* or same-side-of-the-line, configuration.

This effect has recently assumed increased importance. While research in the past has shown that *trans* fatty acids in hydrogenated fats may elevate serum cholesterol significantly in animals, Mensink and Katan (1990) have now shown that the same may be true for humans. *Trans* fatty acids led to almost double the elevation of the total/HDL ratio compared with naturally saturated fat. As you will recall, a *lower* ratio is desirable. The increase in the ratio occurred in large part because the *trans* fatty acids led to a relatively greater

[3]Recently, Manson et al. (1990) showed that as obesity increases in women, so does the incidence of heart disease and death from heart disease.

decrease in the "good," protective HDL component, compared with saturated fat.

Although research subjects in the study consumed more *trans* fatty acids than found in the average diet, the results still caution that using hydrogenated fats to replace butter and meat fat may be of little, if any, value. Indeed, the authors concluded that the effect of *trans* fatty acids on the serum lipid profile may be at least as unfavorable as saturated fatty acids because of the lowering of HDL that accompanied the increase in LDL.

RECENT RESEARCH ON DIETARY FACTORS THAT REDUCE RISK FACTORS FOR ATHEROSCLEROSIS AND HEART DISEASE

As Mattson (1989) stated in a *Journal of the American Dietetic Association* article: The primary recommendation for a healthful diet remains to decrease the intake of saturated fat and cholesterol. Mattson also presents evidence showing that both monounsaturated and polyunsaturated fats are effective in controlling blood lipid levels and may reduce the risk of coronary heart disease. Epidemiological studies in the United States and Australia certainly support these statements, since, beginning a generation ago, there has been a decline in saturated-fat intake and an increase in monounsaturated and polyunsaturated fat consumption in both countries. This change in the fat composition of the diets in both countries has the correct time relationship to a decline in coronary heart disease mortality that also has been noted in both countries (for example, Hetzel et al., 1989).

In reviewing the relationship among diet, lipids, and heart disease and looking at preventive and ameliorative measures, Stone (1990) echoes the call to reduce saturated fat and notes the cholesterol-lowering ability of monounsaturated and polyunsaturated fats. Increasing intake of fiber foods, which can be substituted for some of the fat calories, is also effective. The review also notes that omega-3 fatty acids may be effective in reducing triglycerides and preventing thrombosis. Regular aerobic exercise is recommended for increasing HDL, while it is not clear that use of alcohol offers any protection against heart disease. Regular exercise may help control triglyceride levels and may prove to be a life-style variable that helps facilitate the rate of lipid clearance after meals. As I indicated in the main text, the blood lipid level after eating is a new factor in the scenario for heart disease that is now receiving considerable attention.

That the key to a reduction in serum cholesterol may lie in reducing saturated fat was demonstrated once again by Edington et al. (1989). In this study, eating nine eggs per week versus no eggs had no impact on the already low serum cholesterol levels of persons eating a low-saturated-fat/high-fiber diet. (An average egg contains slightly over 200 milligrams of cholesterol.) The authors concluded that a reduction in dietary cholesterol below 400 milligrams per day produces no further substantial serum cholesterol reduction in persons who already have reduced their saturated-fat intake.[4]

Omega-3 fatty acids and the consumption of fish continue to show up as important factors in the reduction of risk for heart disease. Levine et al. (1989), in an experimental study with hyperlipidemic patients with atherosclerosis, showed that a modest amount of omega-3 fatty acids can have a significant preventive impact on blood platelet activity in persons susceptible to atherothrombotic disorders. In a study using rabbits that were genetically predisposed to hyperlipidemia, Lichtenstein and Chobanian (1990) found several benefits to incorporation of fish oil in the diet: plasma triglycerides and cholesterol decreased, systolic blood pressure decreased, platelet count and response to aggregating agents decreased, and less cholesterol was found deposited in the aorta. They concluded that dietary fish oil resulted in less aortic lipid deposition and that the decrease was due to the lowering of plasma triglycerides, cholesterol, platelet count and aggregability, and systolic blood pressure.

Bulliyya et al. (1990) compared a fish-consuming population with a non-fish-consuming population and found that the fish-consuming population showed lower serum cholesterol, lower triglycerides, and higher levels of HDL cholesterol. Bleeding time and clotting time were also significantly prolonged which protects against thrombosis in the fish-eating population. The authors concluded that the fish-consuming population showed a number of lower risk factors for heart disease.

However, Kromhout (1989) notes that the amount of saturated

[4]The American Heart Association recommends that cholesterol intake be below 300 milligrams per day, and preferably not higher than 100 milligrams per 1,000 calories of energy intake.

fat in the diet is more important in explaining the difference in heart disease mortality between populations than is fish consumption. And, looking at populations traditionally high or low in fish consumption, Simonsen and Nordoy (1989) found a high rate of cardiac mortality in the fish-eating group when saturated fat intake also was high. They concluded that eating fish may not be sufficient to prevent heart disease if the diet is also rich in saturated fat.[5]

IN SUMMARY

Perhaps the best conclusion that one can draw from the above examination of both the predisposing and protective dietary factors in heart disease is that the best approach to prevention is multifaceted. We need to consider the many predisposing factors that I have discussed, and oppose these with appropriate dietary action.

The research on physiological factors relating to heart disease shows that we need to be concerned with (1) plasma lipids (including the various lipoprotein components and triglyceride), (2) blood pressure, (3) coagulation factors, and (4) structural vascular factors, all of which are influenced by diet. The research on predisposing and protective measures suggests five important dietary changes. By *reducing* consumption of (1) total fat, (2) saturated fat, and (3) dietary cholesterol, and *increasing* consumption of (4) plant foods and (5) fish, we remove the predisposing factors and add the protective measures in our diets. I have attempted to incorporate all the dietary actions that can maximize protection from heart disease in the general population in the One Meal at a Time program. And, as the forthcoming discussion of the latest research on diet and cancer will show, these recommendations are consistent with the protective measures you should take against cancer.

DIET AND CANCER

As with heart disease, research in the past two years adds strength to the diet/cancer association. "Diet is one of the major causes of can-

---

[5]Compared with fish raised in commercial fish ponds, fish in the wild contain several times more omega-3 fatty acids and usually much less total fat. Thus, from a health standpoint, it is preferable to choose fish such as salmon and trout (which are normally high in omega-3 fatty acids) with wild origins.

cer" (Miller, 1990). Nine of the leading cancers, with the exception of leukemia, are associated with diet. Some foods predispose; others protect (Greenwald, 1989).

As I pointed out in Chapter 2, there are many kinds of cancers and the precise predisposing or protective elements in the diet associated with different cancers may vary. It's been harder to pinpoint dietary relationships because of this complexity than in the case of heart disease and atherosclerosis.

In this summary I will focus on foods and nutrients such as total fat and saturated fat that continually turn up, study after study, in either a predisposing or a protective role.

FOODS THAT PREDISPOSE TO CANCER

A *high-fat diet* is related to an increased risk for *colon and rectal cancer* (Freudenheim et al., 1990; Shike et al., 1990; Vogel and McPherson, 1989; West et al., 1989), *breast cancer* (Yu et al., 1990), and *prostate cancer* (Miller, 1990). With respect to breast cancer, Van't Veer et al. (1990a) showed that for every 10 percent increase in the energy derived from fat in the diet, breast cancer risk increases by 30 percent.[6]

Among the fatty acids, *saturated fat* in particular appears to have the strongest and most pervasive influence. Diets high in saturated fat are associated with increased risk for *colon cancer* (Benito et al., 1990; Berrino and Muti, 1989; Whittemore et al., 1990; Willett, 1989), *breast cancer* (Berrino and Muti, 1989; Brisson et al., 1989; Howe et al., 1990; Toniolo et al., 1989; Willett, 1989), and *ovarian cancer* (Shu et al., 1989).

When particular foods are examined, people who consume a great deal of *animal foods,* which are high in saturated fat and protein, have an increased risk of several cancers, including *colon cancer* (Benito et al., 1990; Lee et al., 1989; West et al., 1989). Increased risk for *pancreatic cancer* has been found for high consumption of *beef and pork* (Olsen et al., 1989), and high consumption of *meat or animal protein in general* may predispose to *prostate cancer* (Mills et al., 1989), *breast cancer* (Toniolo et al., 1989), and *stomach cancer* (Buiatti et al., 1989;

[6]Subjects in the lowest fat-intake group in this study were eating fewer than 65 grams of fat a day. Subjects in the highest fat-intake group were eating more than 113 grams of fat a day. Thus women following my recommendations in the One Meal at a Time program fall well under the boundary for the group with the lowest fat intake in this study and the lowest risk for breast cancer.

Wu-Williams et al., 1990). *Salt and salty foods* also may promote *gastric cancers* (Buiatti et al., 1989; Demirer et al., 1990).

Total calorie intake and *obesity* are related to colon and rectal cancer (Freudenheim et al., 1990), with people at the higher ends of these two variables having about twice the risk as people at the lower extremes. A higher amount of *total calories* also increases the likelihood of *breast cancer* (Yu et al., 1990).

Finally, at least one study links a very high intake of cholesterol to lung cancer (Jain et al., 1990).

To summarize the general picture, aspects of the diet that consistently predispose to one or more cancers are:

- Too much fat of any kind
- Too much saturated fat in particular
- A high consumption of animal products
- A high caloric intake
- Salt and salty foods

FOODS THAT PROTECT AGAINST CANCER

At the head of the list of foods that protect against cancer are vegetables and fruits, followed by grain and cereal products. A moment's reflection should make some of the reasons intuitively obvious: These foods contain virtually no fat and, ounce per ounce, fewer calories than fat or meat products. They are what nutritionists call "nutrient dense." And generally, the more vegetables people eat, the less meat and fat.

Increased consumption of *vegetables* has been found to protect against *colorectal cancer* (Miller, 1990; Vogel and McPherson, 1989; West et al., 1989; Willett, 1989), with *cruciferous vegetables* (such as broccoli, cauliflower, and cabbage) having some special impact (Benito et al., 1990; Lee et al., 1989).

Increased consumption of *vegetables* also has been linked to reduced risk for *stomach cancer* (Buiatti et al., 1989; Demirer et al., 1990; Graham et al., 1990), *laryngeal cancer* (La Vecchia et al., 1990), *pharyngeal cancer* (Rossing et al., 1989), *breast cancer* (Howe et al., 1990; Willett, 1989), *lung cancer* (Willett, 1990), and *cervical cancer* (Verreault et al., 1989). Cruciferous vegetables may play a special protective role in one or more of these cancers, as well as for colon cancer (Olsen et al., 1989).

Fresh fruit has been found to be protective with respect to *stomach cancer* (Demirer et al., 1990; Wu-Williams et al., 1990), *laryngeal cancer* (La Vecchia et al., 1990), *breast cancer* (Howe et al., 1990), *colon cancer* (Willett, 1989), and *lung cancer* (Willett, 1990), and *fruit juice high in vitamin C* has been found to protect against *cervical cancer* (Verreault et al., 1989).

Cereals and whole-grain foods tend to be protective with respect to several cancers common in the Western world, including breast, colon, prostate, and lung cancers (Kodama and Kodama, 1990; Van't Veer et al., 1990b; Wu-Williams et al., 1990).

Because of their special significance, I'd like to add a few details to my mention of several studies that were published too recently to have been included in the National Research Council's *Diet and Health.*

Yu et al. (1990) studied Chinese women living in Shanghai, who on the average consume a low-fat diet (only about 23 percent of calories from fat). They found that women in the highest quintile of the distribution of fat intake and calorie intake had almost twice the likelihood of breast cancer as women in the lowest quintile, even though the extra calories came from monounsaturated fat. While they urge caution until these results are replicated, the results add to the evidence that total fat intake regardless of kind of fat may be predisposing for breast cancer. These findings for the impact of total fat on breast cancer are in accord with those of Van't Veer et al. (1990a) quoted earlier.

The results relating total fat intake to breast cancer should not, however, be interpreted to mean that saturated fat has any less special significance than I inferred in my earlier discussion. Howe et al. (1990), for example, examined the data from 12 studies that compared the diets of women with breast cancer to non-cancerous control subjects and found consistent significant positive correlations between saturated fat and risk of breast cancer, especially in post-menopausal women. A diet high in saturated fat increased risk by 46 percent. On the other hand, a high intake of vegetables and fruits decreased risk by 31 percent. Studies that look at diet in this way establish relationships—that is, that events occur together. But *if,* indeed, fat has a *causative* role, and fruit and vegetables are protective, then the authors estimate that appropriate dietary changes would prevent about 24 percent of breast cancer in postmenopausal women and 16 percent in premenopausal women.

In a most important study of Chinese men and women living in the

United States and in China, Whittemore et al. (1990) found that saturated fat is the key dietary villain in colorectal cancer, and the effect is especially strong in sedentary persons. The risk increases the longer a person is exposed to a saturated-fat diet and a sedentary life-style in both countries, and the higher risk in the United States compared to China is due to the difference in these two habits between Chinese living in the United States and Chinese living in China. The authors estimate that a saturated-fat intake exceeding 10 grams per day, combined with physical inactivity, could account for 60 percent of the colorectal cancer incidence in men and 40 percent in women. This is one of the highest estimates of a life-style impact on colorectal cancer that I have seen.

The dietary conclusions of this study of the two Chinese populations have recently received additional support in a study of American women (88,751 nurses) whose eating habits were surveyed as part of a large ongoing study of life-style and health among nurses (Willett et al., 1990). At the beginning of this part of the study, all of the women were free of bowel disease. Over a period of six years, women who ate beef, pork, or lamb as a main dish every day had a relative risk of developing colon cancer that was two and a half times greater than those who reported consumption less than once a month. The consumption of fish and chicken *without skin* seemed to have a protective effect. Women in the *highest* quintile of fish and chicken consumption and the *lowest* quintile of meat consumption had the lowest incidence of colon cancer. The authors concluded that it was the saturated-fat content of meat that was responsible for the increased risk, and that it would be wise for people to substitute fish and chicken for meats high in fat. Saturated fat in dairy products was not associated with increased risk.

There is considerable lore concerning the protective impact of allium vegetables (garlic, onions) on cancer and heart disease. Animal research has demonstrated that tumors can be inhibited by allium compounds. You et al. (1989) showed that persons in the highest quartile of consumption of garlic, onions, and other foods in the allium family have only 40 percent the risk of developing gastric cancer as persons in the lowest quartile. I suspect that more research on the effects of allium vegetables, as well as on the more established impact of cruciferous vegetables, will be forthcoming.

Finally, I should point out that cigarette smoking and alcohol play key roles in many cancers in addition to lung cancer. For example,

Young (1989) points out that alcohol consumption (10 or more drinks a week versus no drinks) in early adult years is associated with breast cancer after the age of 35. Both alcohol consumption and cigarette smoking are linked to laryngeal cancer (La Vecchia et al., 1990).

I have limited my presentation to a discussion of foods rather than include material on vitamins and minerals, or on other nutrients that are found in these foods. I have done this for two reasons. First, we don't eat nutrients in isolation and the advantages of supplementation have not been demonstrated. Second, the evidence for any particular vitamin or mineral is a matter of inference and only suggestive. Nevertheless, isolating specific nutrients that have an impact on disease processes is a matter of great scientific interest.

At the present time, research suggests that beta-carotenoids (found in green leafy vegetables, yellow and orange vegetables, and certain yellow and orange fruits), or other carotenoids found in fruits and vegetables, may play key protective roles in several cancers. Similarly, vitamins C and A (again, found abundantly in fruits and vegetables) frequently turn up as likely protective nutrients, and sometimes vitamin E (found in vegetable oils and whole grains). Occasionally, selenium (found in plant foods, fish, lean meat, and cereals) or calcium (low-fat dairy products and green leafy vegetables) seems to be the likely nutrient. And, of course, increased fiber is often given the credit for the relationship found between a high intake of fruits, vegetables, and grains and a protective impact on colon and other cancers. Studies that report the possible relationship between individual nutrients and cancer are included in the bibliography.

CONCLUSIONS

In conclusion, I would like to point out that the first evidence showing a link between cigarette smoking and lung cancer appeared in 1937. The idea was greeted with skepticism and generated a great deal of controversy. After all, physicians had been featured in cigarette advertising, extolling the benefits of smoking up to that time!

It was not until 1963 that the scientific community and the federal government were convinced sufficiently of the relationship between cigarette smoking and cancer to issue a Surgeon General's Report warning that cigarette smoking can cause cancer. In the meantime, millions of people died of lung cancer, caused by cigarette smoking. While the percentage of people smoking in the United States has decreased, millions still contract lung cancer as a result of smoking cigarettes.

As in the first 25 years of research on the relationship of smoking and cancer, controversy still rages in the scientific community over the advisability of supporting strong public health measures to decrease fat consumption and increase the consumption of fruits, vegetables, and grains. The 1990 Federal Nutrition Policy Guidelines are, in fact, more watered down than the 1985 Guidelines. In my opinion, the evidence that a high-fat/low-fiber diet is implicated in heart disease and several cancers is overwhelming. The position taken in the 1989 National Research Council report *Diet and Health* has been considerably strengthened by research appearing since its publication. I'd like to remind you once more that 70 percent of all mortality in the United States is due to heart disease and cancer. At least half of the incidence of these diseases is either premature or unnecessary, and related to dietary factors. Since the cost and inconvenience of cutting fat consumption and increasing your consumption of plant foods are practically nil, once you understand how to do it, I strongly urge you to get ahead of our government's regrettably conservative policy, as smokers should have done in 1937, and make the dietary changes that can help assure you of a happier, healthier, longer life.

REFERENCES

Albers, J.J.; Brunzell, J.D.; and Knopp, R.H. (1989) Apoprotein measurements and their clinical application. *Clinics in Laboratory Medicine,* 9(1), 137–52.

Benito, E.; Obrador, A.; Stiggelbout, A.; Bosch, F.X.; Mulet, M.; Muñoz, N.; and Kaldor, J. (1990) A population-based case-control study of colorectal cancer in Majorca. I. Dietary factors. *International Journal of Cancer,* 45(1), 69–76.

Berns, M.A.; de Vries, J.H.; and Katan, M.B. (1989) Increase in body fatness as a major determinant of changes in serum total cholesterol and high density lipoprotein cholesterol in young men over a 10-year period. *American Journal of Epidemiology,* 130(6), 1109–1122.

Berrino, F., and Muti, P. (1989) Mediterranean diet and cancer. *European Journal of Clinical Nutrition,* 43, Supplement 2, 49–55.

Blankenhorn, D.H.; Johnson, R.L.; Mack, W.J.; el Zein, H.A.; and Vailas, L.I. (1990) The influence of diet on the appearance of new lesions in human coronary arteries. *Journal of the American Medical Association,* 263(12), 1646–1652.

Blankenhorn, D.H., and Kramsch, D.M. (1989) Reversal of atherosis and sclerosis. The two components of atherosclerosis. *Circulation,* 79(1), 1–7.

Brisson, J.; Verreault, R.; Morrison, A.S.; Tennina, S.; and Meyer, F. (1989) Diet, mammographic features of breast tissue, and breast cancer risk. *American Journal of Epidemiology,* 130(1), 14–24.

Buiatti, E.; Palli, D.; Decarli, A.; Amadori, D.; Avellini, C.; Bianchi, S.; Biserni, R.; Cipriani, F.; Cocco, P.; Giacosa, A.; et al. (1989) A case-control study of gastric cancer and diet in Italy. *International Journal of Cancer,* 44(4), 611–616.

Bulliyya, G.; Reddy, K.K.; Reddy, G.P.; Reddy, P.C.; Reddanna, P.; and Kumari, K.S. (1990) Lipid profiles among fish-consuming coastal and non-fish-consuming inland populations. *European Journal of Clinical Nutrition,* 44(6), 481–485.

Cooper, K.H. (1988) *Controlling Cholesterol.* New York: Bantam.

Davidoff, P.; Bruckert, E.; Giral, P.; Doumith, R.; Thervet, F.; Truffert, J.; and de Gennes, J.L. (1989) [Lipoprotein Lp(a): A new risk factor of atherogenesis] La lipoproteine Lp(a): Nouveau facteur de risque atherogene. *Diabete et Metabolisme,* 15(2), 55–60 (published in French).

Demirer, T.; Icli, F.; Uzunalimoglu, O.; and Kucuk, O. (1990) Diet and stomach cancer incidence. A case-control study in Turkey. *Cancer,* 65(10), 2344–2348.

Edington, J.D.; Geekie, M.; Carter, R.; Benfield, L.; Ball, M.; and Mann, J. (1989) Serum lipid response to dietary cholesterol in subjects fed a low-fat, high-fiber diet. *American Journal of Clinical Nutrition,* 50(1), 58–62.

Freudenheim, J.L.; Graham, S.; Marshall, J.R.; Haughey, B.P.; and Wilkinson, G. (1990) A case-control study of diet and rectal cancer in western New York. *American Journal of Epidemiology,* 131(4), 612–624.

Ginsberg, H.N. (1990) Lipoprotein physiology and its relationship to atherogenesis. *Endocrinology and Metabolism Clinics of North America,* 19(2), 211–228.

Graham, S.; Haughey, B.; Marshall, J.; Brasure, J.; Zielezny, M.; Freudenheim, J.; West, D.; Nolan, J.; and Wilkinson, G. (1990) Diet in the epidemiology of gastric cancer. *Nutrition and Cancer,* 13(1–2), 19–34.

Greenwald, P. (1989) Strengths and limitations of methodologic approaches to the study of diet and cancer: Summary and future perspectives with emphasis on dietary fat and breast cancer. *Preventive Medicine,* 18(2), 163–166.

Guthrie, H. A. (1989) *Introductory Nutrition.* St. Louis: Times Mirror/Mosby College Publishing.

Hegele, R.A. (1989) Lipoprotein (a): An emerging risk factor for atherosclerosis. *Canadian Journal of Cardiology,* 5(5), 263–265.

Hetzel, B.S.; Charnock, J.S.; Dwyer, T.; and McLennan, P.L. (1989) Fall in coronary heart disease mortality in U.S.A. and Australia due to sudden death: Evidence for the role of polyunsaturated fat. *Journal of Clinical Epidemiology,* 42(9), 885–893.

Howe, G.R.; Hirohata, T.; Hislop, T.G.; Iscovich, J.M.; Yuan, J.M.; Katsouyanni, K.; Lubin, F.; Marubini, E.; Modan, B.; Rohan, T.; et al. (1990) Dietary factors and risk of breast cancer: Combined analysis of 12 case-control studies. *Journal of the National Cancer Institute,* 82(7), 561–569.

Jain, M.; Burch, J.D.; Howe, G.R.; Risch, H.A.; and Miller, A.B. (1990) Dietary factors and risk of lung cancer: Results from a case-control study, Toronto, 1981–1985. *International Journal of Cancer,* 45(2), 287–293.

Kodama, M., and Kodama, T. (1990) Interrelation between Western type cancers and non-Western type cancers as regards their risk variations in time and space. II. Nutrition and cancer risk. *Anticancer Research,* 10(4), 1043–1049.

Kromhout, D. (1989) N-3 fatty acids and coronary heart disease: Epidemiology from Eskimos to Western populations. *Journal of Internal Medicine Supplement*, 225(731), 47–51.

La Vecchia, C.; Negri, E.; D'Avanzo, B.; Franceschi, S.; Decarli, A.; and Boyle, P. (1990) Dietary indicators of laryngeal cancer risk. *Cancer Research*, 50(15), 4497–4500.

Lee, H.P.; Gourley, L.; Duffy, S.W.; Esteve, J.; Lee, J.; and Day, N.E. (1989) Colorectal cancer and diet in an Asian population—a case-control study among Singapore Chinese. *International Journal of Cancer*, 43(6), 1007–1016.

Levine, P.H.; Fisher, M.; Schneider, P.B.; Whitten, R.H.; Weiner, B.H.; Ockene, I.S.; Johnson, B.F.; Johnson, M.H.; Doyle, E.M.; Riendeau, P.A.; et al. (1989) Dietary supplementation with omega-3 fatty acids prolongs platelet survival in hyperlipidemic patients with atherosclerosis. *Archives of Internal Medicine*, 149(5), 1113–1116.

Lichtenstein, A.H., and Chobanian, A.V. (1990) Effect of fish oil on atherogenesis in Watanabe heritable hyperlipidemic rabbit. *Arteriosclerosis*, 10(4), 597–606.

Manson, J.E.; Colditz, G.A.; Stampfer, M.J.; Willett, W.C.; Rosner, B.; Monson, R.R.; Speizer, F.E.; and Hennekens, C.H. (1990) A prospective study of obesity and risk of coronary heart disease in women. *New England Journal of Medicine*, 322(13), 882–889.

Marckmann, P.; Sandstrom, B.; and Jespersen, J. (1990) Effects of total fat content and fatty acid composition in diet on factor VII coagulant activity and blood lipids. *Atherosclerosis*, 80(3), 227–233.

Mattson, F.H. (1989) A changing role for dietary monounsaturated fatty acids. *Journal of the American Dietetic Association*, 89(3), 387–391.

Mensink, R.P., and Katan, M.B. (1990) Effect of dietary *trans* fatty acids on high-density and low-density lipoprotein cholesterol levels in healthy subjects. *New England Journal of Medicine*, 323(7), 439–445.

Mezdour, H.; Parra, H.J.; Aguie-Aguie, G.; and Fruchart, J.C. (1990) [Lipoprotein (a): An additional marker of atherosclerosis] La lipoproteine (a): Un marqueur additionnel de l'atherosclerose. *Annales de Biologie Clinique* (Paris), 48(3), 139–153 (published in French).

Miller, A.B. (1990) Diet and cancer: A review. *Acta Oncologica*, 29(1), 87–95.

Miller, G.J.; Cruickshank, J.K.; Ellis, L.J.; Thompson, R.L.; Wilkes, H.C.; Stirling, Y.; Mitropoulos, K.A.; Allison, J.V.; Fox, T.E.; and Walker, A.O. (1989) Fat consumption and factor VII coagulant activity in middle-aged men: An association between a dietary and thrombogenic coronary risk factor. *Atherosclerosis*, 78(1), 19–24.

Mills, P.K.; Beeson, W.L.; Phillips, R.L.; and Fraser, G.E. (1989) Cohort study of diet, lifestyle, and prostate cancer in Adventist men. *Cancer*, 64(3), 598–604.

National Research Council (NRC). (1989) *Diet and Health: Implications for Reducing Chronic Disease Risk*. Committee on Diet and Health, Food and Nutrition Board, Commission on Life Sciences, National Research Council. Washington, D.C.: National Academy Press.

National Research Council (NRC). (1989) *Recommended Dietary Allowances*, 10th ed. Washington, D.C.: National Academy Press.

Nestel, P.J. (1989) Current strategies for atherosclerosis and lowering cholesterol. *Clinical and Experimental Hypertension (A)*, 11(5–6), 915–925.

Nordoy, A., and Goodnight, S.H. (1990) Dietary lipids and thrombosis: Relationships to atherosclerosis. *Arteriosclerosis*, 10(2), 149–163.

Olsen, G.W.; Mandel, J.S.; Gibson, R.W.; Wattenberg, L.W.; and Schuman, L.M. (1989) A case-control study of pancreatic cancer and cigarettes, alcohol, coffee and diet. *American Journal of Public Health,* 79(8), 1016–1019.

Rossing, M.A.; Vaughan, T.L.; and McKnight, B. (1989) Diet and pharyngeal cancer. *International Journal of Cancer,* 44(4), 593–597.

Sandkamp, M.; Funke, H.; Schulte, H.; Kohler, E.; and Assmann, G. (1990) Lipoprotein (a) is an independent risk factor for myocardial infarction at a young age. *Clinical Chemistry,* 36(1), 20–23.

Schwenke, D.C., and Carew, T.E. (1989) Initiation of atherosclerotic lesions in cholesterol-fed rabbits. I. Focal increases in arterial LDL concentration precede development of fatty streak lesions. *Arteriosclerosis,* 9(6), 895–907.

Shekelle, R.B., and Stamler, J. (1989) Dietary cholesterol and ischaemic heart disease. *Lancet,* 1(8648), 1177–1179.

Shike, M.; Winawer, S.J.; Greenwald, P.H.; Bloch, A.; Hill, M.J.; and Swaroop, S.V. (1990) Primary prevention of colorectal cancer. The WHO Collaborating Centre for the Prevention of Colorectal Cancer. *Bulletin of the World Health Organization,* 68(3), 377–385.

Shu, X.O.; Gao, Y.T.; Yuan, J.M.; Ziegler, R.G.; and Brinton, L.A. (1989) Dietary factors and epithelial ovarian cancer. *British Journal of Cancer,* 59(1), 92–96.

Simonsen, T., and Nordoy, A. (1989) Ischaemic heart disease, serum lipids and platelets in Norwegian populations with traditionally low or high fish consumption. *Journal of Internal Medicine, Supplement,* 225(731), 83–89.

Stam, H.; Hulsmann, W.C.; Jongkind, J.F.; van der Kraaij, A.M.; and Koster, J.F. (1989) Endothelial lesions, dietary composition and lipid peroxidation. *Eicosanoids,* 2(1), 1–14.

Stein, O., and Stein, Y. (1990) Recent developments in atherogenesis. *Arzneimittel-Forschung,* 40(3A), 348–350.

Stone, N.J. (1990) Diet, lipids, and coronary heart disease. *Endocrinology and Metabolism Clinics of North America,* 19(2), 321–344.

Tertov, V.V.; Orekhov, A.N.; Kacharava, A.G.; Sobenin, I.A.; Perova, N.V.; and Smirnov, V.N. (1990) Low density lipoprotein-containing circulating immune complexes and coronary atherosclerosis. *Experimental and Molecular Pathology,* 52(3), 300–308.

Toniolo, P.; Riboli, E.; Protta, F.; Charrel, M.; and Cappa, A.P. (1989) Calorie-providing nutrients and risk of breast cancer. *Journal of the National Cancer Institute,* 81(4), 278–286.

Trevisan, M.; Krogh, V.; Freudenheim, J.; Blake, A.; Muti, P.; Panico, S.; Farinaro, E.; Mancini, M.; Menotti, A.; and Ricci, G. (1990a) Consumption of olive oil, butter, and vegetable oils and coronary heart disease risk factors. The Research Group ATS-RF2 of the Italian National Research Council. *Journal of the American Medical Association,* 263(5), 688–692.

Trevisan, M.; Krogh, V.; Freudenheim, J.L.; Blake, A.; Muti, P.; Panico, S.; Farinaro, E.; Mancini, M.; Menotti, A.; and Ricci, G. (1990b) Diet and coronary heart disease risk factors in a population with varied intake. The Research Group ATS-RF2 of the Italian National Research Council. *Preventive Medicine,* 19(3), 231–241.

Utermann, G. (1989) The mysteries of lipoprotein (a). *Science,* 246(4932), 904–910.

Van't Veer, P.; Kok, F.P.; Brants, H.A.; Ockhuizen, T.; Sturmans, F.; and Hermus, R.J. (1990a) Dietary fat and the risk of breast cancer. *International Journal of Epidemiology,* 19(1), 12–18.

Van't Veer, P.; Kolb, C.M.; Verhoef, P.; Kok, F.J.; Schouten, E.G.; Hermus, R.J.; and Sturmans, F. (1990b) Dietary fiber, beta-carotene and breast cancer: Results from a case-control study. *International Journal of Cancer,* 45(5), 825–828.

Verreault, R.; Chu, J.; Mandelson, M.; and Shy, K. (1989) A case-control study of diet and invasive cervical cancer. *International Journal of Cancer,* 43(6), 1050–1054.

Vogel, V.G., and McPherson, R.S. (1989) Dietary epidemiology of colon cancer. *Hematology/Oncology Clinics of North America,* 3(1), 35–63.

West, D.W.; Slattery, M.L.; Robison, L.M.; Schuman, K.L.; Ford, M.H.; Mahoney, A.W.; Lyon, J.L.; and Sorensen, A.W. (1989) Dietary intake and colon cancer: Sex- and anatomic site-specific associations. *American Journal of Epidemiology,* 130(5), 883–894.

Whittemore, A.S.; Wu-Williams, A.H.; Lee, M.; Zheng, S.; Gallagher, R.P.; Jiao, D.A.; Zhou, L.; Wang, X.H.; Chen, K.; Jung, D.; et al. (1990) Diet, physical activity, and colorectal cancer among Chinese in North America and China. *Journal of the National Cancer Institute,* 82(11), 915–926.

Willett, W.C. (1989) The search for the causes of breast and colon cancer. *Nature,* 338(6214), 389–394.

Willett, W.C. (1990) Vitamin A and lung cancer. *Nutrition Reviews,* 48(5), 201–211.

Willett, W.C.; Stampfer, M.J.; Colditz, G.A.; Rosner, B.A.; and Speizer, F.E. (1990) Relation of meat, fat and fiber intake to the risk of colon cancer in a prospective study among women. *New England Journal of Medicine,* 323(24), 1664–1672.

Wong, W.L.; Eaton, D.L.; Berloui, A.; Fendly, B.; and Hass, P.E. (1990) A mono-clonal-antibody-based enzyme-linked immunosorbent assay of lipoprotein (a). *Clinical Chemistry,* 36(2), 192–197.

Wu-Williams, A.H.; Yu, M.C.; and Mack, T.M. (1990) Life-style, workplace, and stomach cancer by subsite in young men of Los Angeles County. *Cancer Research,* 50(9), 2569–2576.

You, W.C.; Blot, W.J.; Chang, Y.S.; Ershow, A.; Yang, Z.T.; An, Q.; Henderson, B.E.; Fraumeni, J.F., Jr.; and Wang, T.G. (1989) Allium vegetables and reduced risk of stomach cancer. *Journal of the National Cancer Institute,* 81(2), 162–164.

Young, T.B. (1989) A case-control study of breast cancer and alcohol consumption habits. *Cancer,* 64(2), 552–558.

Yu, S.Z.; Lu, R.F.; Xu, D.D.; and Howe, G.R. (1990) A case-control study of dietary and nondietary risk factors for breast cancer in Shanghai. *Cancer Research,* 50(16), 5017–5021.

BIBLIOGRAPHY

Armstrong, V.W. (1990) [Lipoprotein (a): Characteristics of a special lipoprotein and its potential clinical significance] Lipoprotein (a): Charakteristik eines besonderen Lipoproteins und dessen mögliche klinische Bedeutung. *Therapeutische Umschau,* 47(6), 475–481 (published in German).

Austin, M.A.; King, M.C.; Vranizan, K.M.; and Krauss, R.M. (1990) Atherogenic lipoprotein phenotype: A proposed genetic marker for coronary heart disease risk. *Circulation,* 82(2), 495–506.

Banks, T.; Ali, N.; and Dais, K. (1989) Dietary management of the patient with atherosclerosis: Are the new National Cholesterol Education Panel recommendations enough? *Journal of the National Medical Association,* 81(5), 493–495.

Berns, M.A.; de Vries, J.H.; and Katan, M.B. (1990) Dietary and other determinants of lipoprotein levels within a population of 315 Dutch males aged 28 and 29. *European Journal of Clinical Nutrition,* 44(7), 535–544.

Buiatti, E.; Palli, D.; Decarli, A.; Amadori, D.; Avellini, C.; Bianchi, S.; Bonaguri, C.; Cipriani, F.; Cocco, P.; Giacosa, A.; et al. (1990) A case-control study of gastric cancer and diet in Italy. II. Association with nutrients. *International Journal of Cancer,* 45(5), 896–901.

Goodnight, S.H., Jr. (1989) The vascular effects of omega-3 fatty acids. *Journal of Investigative Dermatology,* 93, Supplement 2, 102S–106S.

Gutierrez Fuentes, J.A.; Gutierrez Yago, J.J.; Diez Monedero, E.; Alvarez Berceruelo, J.; Zamorano Curiel, P.; and Tejerina Abanades, L. (1989) [Lipoprotein Lp(a): A risk factor for atherosclerosis] Lipoproteina Lp(a): Factor de riesgo para la aterosclerosis. *Medicina Clinica* (Barcelona), 93(15), 565–567 (published in Spanish).

Hajjar, K.A.; Gavish, D.; Breslow, J.L.; and Nachman, R.L. (1989) Lipoprotein (a) modulation of endothelial cell surface fibrinolysis and its potential role in atherosclerosis. *Nature,* 339(6222), 303–305.

Heilbrun, L.K.; Nomura, A.; Hankin, J.H.; and Stemmermann, G.N. (1989) Diet and colorectal cancer with special reference to fiber intake. *International Journal of Cancer,* 44(1), 1–6.

Hocman, G. (1989) Prevention of cancer: Vegetables and plants. *Comparative Biochemistry and Physiology (B),* 93(2), 201–212.

Iscovich, J.M.; Iscovich, R.B.; Howe, G.; Shiboski, S.; and Kaldor, J.M. (1989) A case-control study of diet and breast cancer in Argentina. *International Journal of Cancer,* 44(5), 770–776.

James, R.W., and Borghini, I. (1990) [A favorable hyperlipoproteinemia: High-density lipoproteins and atherosclerosis] Eine günstige Hyperlipoproteinamie: Lipoproteine hoher Dichte und Atherosklerose. *Therapeutische Umschau,* 47(6), 448–455 (published in German).

James, W.P.; Duthie, G.G.; and Wahle, K.W. (1989) The Mediterranean diet: Protective or simply non-toxic? *European Journal of Clinical Nutrition,* 43, Supplement 2, 31–41.

Kostner, G. (1990) [Recent pathophysiologic aspects of atherogenesis] Neuere pathophysiologische Aspekte der Atherogenese. *Wiener Medizinische Wochenschrift,* 140(4), 101–109 (published in German).

Laakso, M., and Barrett-Connor, E. (1989) Asymptomatic hyperglycemia is associated with lipid and lipoprotein changes favoring atherosclerosis. *Arteriosclerosis,* 9(5), 665–672.

Laakso, M.; Sarlund, H.; and Mykkanen, L. (1990) Insulin resistance is associated with lipid and lipoprotein abnormalities in subjects with varying degrees of glucose tolerance. *Arteriosclerosis,* 10(2), 223–231.

LaRosa, J.C.; Hunninghake, D.; Bush, D.; Criqui, M.H.; Getz, G.S.; Gotto, A.M., Jr.; Grundy, S.M.; Rakita, L.; Robertson, R.M.; Weisfeldt, M.L.; et al. (1990) The cholesterol facts: A summary of the evidence relating dietary fats, serum cholesterol, and coronary heart disease. A joint statement by the American Heart Association and the National Heart, Lung, and Blood Institute. The Task Force on Cholesterol Issues, American Heart Association. *Circulation,* 81(5), 1721–1733.

La Vecchia, C.; Negri, E.; Parazzini, F.; Marubini, E.; and Trichopolous, D. (1990)
Diet and cancer risk in northern Italy: An overview from various case-control
studies. *Tumori,* 76(4), 306–310.

Leren, P. (1989) Prevention of coronary heart disease: Some results from the Oslo
secondary and primary intervention studies. *Journal of the American College of Nutrition,* 8(5), 407–410.

McCann, B.S.; Warnick, G.R.; and Knopp, R.H. (1990) Changes in plasma lipids and
dietary intake accompanying shifts in perceived workload and stress. *Psychosomatic
Medicine,* 52(1), 97–108.

Mensink, R.P., and Katan, M.B. (1989) An epidemiological and an experimental
study on the effect of olive oil on total serum and HDL cholesterol in healthy
volunteers. *European Journal of Clinical Nutrition,* 43, Supplement 2, 43–48.

Mensink, R.P., and Katan, M.B. (1989) Effect of a diet enriched with monounsaturated or polyunsaturated fatty acids on levels of low-density and high-density
lipoprotein cholesterol in healthy women and men. *New England Journal of Medicine,*
321(7), 436–441.

Mensink, R.P.; de Groot, M.J.; van den Broeke, L.T.; Severijnen-Nobels, A.P.; Demacker, P.N.; and Katan, M.B. (1989) Effects of monounsaturated fatty acids vs.
complex carbohydrates on serum lipoproteins and apoproteins in healthy men and
women. *Metabolism,* 38(2), 172–178.

Micozzi, M.S.; Beecher, G.R.; Taylor, P.R.; and Khachik, F. (1990) Carotenoid analyses of selected raw and cooked foods associated with a lower risk for cancer.
Journal of the National Cancer Institute, 82(4), 282–285.

Mitchell, J.R. (1990) What do we gain by modifying risk factors for coronary disease?
Schweizerische Medizinische Wochenschrift, 120(11), 359–364.

Niendorf, A.; Rath, M.; Wolf, K.; Peters, S.; Arps, H.; and Dietel, M. (1990) Morphological detection and quantification of lipoprotein (a) deposition in atheromatous lesions of human aorta and coronary arteries. *Virchows Archives,* A, 417(2),
105–111.

Osterud, B., and Hansen, J.B. (1989) Fatty acids, platelets and monocytes: Something
to do with atherogenesis. *Annals of Medicine,* 21(1), 47–51.

Perez, G.O.; Mendez, A.J.; Goldberg, R.B.; Duncan, R.; Palomo, A.; DeMarchena,
E.; and Hsia, S.L. (1990) Correlates of atherosclerosis in coronary arteries of patients undergoing angiographic evaluation. *Angiology,* 41(7), 525–532.

Ran, B.F. (1989) [The inhibitory effect of apolipoproteins in HDL on experimental
atherosclerosis in rabbits.] *Chung-hua Ping Li Hsueh Tsa Chih [Chinese Journal of
Pathology],* 18(4), 257–261 (published in Chinese; English summary furnished by
MEDLINE).

Renaud, S., and de Lorgeril, M. (1989) Dietary lipids and their relation to ischaemic
heart disease: From epidemiology to prevention. *Journal of Internal Medicine Supplement,* 225(731), 39–46.

Segal, D.L. (1990) The rationale for controlling dietary lipids in the prevention of
coronary heart disease. *Bulletin of the Pan American Health Organization,* 24(2), 197–
209.

Slattery, M.L.; Schuman, K.L.; West, D.W.; French, T.K.; and Robison, L.M. (1989)
Nutrient intake and ovarian cancer. *American Journal of Epidemiology,* 130(3), 497–
502.

Stein, E.A. (1990) Lipid risk factors and atherosclerosis: What do we measure? *Scandinavian Journal of Clinical and Laboratory Investigation,* Supplement 198, 3–8.

Van't Veer, P.; Dekker, J.M.; Lamers, J.W.; Kok, F.J.; Schouten, E.G.; Brants, H.A.; Sturmans, F.; and Hermus, R.J. (1989) Consumption of fermented milk products and breast cancer: A case-control study in the Netherlands. *Cancer Research,* 49(14), 4020–4023.

RECOMMENDED READINGS

Connor, S.L., and Conner, W.E. (1986) *The New American Diet.* New York: Simon and Schuster.

Cooper, K.H. (1983) *The Aerobics Program for Total Well-being.* New York: Bantam.

Cooper, K.H. (1988) *Controlling Cholesterol.* New York: Bantam.

Gershoff, S. (1990) *The Tufts University Guide to Total Nutrition.* New York: Harper & Row.

Hittleman, R. (1973) *Yoga: 28 Day Exercise Plan.* New York: Bantam.

Kwiterovich, P. (1990) *Beyond Cholesterol.* Baltimore: Johns Hopkins University Press.

APPENDIX B

NUTRIENT COUNTER[1]

HOW TO USE THIS COUNTER

The food items listed in this Counter are in alphabetical order within a number of different food categories. We include many of the new "lite" or reduced-fat products and an extensive list of combination foods. The latter include representative items from different food manufacturers, or an average from several manufacturers without naming them. Combination foods may be listed as "hmde" (home-made) or "frzn" (frozen). Values for these dishes, soups, salads, and sandwiches represent combinations of ingredients from traditional recipes.

We also include a wide sampling of items from fast-food chains and other popular restaurants. Additional information and complete nutrition listings are often available for the asking at these establish-ments. Because many fast-food menu items change frequently, it is a

[1]Nutrient values in this appendix were obtained from materials provided by the U.S. Department of Agriculture as well as from the food industry, journal articles, and computer data banks, in which information is assumed to be public domain. When nutrient values from different sources do not agree because of variations in the food samples tested (for example, in the beef section), we have entered an average value.

good idea to ask for nutrition information periodically. Also take advantage of the nutrition labeling on food products when you shop. Recent legislation assures us that we will have nutrition labeling on virtually everything in the near future.

In the meat, fish, and poultry categories, values are for cooked portions, without added fat, unless otherwise specified. In some cases, where values vary according to cooking method, the cooking method is specified. Beef entries are grouped according to their percentage of fat; the term "lean" refers to trimmed cuts with minimal marbling. The Counter contains the most up-to-date values for cuts of beef and pork that had just been made available in late 1990, when this book went to press.

Food items are listed in commonly consumed portion sizes. Information is given for total fat in grams, saturated fat in grams, milligrams (mg) of cholesterol, total calories, grams of fiber, and milligrams (mg) of sodium (NA = not available). Instructions for keeping a food diary are given in Chapter 4 of the main text, and a table showing the number of fat grams for different percentages of total calories from fat depending on total calories consumed appears in Chapter 3 (Table 3–1).

ORGANIZATION OF THIS COUNTER

The categories of foods are organized as follows, with the page numbers of their beginnings:

Item	Serving	Total Fat (grams)	Saturated Fat (grams)	Cholesterol (mg)	Calories	Fiber (grams)	Sodium (mg)
BEVERAGES							
apple juice	6 fl. oz.	0	0	0	92	1	6
beer							
regular*	12 fl. oz.	0	0	0	148	0	19
light*	12 fl. oz.	0	0	0	100	0	10
low alcohol	12 fl. oz.	0	0	0	112	0	11
carbonated drink							
regular	12 fl. oz.	0	0	0	152	0	14
sugar free	12 fl. oz.	0	0	0	1	0	8
club soda/seltzer	12 fl. oz.	0	0	0	0	0	75
coffee, brewed or instant	8 fl. oz.	0	0	0	4	0	4
coffee, flavored mixes, instant	6 fl. oz.	2.4	1.9	0	55	0	192
cordials and liqueurs, 54 proof*	1 fl. oz.	0	0	0	97	0	3
daiquiri*	3.5 fl. oz.	0	0	0	122	0	0
eggnog, nonalcoholic, commercial	8 fl. oz.	19.0	11.2	149	342	0	138
Gatorade	8 fl. oz.	0	0	0	60	0	96
gin*	1 fl. oz.	0	0	0	39	0	0
grape juice drink, canned	6 fl. oz.	0	0	0	89	0	12
Hawaiian punch	8 fl. oz.	0	0	0	120	0	25
Kool-Aid, from mix, any flavor	8 fl. oz.	0	0	0	95	0	8
lemonade, mix or frzn	8 fl. oz.	0	0	0	102	0	13
orange juice, unsweetened	6 fl. oz.	0	0	0	83	0	2
pineapple-orange juice	6 fl. oz.	0	0	0	99	0	8
rum*	1 fl. oz.	0	0	0	70	0	0
Tang, orange or grape	8 fl. oz.	0	0	0	117	0	2
tea, brewed or instant	8 fl. oz.	0	0	0	0	0	3
vodka*	1 fl. oz.	0	0	0	70	0	0
whiskey*	1 fl. oz.	0	0	0	70	0	0
wine*							
dessert and apertif	4 fl. oz.	0	0	0	184	0	0
table, all types	4 fl. oz.	0	0	0	83	0	0
wine cooler	8 fl. oz.	0	0	0	83	0	9
BREADS AND FLOURS							
bagel, plain	1 medium	1.4	0.2	0	163	2	198
barley flour	1 cup	0.5	0.3	0	698	31	6
biscuit							
baking powder	1 medium	6.6	1.9	3	156	1	344
buttermilk	1 medium	4.8	1.2	2	103	1	366
from mix	1 medium	4.3	1.2	3	121	1	341
Bisquick mix	1 cup	17.0	4.1	0	511	2	1703
Boston brown bread							
canned	1/2-in. slice	0.6	0.2	NA	85	2	100
w/raisins, canned	1/2-in. slice	0.6	0.2	NA	88	2	130
breadsticks							
plain	1 piece	0.2	0.1	NA	23	0	70
sesame	1 piece	3.7	1.2	NA	56	0	85
soft type	1 medium	0.1	0	NA	28	0	79
bread							
buttermilk	1 slice	1.1	NA	5	71	1	160

*Although alcohol contains no fat, scientific evidence suggests that it may facilitate fat storage and hamper your weight-loss efforts. Excessive alcohol intake is detrimental to your health. We concur with other health organizations in recommending discretion in the use of alcoholic beverages.

Item	Serving	Total Fat (grams)	Saturated Fat (grams)	Cholesterol (mg)	Calories	Fiber (grams)	Sodium (mg)
bread *(cont.)*							
French/Vienna	1 slice	1.0	NA	0	70	1	138
fruit w/nuts	1 slice	7.0	NA	NA	160	1	162
fruit w/o nuts	1 slice	3.4	NA	NA	127	1	126
honey wheatberry	1 slice	1.1	NA	2	70	2	205
Italian	1 slice	0.5	NA	NA	78	1	151
"lite" varieties	1 slice	0.5	0.1	3	40	1	80
mixed grain	1 slice	0.9	NA	NA	70	2	103
pita, plain	1 large	0.8	NA	NA	240	2	430
pita, whole wheat	1 large	1.2	0.2	0	236	7	510
raisin	1 slice	1.0	NA	1	70	1	94
Roman meal	1 slice	1.0	NA	5	68	1	57
rye, American	1 slice	0.9	NA	NA	66	2	174
rye, pumpernickel	1 slice	0.8	NA	NA	82	2	173
sourdough	1 slice	0.5	NA	0	68	1	140
wheat, commercial	1 slice	1.0	NA	0	61	1	129
white, commercial	1 slice	0.9	NA	NA	64	0	123
white, hmde	1 slice	1.7	NA	NA	72	0	102
whole wheat, commercial	1 slice	1.1	NA	NA	61	2	159
whole wheat, hmde	1 slice	1.6	NA	NA	67	2	89
breadcrumbs	1 cup	4.6	1.1	NA	392	3	736
bulgur, dry	1 cup	2.3	NA	0	548	14	6
coffee cake	1 piece	7.0	2.1	19	233	1	160
cornflake crumbs	1 oz.	0	0	0	110	1	290
cornmeal, dry	1 cup	1.6	0.3	0	502	10	201
cornstarch	1 T	0	0	0	35	0	0
cornbread							
from mix	1/8 mix	4.0	1.3	15	160	1	250
hmde	1 piece	7.3	2.2	17	198	2	232
crackers							
Captain's Wafers	2 crackers	1.0	0.4	0	30	0	88
cheese	5 pieces	4.9	1.6	4	81	0	180
Cheese Nips	13 crackers	3.0	1.1	3	70	0	130
cheese w/peanut butter	2-oz. pkg.	13.5	3.0	7	283	0	600
Chicken in a Biskit	7 crackers	4.0	1.2	3	70	0	115
Goldfish, any flavor	12 crackers	2.0	0.7	1	34	0	45
graham	2 squares	1.3	0.5	0	60	0	66
graham, crumbs	1/2 cup	4.5	2.0	1	180	2	180
Harvest Wheats	4 crackers	3.6	1.1	0	72	0	112
Hi Ho	4 crackers	4.4	1.3	1	82	0	31
matzohs	1 board	0.9	0.2	0	115	0	75
melba toast	1 piece	0.2	0	0	15	0	12
Norwegian flatbread	2 thin	0.3	0	0	40	0	32
oyster	33 crackers	3.3	0.7	0	120	0	250
Premium Fat Free	5 crackers	0	0	0	50	0	115
rice cakes	1 piece	0.3	0	0	35	0	10
rice wafer	3 wafers	0	0	0	31	0	195
Ritz	3 crackers	2.9	1.1	1	54	0	90
Ritz Bits	22 pieces	5.0	1.6	1	80	0	140
Ritz cheese	3 crackers	2.9	1.1	1	0	0	72
rye w/cheese	1.5-oz. pkg.	9.5	3.0	3	205	0	588
Ryekrisp, plain	2 crackers	0.2	0	0	50	0	100
Ryekrisp, sesame	2 crackers	1.5	0.4	0	60	0	141
saltines	2 crackers	0.6	0.1	0	26	0	80
sesame wafers	3 crackers	3.0	0.8	0	70	0	190
Sociables	6 crackers	3.0	1.1	0	70	0	130
soda	5 crackers	1.6	0.4	0	42	0	156

Item	Serving	Total Fat (grams)	Saturated Fat (grams)	Cholesterol (mg)	Calories	Fiber (grams)	Sodium (mg)
crackers *(cont.)*							
Triscuit	2 crackers	1.3	0.2	0	42	0	60
toasted w/peanut butter	1.5-oz. pkg.	10.5	2.9	2	212	0	405
Uneeda	2 crackers	1.0	0.3	0	42	0	67
Vegetable Thins	7 crackers	4.0	1.0	0	70	0	100
Wasa crispbread	1 piece	1.0	0.2	0	45	1	50
Waverly Wafers	2 crackers	1.6	0.6	0	36	0	80
Wheat Thins	4 crackers	1.4	0.5	0	36	0	60
Wheat Thins, nutty	4 crackers	2.8	0.9	0	45	0	142
wheat w/cheese	1.5-oz. pkg.	10.9	3.0	1	212	0	490
Wheatsworth	5 crackers	3.0	1.0	0	70	0	135
zwieback	2 crackers	0.7	0.2	0	40	0	20
crepe	1 medium	1.5	0.5	37	48	0	130
croissant	1 medium	11.5	6.9	30	167	1	126
croutons, commercial	¼ cup	1.9	1.6	0	44	1	115
Danish pastry	1 medium	19.3	6.8	30	256	1	103
doughnut							
cake	1	7.6	3.4	27	182	0	152
yeast	1	14.3	6.5	24	239	1	144
English muffin							
plain	1	1.1	0.2	0	135	1	291
w/raisins	1	1.2	0.2	0	150	1	203
whole wheat	1	2.5	0.5	0	139	2	147
flour							
carob	1 cup	2.0	NA	0	452	11	NA
rice	1 cup	1.3	0.5	0	428	3	45
rye, medium	1 cup	1.5	0.2	0	308	13	1
soybean	1 cup	18.0	2.5	0	380	2	11
wheat, cake	1 cup	0.8	0.1	0	349	4	2
white, bread	1 cup	1.2	0.2	0	409	4	2
white, all purpose	1 cup	1.2	0.2	0	418	4	2
white, self-rising	1 cup	1.2	0	0	436	4	1290
whole wheat	1 cup	2.4	0	0	399	11	4
French toast							
frzn variety	1 slice	6.0	1.0	54	139	0	257
hmde	1 slice	10.7	2.6	75	172	1	250
hushpuppy	1 medium	11.4	3.0	18	146	1	109
matzoh ball	1	7.6	2.2	76	121	0	202
muffins							
all types, commercial	1 large	10.3	4.3	24	187	1	263
banana nut	1 medium	5.0	2.2	20	135	2	175
blueberry, from mix	1 medium	4.3	1.9	9	126	0	185
bran, hmde	1 medium	5.1	2.1	16	112	2	160
corn	1 medium	4.2	1.2	18	130	1	192
white, plain	1 medium	4.0	2.2	12	118	0	132
pancakes							
blueberry, from mix	3 medium	15.0	4.3	85	320	4	438
buckwheat, from mix	3 medium	12.3	3.9	90	270	3	340
buttermilk, from mix	3 medium	10.0	3.2	105	270	2	463
hmde	3 medium	9.6	3.0	79	312	2	227
"lite," from mix	3 medium	2.0	NA	10	130	5	570
popover	1	5.0	2.6	51	170	0	176
rice bran	1 oz.	0.4	0.1	0	80	2	4
rolls							
brown & serve	1	2.2	NA	5	92	0	140
cloverleaf	1	3.2	0.6	21	89	0	155
crescent	1	5.6	2.8	6	102	1	256

Item	Serving	Total Fat (grams)	Saturated Fat (grams)	Cholesterol (mg)	Calories	Fiber (grams)	Sodium (mg)
rolls *(cont.)*							
croissant	1 small	6.1	3.5	21	109	0	106
French	1	0.4	0.1	0	137	1	287
hamburger	1	3.0	0.8	1	180	1	304
hard	1	1.2	0.3	1	115	1	231
hot dog	1	2.1	0.5	1	116	1	241
kaiser/hoagie	1 medium	1.6	0.4	2	156	1	312
parkerhouse	1	2.1	0.9	1	59	0	100
raisin	1 large	1.7	0.4	0	165	1	235
rye, dark	1	1.6	0.1	0	55	2	125
rye, light, hard	1	1.0	0.1	0	79	2	235
sandwich	1	3.1	0.4	2	162	1	312
sesame seed	1	2.1	0.6	1	59	1	210
submarine	1 medium	3.0	0.8	3	290	2	580
wheat	1	1.7	0.4	0	52	1	130
white, commercial	1	2.0	1.0	1	110	0	175
white, hmde	1	3.1	0.5	2	119	1	202
whole wheat	1	1.1	0.2	1	85	3	184
yeast, sweet	1	7.9	2.1	20	198	1	106
scone	1	5.5	1.5	38	120	1	189
stuffing							
Stove Top	1/2 cup	9.0	5.0	21	176	0	560
bread, from mix	1/2 cup	12.2	6.0	0	198	0	500
cornbread, from mix	1/2 cup	4.8	2.5	43	175	0	568
sweet roll, iced	1 medium	7.9	2.1	20	198	1	100
toaster pastry, any flavor	1	5.0	NA	NA	195	0	229
tortilla							
corn (unfried)	1 medium	0.8	0.1	0	48	1	38
flour	1 medium	2.5	1.1	0	59	1	63
turnover, fruit filled	1	19.3	NA	NA	225	1	240
waffle							
frozen, Eggo	1	5.0	NA	NA	120	1	300
frozen, other	1 medium	2.6	0.7	11	95	1	235
hmde	1 large	12.6	4.1	61	245	1	303
weiner wrap, plain/cheese	1 wrap	2.0	NA	NA	60	0	373
CANDY							
butterscotch							
candy	6 pieces	2.5	0.5	0	116	0	19
chips	1 oz.	6.7	NA	0	234	0	15
candied fruit							
apricot	1 oz.	0.1	0	0	94	1	5
cherry	1 oz.	0.1	0	0	96	1	5
citrus peel	1 oz.	0.1	0	0	90	1	5
figs	1 oz.	0.1	0	0	84	2	5
candy bar							
Almond Joy	1 oz.	7.8	5.3	1	136	2	58
Baby Ruth	1 oz.	6.6	2.4	1	141	1	60
Bit-o-Honey	1 oz.	2.2	NA	NA	121	0	80
Butterfinger	1 oz.	5.5	2.6	0	131	1	46
Chunky, milk choc.	1 oz.	4.4	NA	NA	120	1	15
Chunky, original	1 oz.	7.1	NA	NA	143	1	15
Golden Almond, Hershey	1 oz.	11.0	2.1	5	161	2	17
Heath	1 oz.	8.9	4.1	2	142	1	109
Kit Kat	1.13 oz.	8.5	NA	0	162	1	40
Krackle, Hershey	1 oz.	8.4	4.7	5	145	1	35
Mars	1.7 oz.	11.0	NA	NA	230	1	80

Item	Serving	Total Fat (grams)	Saturated Fat (grams)	Cholesterol (mg)	Calories	Fiber (grams)	Sodium (mg)
candy bar *(cont.)*							
milk choc., Hershey	1 oz.	9.2	5.0	6	147	1	27
milk choc., Nestle	1 oz.	9.0	5.0	6	146	1	18
milk choc. w/almonds	1 oz.	10.1	4.8	5	151	2	17
Milky Way	1 oz.	3.9	2.2	2	118	0	49
Mounds	1 oz.	7.3	5.3	0	131	2	52
Mr. Goodbar	1 oz.	10.8	4.7	4	154	2	19
Nestle's Crunch	1.06 oz.	8.0	4.5	4	160	1	35
Snickers	1 oz.	6.5	NA	3	135	1	70
Special Dark, Hershey	1.02 oz.	8.6	NA	NA	157	1	5
Three Musketeers	1 oz.	4.0	1.8	2	140	0	67
Twix	1 oz.	7.0	NA	NA	140	0	60
candy-coated almonds	1 oz.	5.3	0.4	0	129	1	6
caramel popcorn	1 cup	7.1	1.8	0	154	1	107
caramels							
plain or choc. w/nuts	1 oz.	6.9	2.5	10	120	0	10
plain or choc. w/o nuts	1 oz.	5.8	2.4	9	114	0	10
carob-coated raisins	1/2 cup	13.5	1.9	0	387	5	83
choc. chips							
milk choc.	1/4 cup	11.0	6.2	0	218	1	60
semi-sweet	1/4 cup	12.2	6.9	0	220	1	10
choc.-covered cherries	1 oz.	4.9	2.9	1	123	1	52
choc.-covered cream center	1 oz.	4.9	2.6	1	123	1	52
choc.-covered peanuts	1 oz.	11.7	4.6	0	159	2	17
choc.-covered raisins	1 oz.	4.9	2.9	3	120	1	18
choc. kisses	6 pieces	9.0	5.0	6	154	1	25
choc. stars	7 pieces	8.1	4.7	5	160	1	35
creme eggs, Cadbury	1 oz.	6.0	NA	NA	136	0	NA
English toffee	1 oz.	2.8	1.7	5	113	0	8
fondant	1 piece	0.2	NA	NA	116	0	52
fudge							
choc.	1 oz.	3.4	1.5	1	112	0	45
choc. w/nuts	1 oz.	4.9	1.2	1	119	0	48
Good & Plenty	1 oz.	0.1	0	0	106	0	10
gumdrops	28 pieces	0.2	0	0	97	0	15
hard candy	6 pieces	0.3	0	0	108	0	9
jelly beans	1 oz.	0	0	0	104	0	3
licorice	1 oz.	0.1	0	0	35	0	10
Life Savers	5 pieces	0.1	0	0	39	0	1
M&M's							
choc. only	1 oz.	5.6	2.4	3	132	1	20
peanut	1 oz.	7.8	2.4	4	145	1	18
malted-milk balls	1 oz.	7.1	4.2	3	137	1	28
marshmallow	1 large	0	0	0	25	0	0
mints	14 pieces	0.6	0	0	104	0	10
peanut brittle	1 oz.	7.7	1.2	0	149	1	44
Peanut Butter Cups, Reese's	1 oz.	9.2	3.6	3	156	1	82
Peppermint Pattie	1 oz.	4.8	2.6	1	124	1	52
Reese's Pieces	1.7-oz. pkg.	13.0	NA	NA	240	0	108
taffy	1 oz.	1.5	0.4	0	99	0	131
Tootsie roll	1 oz.	2.3	0.6	0	112	1	56
yogurt-covered raisins	1/2 cup	14.0	11.4	2	313	2	36
CEREALS							
All Bran	3/4 cup	1.1	0.2	0	159	19	719
Alpha-Bits	1 cup	0.6	0.2	0	111	1	170
Apple Jacks	1 cup	0.1	0	0	110	1	200

Item	Serving	Total Fat (grams)	Saturated Fat (grams)	Cholesterol (mg)	Calories	Fiber (grams)	Sodium (mg)
Bran Buds	⅓ cup	0.7	0.1	0	72	10	172
Bran Chex	1 cup	1.2	0.2	0	136	9	448
Bran Flakes, 40%	1 cup	0.7	0.1	0	127	6	303
Bran, 100%	½ cup	1.9	0.3	0	84	9	189
bran, unprocessed, dry	¼ cup	0.6	0.1	0	29	6	1
Cap'n Crunch	¾ cup	3.4	1.7	0	121	0	185
Cheerios	1 cup	1.6	0.3	0	90	2	233
Corn Chex	1 cup	0.1	0	0	111	1	271
cornflakes	1 cup	0.1	0	0	108	1	279
corn grits w/o added fat	½ cup	0.5	0	0	71	1	0
Cracklin' Oat Bran	⅓ cup	2.7	1.3	0	72	3	116
Cream of Wheat w/o added fat	½ cup	0.3	0	0	67	0	3
Fiber One	1 cup	2.2	0.4	0	128	21	463
Fruit Loops	1 cup	0	0	0	111	1	200
Frosted Mini-Wheats	4 biscuits	0.3	0	0	102	1	8
Fruit & Fibre							
w/apples & cinn.	½ cup	0.3	0	0	90	3	160
w/dates, raisins, walnuts	½ cup	0.7	0.1	0	89	4	162
Golden Grahams	¾ cup	1.1	0.1	0	109	1	178
granola							
commercial brands	⅓ cup	6.9	3.3	0	186	3	58
hmde	⅓ cup	10.0	4.8	0	184	2	80
Grapenut Flakes	1 cup	0.4	0.2	0	116	2	158
Grapenuts	¼ cup	0.2	0	0	104	2	188
Honeynut Cheerios	¾ cup	0.7	0.1	0	107	1	250
Kix	1½ cup	0.7	0.2	0	110	0	290
Life, plain or cinn.	1 cup	2.6	0.5	0	162	4	241
Most	⅔ cup	0.3	0	0	95	2	150
Mueslix, Kellogg's	½ cup	1.0	0.8	0	140	4	94
Nutri-Grain							
barley	¾ cup	0.2	NA	0	106	2	192
corn	⅔ cup	0.7	NA	0	108	2	187
wheat	¾ cup	0.3	NA	0	102	2	193
oat bran, cooked cereal w/o added fat	½ cup	1.2	0.4	0	55	2	256
oat bran, dry	¼ cup	1.6	0.3	0	82	3	1
oats							
instant	1 packet	1.7	0.2	0	108	1	105
w/o added fat	½ cup	1.2	0.2	0	72	1	1
Product 19	1 cup	0.2	0	0	108	1	325
puffed rice	1 cup	0	0	0	56	0	0
puffed wheat	1 cup	0.1	0	0	44	1	1
Raisin Bran	1 cup	0.8	0.1	0	156	5	296
Rice Chex	1 cup	0.1	0	0	111	1	271
Rice Krispies	1 cup	0.2	0	0	110	0	291
shredded wheat	1 cup	0.5	0.1	0	85	2	3
Shredded Wheat Squares, fruit filled	½ cup	0	0	0	90	3	5
Special K	1 cup	0.1	0	0	111	0	265
Sugar Frosted Flakes	1 cup	0	0	0	147	1	267
Sugar Smacks	¾ cup	0.5	0	0	106	1	70
Team	1 cup	0.5	0.1	0	111	1	175
Total	1 cup	0.7	0.1	0	100	2	280
Wheat Chex	1 cup	1.2	0.2	0	169	6	308
wheat germ, toasted	¼ cup	3.0	0.5	0	108	4	1
Wheaties	1 cup	0.5	0.1	0	99	2	270

Item	Serving	Total Fat (grams)	Saturated Fat (grams)	Cholesterol (mg)	Calories	Fiber (grams)	Sodium (mg)
whole-wheat, natural, w/o added fat	½ cup	0.7	0.1	0	71	2	10

CHEESES

Item	Serving	Total Fat (grams)	Saturated Fat (grams)	Cholesterol (mg)	Calories	Fiber (grams)	Sodium (mg)
Alpine Lace, Free 'n' Lean							
mozzarella	1 oz.	0	0	5	35	0	290
American	1 oz.	0	0	5	35	0	290
cheddar	1 oz.	0	0	5	35	0	290
American							
processed	1 oz.	8.9	5.6	27	106	0	406
reduced calorie	1 oz.	2.2	2.3	12	50	0	400
blue	1 oz.	8.2	5.3	21	100	0	396
brick	1 oz.	8.4	5.3	27	105	0	159
Brie	1 oz.	7.9	4.9	28	95	0	178
caraway	1 oz.	8.3	5.4	30	107	0	196
cheddar							
grated	¼ cup	9.4	6.0	30	114	0	176
sliced	1 oz.	9.4	6.0	30	114	0	176
Cheez Whiz	1 oz.	6.0	3.1	16	80	0	370
cheese fondue	¼ cup	11.7	7.2	37	170	0	109
cheese food, cold pack	2 T	7.8	4.4	18	94	0	274
cheese sauce	¼ cup	9.8	NA	NA	132	0	576
cheese spread (Kraft)	1 oz.	6.0	3.8	16	82	0	381
Colby	1 oz.	9.1	5.7	27	112	0	171
cottage cheese							
1% fat	½ cup	1.2	0.8	5	82	0	459
2% fat	½ cup	2.2	1.4	10	101	0	459
creamed	½ cup	5.1	3.2	17	117	0	457
cream cheese							
"lite" (Neufchâtel)	1 oz. (2 T)	6.6	4.2	20	74	0	113
regular	1 oz. (2 T)	9.9	6.2	31	99	0	84
Weight Watchers	1 oz. (2 T)	2.0	NA	NA	35	0	40
Edam	1 oz.	7.9	5.0	25	101	0	274
feta	1 oz.	6.0	4.2	25	75	0	316
Gouda	1 oz.	7.8	5.0	32	101	0	232
hot pepper cheese	1 oz.	6.9	4.3	18	92	0	357
Jarlsberg	1 oz.	6.9	4.2	16	100	0	130
Kraft American Singles	1 oz.	7.0	4.0	25	90	0	390
Kraft Free	1 oz.	0	0	5	45	0	430
Kraft Light 'n' Lively	1 oz.	4.0	2.0	15	70	0	410
Limburger	1 oz.	7.7	4.8	26	93	0	227
Monterey Jack	1 oz.	8.6	5.0	30	106	0	152
mozzarella							
part skim	1 oz.	4.5	2.4	16	72	0	132
part skim, low moisture	1 oz.	4.9	3.1	15	79	0	150
whole milk	1 oz.	6.1	3.7	22	80	0	106
whole milk, low moisture	1 oz.	7.0	4.4	25	90	0	118
Muenster	1 oz.	8.5	5.4	27	104	0	178
Parmesan							
grated	1 T	1.5	1.0	4	23	0	93
hard	1 oz.	7.3	4.7	19	111	0	454
pimento cheese spread	1 oz.	9.4	5.6	27	106	0	405
port wine, cold pack	1 oz.	9.0	4.7	35	100	0	151
provolone	1 oz.	7.6	4.8	20	100	0	248
ricotta							
"lite" reduced fat	½ cup	4.0	NA	15	109	0	132

Item	Serving	Total Fat (grams)	Saturated Fat (grams)	Cholesterol (mg)	Calories	Fiber (grams)	Sodium (mg)
ricotta *(cont.)*							
part skim	1/2 cup	9.8	6.1	38	171	0	155
whole milk	1/2 cup	16.1	10.3	63	216	0	104
Romano	1 oz.	7.6	NA	29	110	0	340
Roquefort	1 oz.	8.7	5.5	26	105	0	513
smoked cheese product	1 oz.	6.7	NA	20	91	0	220
Swiss							
processed	1 oz.	7.1	2.9	15	95	0	388
sliced	1 oz.	7.8	5.0	26	107	0	74

COMBINATION FOODS

Item	Serving	Total Fat (grams)	Saturated Fat (grams)	Cholesterol (mg)	Calories	Fiber (grams)	Sodium (mg)
baked beans w/pork	1/2 cup	1.8	0.8	8	134	4	524
beans & franks, canned	1 cup	16.0	6.0	15	366	7	1105
beans							
refried, canned	1/2 cup	1.4	0.5	0	135	7	530
refried w/fat	1/2 cup	13.2	5.2	12	271	7	1071
refried w/sausage, canned	1/2 cup	13.0	6.0	25	194	8	825
beef & vegetable stew	1 cup	10.5	4.9	NA	218	2	292
beef burgundy	1 cup	21.2	8.0	72	336	1	467
beef noodle casserole	1 cup	19.2	6.5	81	329	2	1205
beef Oriental, Lean Cuisine	9 1/8 oz.	9.0	NA	NA	270	2	295
beef pie							
frzn	8 oz.	23.0	5.9	41	430	2	1093
hmde	8 oz.	30.0	8.0	42	515	3	596
beef stew, frzn	1 cup	8.0	NA	NA	184	2	977
beef teriyaki, Stouffer's	10 oz.	11.0	NA	NA	365	2	1265
beef vegetable stew, hmde	1 cup	13.8	5.3	46	244	2	649
beef							
chipped, creamed	1/2 cup	11.0	3.7	21	175	0	681
chipped, creamed, frzn	5 1/2 oz.	16.0	NA	NA	235	0	1082
short ribs w/gravy, frzn	5 3/4 oz.	25.0	NA	59	350	0	702
sloppy joe	5 oz.	12.4	NA	NA	199	0	NA
burrito							
bean w/cheese	1 large	9.7	5.4	26	230	4	642
bean w/o cheese	1 large	2.8	0.9	3	142	4	510
beef	1 large	24.9	10.1	86	424	2	712
with guacamole, frzn	6 oz.	16.0	NA	NA	354	2	823
cabbage roll w/beef & rice	1 medium	8.2	2.9	26	172	2	386
cannelloni, meat & cheese	1 piece	29.7	13.5	185	420	1	597
casserole, meat, veg., rice, sauce	1 cup	12.2	4.7	62	276	3	238
cheese soufflé	1 cup	11.0	3.2	132	174	0	118
chicken, glazed, Lean Cuisine	8 1/2 oz.	7.0	NA	55	270	1	750
chicken à la king							
Stouffer's	9 1/2 oz.	11.0	NA	NA	330	1	840
Swanson	5 1/4 oz.	12.0	NA	NA	180	1	690
hmde	1 cup	18.3	4.9	67	318	1	727
chicken & dumplings	1 cup	10.5	2.7	103	298	1	611
chicken & noodles, Stouffer's	5 3/4 oz.	15.0	2.9	55	250	1	809
chicken & rice casserole	1 cup	18.0	5.1	103	365	1	600
chicken & veg. stir-fry	1 cup	6.9	1.2	26	142	3	482
chicken cacciatore, Stouffer's	11 1/4 oz.	11.0	NA	NA	310	1	770
chicken divan, Stouffer's	8 1/2 oz.	22.0	NA	NA	335	0	850
chicken fricassee, hmde	1 cup	20.9	7.2	NA	328	1	370
chicken-fried steak	3 1/2 oz.	23.4	6.8	115	355	0	365
chicken noodle casserole	1 cup	10.7	3.2	59	269	2	866

Item	Serving	Total Fat (grams)	Saturated Fat (grams)	Cholesterol (mg)	Calories	Fiber (grams)	Sodium (mg)
chicken paprikash, Stouffer's	10½ oz.	15.0	NA	NA	390	1	1250
chicken parmigiana, hmde	7 oz.	14.8	4.5	11	308	2	620
chicken pie							
frzn	8 oz.	23.0	7.6	40	430	1	906
hmde	8 oz.	31.4	10.3	56	546	2	594
chicken salad							
regular	½ cup	21.2	9.1	56	271	0	316
chicken w/almonds, Chinese	1 cup	10.9	2.3	22	203	3	1228
chili							
w/beans	1 cup	14.8	5.9	52	302	6	915
w/o beans	1 cup	19.3	7.8	70	302	3	1030
chitterlings, cooked	3½ oz.	29.4	10.1	143	303	0	39
chop suey w/o rice							
beef	1 cup	17.0	8.5	NA	300	3	1053
fish or poultry	1 cup	6.7	1.7	10	124	4	1564
chow mein							
beef, canned, La Choy	1 cup	2.3	NA	NA	72	2	900
chicken, canned, La Choy	1 cup	2.3	NA	NA	68	2	800
hmde	1 cup	8.8	2.4	NA	224	2	718
pepper, La Choy	1 cup	1.4	NA	NA	89	2	720
corned-beef hash	1 cup	24.4	7.5	80	374	2	1158
crab cake	1 small	3.8	1.4	39	61	0	132
creamed chipped beef	1 cup	22.0	NA	55	332	0	1608
curry w/o meat	1 cup	6.6	2.8	15	138	2	294
deviled crab	½ cup	15.4	4.1	50	231	1	468
deviled egg	1 large	5.3	1.2	109	63	0	140
egg foo yung w/sauce	1 piece	11.5	3.0	107	129	1	492
egg salad	½ cup	17.4	3.7	327	212	0	354
eggplant Parmesan,							
traditional	1 cup	24.0	8.7	31	356	3	1196
egg roll							
restaurant	1 (3½ oz.)	10.5	2.6	52	153	1	469
frzn, La Choy	4	4.5	NA	NA	112	1	168
enchilada							
bean, beef, & cheese	1 piece	14.1	7.3	38	243	3	756
beef, frzn	7½ oz.	16.0	NA	NA	250	1	1200
cheese, frzn	8 oz.	21.0	NA	NA	366	1	1175
chicken, frzn	7½ oz.	11.0	NA	NA	247	1	1105
falafel	1 small	5.0	0.8	9	74	1	36
fettuccine Alfredo	1 cup	29.7	NA	NA	461	1	912
fillet of fish divan, frzn	12⅜ oz.	3.0	NA	85	240	0	700
fish creole	1 cup	5.4	NA	NA	172	2	NA
fritter, corn	1 medium	8.5	2.0	0	132	1	167
frzn dinner							
chopped beefsteak	11 oz.	26.5	NA	NA	443	2	NA
chopped steak	18 oz.	41.0	NA	NA	730	3	NA
fried chicken	11 oz.	31.0	NA	NA	590	2	1831
meat loaf	19 oz.	57.7	NA	NA	916	3	3050
meat loaf	11 oz.	29.0	NA	NA	530	2	1525
Salisbury steak	11 oz.	29.0	NA	NA	500	2	1340
turkey	11 oz.	11.0	NA	NA	360	2	1416
green pepper stuffed w/rice							
& beef	1 average	13.5	5.8	52	262	2	986
ham salad w/mayo	½ cup	20.2	4.4	54	277	0	1300
ham spread, Spreadables	½ cup	19.7	10.4	45	271	0	1156
Hamburger Helper, all							
varieties	1 cup	18.9	7.2	76	375	1	1037

Item	Serving	Total Fat (grams)	Saturated Fat (grams)	Cholesterol (mg)	Calories	Fiber (grams)	Sodium (mg)
hamburger rice casserole	1 cup	21.0	7.7	57	376	3	755
lasagna							
cheese, frzn	10½ oz.	14.0	NA	NA	385	2	800
hmde w/beef & cheese	1 piece	19.8	10.0	81	400	2	1316
zucchini lasagna, Lean							
Cuisine	11 oz.	6.0	NA	NA	260	2	975
lo mein, Chinese	1 cup	7.2	1.4	11	185	1	368
lobster							
Cantonese	1 cup	19.6	5.6	240	334	0	1586
Newburg	7 oz.	21.2	NA	NA	388	0	850
salad	½ cup	7.0	1.5	36	119	0	432
macaroni & cheese							
from package	1 cup	17.3	NA	22	386	0	1087
frzn	6 oz.	12.0	NA	17	260	0	800
manicotti, cheese & tomato	1 piece	11.8	6.0	61	238	2	610
meatball (reg. ground beef)	1 medium	5.1	2.0	30	72	0	94
meat loaf, w/reg. ground							
beef	2½ oz.	14.6	6.1	73	237	0	497
moo goo gai pan	1 cup	17.2	3.1	66	304	1	595
onion rings	10 average	17.0	6.0	0	234	1	263
oysters Rockefeller,							
traditional	6–8 oysters	14.0	NA	NA	230	1	NA
pepper steak (w/trimmed							
sirloin)	1 cup	9.3	NA	35	213	2	788
pizza rolls, Jeno's	3 pieces	6.9	2.0	10	129	1	229
pizza							
cheese	1 slice	10.1	5.2	40	183	1	680
cheese, French bread, frzn	5⅛ oz.	13.0	6.7	37	330	1	840
combination w/meat	1 slice	17.5	9.0	56	272	1	1000
deep dish, cheese	1 slice	13.5	6.9	45	426	4	1170
pepperoni, frzn	¼ pizza	18.0	9.3	47	364	2	825
pork, sweet & sour	1½ cup	21.7	NA	80	386	1	850
quiche							
Lorraine (bacon)	1 slice	20.5	NA	140	360	1	875
plain or vegetable	1 slice	17.6	NA	135	312	1	539
ratatouille	½ cup	7.5	NA	0	87	2	880
ravioli, canned	1 cup	7.3	3.6	20	240	3	1002
ravioli w/meat & tomato							
sauce	1 piece	3.0	0.9	19	49	0	96
Salisbury steak w/gravy	8 oz.	27.3	12.3	126	364	1	1261
salmon patty,							
traditional	3½ oz.	12.4	4.1	94	239	1	783
sandwiches							
BLT w/mayo	1	15.6	4.1	23	282	1	935
chicken w/mayo & lettuce	1	14.4	1.8	119	303	1	256
club w/mayo	1	20.8	5.4	52	590	3	1396
corned beef on rye	1	10.8	3.2	34	296	1	774
cream cheese & jelly	1	16.0	10.8	38	368	1	421
egg salad	1	12.5	2.5	228	279	1	482
ham & mayo	1	9.8	2.3	29	281	1	412
ham salad	1	16.9	4.2	40	321	1	372
peanut butter & jelly	1	15.1	2.3	10	374	3	406
Reuben	1	33.3	11.8	77	531	6	1535
roast beef & gravy	1	24.5	NA	55	429	1	785
roast beef & mayo	1	22.6	NA	60	328	1	800
sub w/salami & cheese	1	41.3	17.7	109	766	3	1842
tuna salad	1	14.2	1.3	10	278	1	443

Item	Serving	Total Fat (grams)	Saturated Fat (grams)	Cholesterol (mg)	Calories	Fiber (grams)	Sodium (mg)
sandwiches *(cont.)*							
turkey & mayo	1	18.4	1.9	17	402	1	517
turkey breast & mustard	1	5.2	1.2	15	285	1	473
turkey ham on rye	1	9.0	1.9	34	239	3	986
shepherd's pie	1 cup	24.0	7.6	41	407	3	1158
shrimp creole w/o rice	1 cup	6.1	1.2	123	146	2	962
shrimp salad	1/2 cup	9.5	1.6	69	136	1	1087
spaghetti							
w/meat sauce	1 cup	16.7	NA	56	317	2	1320
w/tomato sauce	1 cup	1.5	0.4	5	179	2	910
SpaghettiOs, Franco							
American	1 cup	2.0	NA	NA	160	2	910
spanakopita	1 piece	24.1	7.0	79	259	2	354
spinach soufflé	1 cup	14.8	7.1	184	212	2	763
stroganoff							
beef, Stouffer's	9 3/4 oz.	20.0	NA	72	390	1	1180
beef w/o noodles	1 cup	44.4	19.4	8	568	1	634
sweet & sour pork	1 cup	21.7	NA	51	386	1	1068
taco, beef	1 medium	17.0	8.5	54	272	2	355
tamale w/sauce	1 piece	6.0	1.6	3	114	1	356
tortellini, meat or cheese	1 cup	15.4	5.4	238	363	1	764
tostada w/refried beans	1 medium	16.3	6.7	20	294	6	249
Tuna Helper	1 cup	9.7	2.1	30	295	1	866
tuna noodle casserole	1 cup	13.3	3.1	38	315	2	1209
tuna salad							
oil pack, w/mayo	1/2 cup	16.3	2.7	20	226	0	351
water pack, w/mayo	1/2 cup	10.5	1.6	14	170	0	112
veal parmigiana							
hmde	1 cup	25.5	9.2	102	485	2	1028
frzn	5 oz.	16.2	NA	67	287	0	858
veal scallopini	1 cup	20.4	7.3	132	429	2	160
Welsh rarebit	1 cup	31.6	17.3	NA	415	0	770
wonton w/pork, fried	1 piece	4.3	1.1	21	82	0	147
Yorkshire pudding	1 piece	2.4	1.0	30	56	0	83
DESSERTS AND TOPPINGS							
apple betty, fruit crisps	1/2 cup	13.3	2.7	0	347	3	114
baklava	1 piece	29.2	7.2	7	426	2	228
brownie							
butterscotch	1	1.8	0.7	8	52	0	22
choc., Little Debbie	2 small	7.3	NA	NA	219	0	135
choc., plain	1 small	3.4	1.5	14	64	0	42
choc., w/nuts & icing	1	5.0	1.3	NA	64	0	40
Hostess	1 small	6.0	NA	NA	151	0	50
Pepperidge Farm	1	8.7	NA	NA	168	0	70
cake							
angel food	1/12 cake	0.2	0	0	161	0	161
banana w/frosting	1/12 cake	16.0	2.7	60	410	1	290
black forest	1/12 cake	14.3	2.1	57	279	1	150
butter w/frosting	1/12 cake	13.0	1.9	61	380	1	400
carrot w/frosting	1/12 cake	19.0	3.8	66	420	3	197
choc. w/frosting	1/12 cake	17.0	4.2	87	388	2	648
coconut w/frosting	1/12 cake	18.1	5.9	53	395	2	177
German choc. w/frosting	1/12 cake	18.5	4.4	82	407	2	600
gingerbread	2 1/2" slice	2.9	1.8	2	267	0	225
lemon chiffon	1/12 cake	4.0	0.8	5	190	0	15

Item	Serving	Total Fat (grams)	Saturated Fat (grams)	Cholesterol (mg)	Calories	Fiber (grams)	Sodium (mg)
cake *(cont.)*							
lemon w/frosting	$^1/_{12}$ cake	16.0	2.8	61	410	1	160
marble w/frosting	$^1/_{12}$ cake	16.0	2.9	69	408	1	172
pineapple upside-down	$2^1/_2''$ slice	9.2	1.9	48	236	2	165
pound	$^1/_{12}$ cake	9.0	4.4	53	200	1	110
pound, Entenmann fat-free	1-oz. slice	0	0	0	70	0	100
shortbread w/fruit	1 piece	8.9	2.1	60	344	1	165
spice w/frosting	$^1/_{12}$ cake	10.9	2.3	52	325	1	155
sponge	1 piece	3.7	0	137	194	0	210
streusel swirl	$^1/_{12}$ cake	11.0	2.0	40	260	1	163
white w/frosting	$^1/_{12}$ cake	14.6	3.6	5	369	1	420
yellow w/frosting	$^1/_{12}$ cake	16.4	5.9	55	391	1	108
cheesecake, traditional	$^1/_8$ pie	22.0	10.4	36	372	0	455
cobbler							
w/biscuit topping	$^1/_2$ cup	6.0	1.7	2	209	3	208
w/pie-crust topping	$^1/_2$ cup	9.3	3.6	5	236	3	151
cookie							
animal	15 cookies	2.9	0.9	NA	120	0	110
anise-seed	1	4.0	1.6	8	63	0	30
anisette toast	1 slice	3.4	0.6	21	95	0	81
arrowroot	1	0.9	NA	NA	24	0	28
Bordeaux, Pepperidge Farm	1	1.8	NA	NA	39	0	32
Capri, Pepperidge Farm	1	4.6	NA	NA	82	0	45
choc. chip, hmde	1	3.7	2.0	8	68	0	26
choc. chip, Pepperidge Farm	1 large	7.4	NA	NA	161	0	75
choc. sandwich (Oreo type)	1	2.1	0	0	49	0	0
choc.	1	3.3	1.0	6	56	0	43
fig bar	1	0.9	0.3	6	56	1	40
gingersnap	1	1.6	0.1	NA	34	0	40
graham cracker, choc. covered	1	3.1	0.9	NA	62	0	53
lemon nut, Pepperidge Farm	1 large	9.0	NA	NA	168	1	75
Lido, Pepperidge Farm	1	5.3	NA	NA	90	0	40
macaroon, coconut	1	1.4	1.3	0	49	0	27
Milano, Pepperidge Farm	1	3.6	NA	NA	63	0	30
molasses	1	2.0	0.9	NA	71	0	100
oatmeal	1	3.2	NA	0	80	0	100
oatmeal raisin	1	3.0	0.8	NA	83	0	28
oatmeal, Pepperidge Farm	1 large	6.4	NA	NA	153	1	150
Orleans, Pepperidge Farm	1	1.8	NA	NA	31	0	10
peanut butter	1	3.2	1.0	6	72	1	36
Rice Krispie bar	1	0.9	0.3	0	36	0	38
shortbread	1	2.3	0.4	NA	42	0	36
Social Tea biscuit	1	0.6	0.1	NA	22	0	18
sugar	1	3.4	1.0	NA	89	0	60
sugar wafers	2 small	2.1	0.5	NA	53	0	30
vanilla-creme sandwich	1	3.1	1.3	0	69	0	75
vanilla wafers	3	1.8	0.7	NA	51	0	30
cream puff w/custard	1	14.6	3.7	60	245	0	112
Creamsicle	1 bar	3.1	NA	0	103	0	27

Item	Serving	Total Fat (grams)	Saturated Fat (grams)	Cholesterol (mg)	Calories	Fiber (grams)	Sodium (mg)
cupcake							
choc. w/icing	1	5.5	2.1	22	159	1	110
yellow w/icing	1	6.0	2.3	23	160	1	108
custard, baked	1/2 cup	6.9	3.4	123	148	0	104
date bar	1 bar	3.1	1.2	2	93	1	49
Dreamsicle	1 bar	6.2	3.9	17	207	0	137
dumpling, fruit	1 piece	15.1	5.5	8	324	2	256
eclair							
w/choc. icing & custard	1 small	15.4	5.7	NA	316	0	147
w/choc. icing & whipped cream	1 small	25.7	11.3	NA	296	0	139
frosting/icing							
choc.	3 T	5.3	2.7	6	148	0	50
cream cheese	3 T	6.8	2.6	11	170	0	43
ready-to-spread	1/12 tub	6.9	2.5	4	169	0	30
seven-minute	3 T	0	0	0	135	0	25
vanilla or lemon	3 T	4.0	1.9	6	140	0	80
fruit ice, Italian	1/2 cup	0	0	0	123	0	0
fruitcake	1 piece	6.2	1.4	11	154	1	37
Fudgesicle	1 bar	0.4	0.2	3	196	1	248
gelatin							
low-cal.	1/2 cup	0	0	0	8	0	4
regular, sweetened	1/2 cup	0	0	0	70	0	50
granola bar	1 bar	6.8	1.5	0	141	1	79
Hostess							
cupcake	1	7.4	3.7	3	206	1	250
Ding Dong	1	8.7	4.0	6	170	0	130
fruit snack pie	1	20.2	6.9	12	403	2	449
Ho Ho	1	6.8	2.8	8	133	1	70
honey bun	1	33.3	NA	30	572	2	675
Snoball	1	2.1	1.1	1	137	0	93
Twinkie	1	3.8	0.8	8	144	0	181
ice cream bar							
choc. coated	1 bar	11.5	10.0	23	178	0	28
toffee krunch	1 bar	10.2	7.0	9	149	1	52
ice cream cake roll	1 slice	6.9	4.0	52	159	0	88
ice cream cone (cone only)	1 medium	0.3	0.1	0	45	0	26
ice cream drumstick	1	10.0	4.1	14	188	1	58
ice cream sandwich	1	6.2	3.6	12	169	0	53
ice cream							
choc. (10% fat)	1/2 cup	7.2	4.5	30	134	1	58
choc. (16% fat)	1/2 cup	11.9	7.4	44	174	0	54
dietetic	1/2 cup	7.0	4.4	27	134	0	48
French vanilla soft serve	1/2 cup	11.5	6.8	76	189	0	76
imitation, Tofutti	1/2 cup	8.0	NA	0	158	1	54
Simple Pleasures	1/2 cup	0.5	0	10	120	0	65
strawberry (10% fat)	1/2 cup	6.0	4.0	28	128	0	55
vanilla (10% fat)	1/2 cup	7.2	4.5	30	134	0	58
vanilla (16% fat)	1/2 cup	11.9	7.4	44	175	0	54
Weight Watchers (1% fat)	1/2 cup	0.8	0.5	2	81	0	57
ice milk							
choc.	1/2 cup	3.1	1.8	9	91	0	52
soft serve, all flavors	1/2 cup	2.3	1.4	7	112	0	82
strawberry	1/2 cup	2.5	1.2	7	106	0	60
vanilla	1/2 cup	2.8	1.5	8	92	0	60
ladyfinger	1	2.0	0.5	NA	79	0	15
lemon bars	1 bar	3.2	0.7	13	70	0	49

Item	Serving	Total Fat (grams)	Saturated Fat (grams)	Cholesterol (mg)	Calories	Fiber (grams)	Sodium (mg)
Little Debbie							
devil square	1 square	5.2	NA	NA	131	0	75
Dutch apple bar	2 oz.	5.3	NA	NA	207	0	70
fudge krispie	2 oz.	7.1	NA	NA	256	1	70
oatmeal cremes	2 pieces	12.6	NA	NA	332	1	250
peanut-butter bar	2 bars	13.5	NA	NA	265	1	200
mousse, choc.	1/2 cup	15.5	8.7	124	189	1	37
napoleon	1 piece	5.3	2.6	10	85	0	35
pie							
apple	1/8 pie	16.9	2.3	3	347	3	195
banana cream or custard	1/8 pie	14.0	10.0	35	353	1	300
blueberry	1/8 pie	17.3	4.0	NA	387	3	350
Boston cream pie	1/8 pie	8.4	2.8	20	260	1	225
cherry	1/8 pie	18.1	5.0	NA	418	2	150
choc. cream	1/8 pie	13.0	4.5	15	311	3	427
choc. meringue, traditional	1/8 pie	18.0	6.5	NA	378	1	325
coconut cream or custard	1/8 pie	19.0	7.0	NA	365	1	300
key lime	1/8 pie	19.0	6.8	10	388	1	290
lemon chiffon	1/8 pie	13.5	3.7	NA	335	1	300
lemon meringue, traditional	1/8 pie	13.1	5.1	8	350	1	260
mincemeat	1/8 pie	18.4	5.0	NA	434	3	400
peach	1/8 pie	17.7	4.6	3	421	3	425
pecan	1/8 pie	23.0	3.5	NA	510	2	250
pumpkin	1/8 pie	16.8	5.7	109	367	5	338
raisin	1/8 pie	12.9	3.1	NA	325	1	336
rhubarb	1/8 pie	17.1	4.5	2	405	3	400
strawberry	1/8 pie	9.1	4.5	2	228	1	250
sweet potato	1/8 pie	18.2	6.0	70	342	2	300
pie tart, fruit filled	1	18.7	NA	NA	362	2	NA
Popsicle	1 bar	0	0	0	96	0	0
pudding							
any flavor except choc.	1/2 cup	5.5	2.9	70	168	0	142
bread	1/2 cup	8.1	3.2	78	219	1	286
choc. w/whole milk	1/2 cup	8.6	4.9	47	247	1	140
choc., D-Zerta	1/2 cup	0.5	0.3	2	65	0	68
from mix w/skim milk	1/2 cup	0	0	0	124	0	125
noodle	1/2 cup	5.3	1.1	72	141	0	158
rice	1/2 cup	5.7	2.0	98	181	0	103
tapioca	1/2 cup	4.6	2.2	82	126	0	150
pudding pop, frzn	1 bar	2.0	1.0	2	75	0	80
sherbet	1/2 cup	1.8	1.2	7	135	0	44
sopaipilla	1 piece	6.0	0.8	0	88	0	68
soufflé, choc.	1/2 cup	3.9	1.4	42	63	0	31
strudel, fruit	1/2 cup	1.2	0.1	2	47	1	12
Tasty Kake							
butterscotch Krimpet	1	2.1	0.9	7	118	0	94
choc. junior	1	12.2	3.5	4	306	1	298
coconut cream	1	31.2	10.2	39	482	1	286
fruit pie	1	14.3	5.1	48	362	2	370
jelly Krimpet	1	1.3	0.3	3	96	0	88
toppings							
butterscotch/caramel	3 T	0.1	0	0	156	0	109
cherry	3 T	0.1	0	0	147	0	10
choc. fudge	2 T	3.8	2.5	0	97	1	36
choc. syrup, Hershey	2 T	0.4	0.2	0	73	1	36
custard sauce, hmde	3 T	2.9	1.0	59	64	0	18

Item	Serving	Total Fat (grams)	Saturated Fat (grams)	Cholesterol (mg)	Calories	Fiber (grams)	Sodium (mg)
toppings *(cont.)*							
lemon sauce, hmde	3 T	2.1	0.4	10	100	0	20
marshmallow creme	3 T	0	0	0	158	0	17
milk choc. fudge	2 T	5.0	2.9	NA	124	0	33
pecans in syrup	3 T	2.8	1.1	0	168	0	40
pineapple	3 T	0.2	0	0	146	0	20
raisin sauce, hmde	3 T	3.0	0.8	0	126	0	18
strawberry	3 T	0.1	0	0	139	0	10
whipped topping							
aerosol	¼ cup	3.9	1.4	NA	46	0	3
from mix	¼ cup	2.0	1.2	4	32	0	12
frzn	¼ cup	4.8	3.6	0	59	0	4
whipping cream							
heavy, fluid	1 T	5.6	3.5	21	52	0	6
light, fluid	1 T	4.6	2.9	17	44	0	5
trifle	½ cup	19.5	9.1	88	289	1	81
turnover, fruit filled	1	19.3	5.4	2	226	1	141
yogurt, frozen							
low fat	½ cup	3.0	2.0	10	115	0	55
nonfat	½ cup	0.2	0	0	81	0	39
EGGS							
boiled-poached	1	5.6	1.6	213	79	0	69
fried w/½ T fat	1 large	7.8	2.9	246	104	0	144
omelet							
2 oz. cheese, 3 egg	1	37.0	12.3	480	510	0	838
plain, 3 egg	1	21.3	5.2	430	271	0	330
Spanish, 2 egg	1	18.0	5.9	375	250	1	225
scrambled w/milk	1 large	8.0	2.8	248	99	0	155
substitute, frzn							
Egg Beaters	¼ cup	0	0	0	30	0	80
others	¼ cup	6.7	1.2	1	96	0	120
white	1 large	0	0	0	16	0	50
yolk	1 large	5.6	1.6	213	63	0	8
FAST FOODS/RESTAURANTS (all listings are for standard servings for the given establishment unless otherwise noted)							
Arby's							
beef 'n' cheddar burger	1	26.8	7.6	63	455	NA	955
chicken breast sandwich	1	25.0	5.1	91	493	NA	1091
french fries	1 order	13.2	3.0	0	246	NA	114
ham & cheese sandwich	1	13.7	4.7	45	292	NA	1350
jamocha shake	1	10.5	2.5	35	368	NA	262
junior roast-beef sandwich	1	9.0	4.5	20	220	NA	345
potato cakes	1 order	12.0	2.2	0	204	NA	397
roast-beef sandwich	1	14.8	7.3	39	353	NA	588
roast-chicken club	1	33.0	8.0	80	610	NA	1500
super roast-beef sandwich	1	22.1	8.5	40	501	NA	798
turkey deluxe sandwich	1	16.6	4.1	39	375	NA	1047
Burger King							
apple pie	1	14.0	4.0	4	311	NA	412
bacon double cheeseburger	1	31.0	14.0	105	515	NA	748
bacon double cheeseburger deluxe	1	39.0	16.0	111	592	NA	804
bagel	1	6.0	1.0	29	272	NA	438
bagel w/cream cheese	1	16.0	6.0	58	370	NA	523
bagel w/egg & cheese	1	16.0	5.0	247	407	NA	759

Item	Serving	Total Fat (grams)	Saturated Fat (grams)	Cholesterol (mg)	Calories	Fiber (grams)	Sodium (mg)
Burger King *(cont.)*							
bagel w/bacon, egg, cheese	1	20.0	7.0	252	453	NA	872
bagel w/sausage, egg, cheese	1	36.0	12.0	293	626	NA	1137
bagel w/ham, egg, cheese	1	17.0	6.0	266	438	NA	1114
biscuit	1	17.0	3.0	2	332	NA	754
biscuit w/bacon	1	20.0	5.0	8	378	NA	867
biscuit w/bacon, egg	1	27.0	7.0	213	467	NA	1033
biscuit w/sausage	1	29.0	8.0	33	478	NA	1007
biscuit w/sausage, egg	1	36.0	10.0	238	568	NA	1172
BK Broiler chicken sandwich	1	18.0	3.0	53	379	NA	764
cheeseburger	1	15.0	7.0	50	318	NA	661
cheeseburger, deluxe	1	23.0	8.0	56	390	NA	652
cheeseburger, double	1	27.0	13.0	100	483	NA	851
chicken sandwich	1	40.0	8.0	82	685	NA	1417
Chicken Tenders	1 order	13.0	3.0	46	236	NA	541
choc. shake	1	10.0	6.0	31	326	NA	198
Croissandwich w/bacon, egg, cheese	1	24.0	8.0	227	361	NA	719
Croissandwich w/sausage, egg, cheese	1	40.0	13.0	268	534	NA	985
Danish	1	36.0	23.0	6	500	NA	288
Fish Tenders	1 order	16.0	3.0	28	267	NA	870
french fries, medium	1 order	20.0	10.0	21	341	NA	241
french toast sticks	1 order	32.0	5.0	80	538	NA	537
garden salad w/o dressing	1	5.0	3.0	15	95	NA	125
hamburger	1	11.0	4.0	37	272	NA	505
hamburger, deluxe	1	19.0	6.0	43	344	NA	496
mushroom swiss double cheeseburger	1	27.0	12.0	95	473	NA	746
Ocean Catch fish fillet	1	27.0	4.0	57	495	NA	879
onion rings, regular	1 order	17.0	4.0	3	302	NA	559
scrambled-egg platter							
no meat	1	34.0	9.0	365	549	NA	893
w/bacon	1	39.0	11.0	373	610	NA	1043
w/sausage	1	53.0	15.0	412	768	NA	1271
side salad							
w/diet dressing	1	0	0	0	42	NA	750
w/regular dressing	1	22.0	3.0	10	332	NA	400
vanilla shake	1	10.0	6.0	33	334	NA	213
Whopper	1	36.0	12.0	90	614	NA	865
Whopper w/cheese	1	44.0	16.0	115	706	NA	1177
Whopper, double beef	1	53.0	19.0	169	844	NA	933
Whopper, double beef w/cheese	1	61.0	24.0	194	935	NA	1245
Whopper Junior	1	17.0	6.0	41	322	NA	486
Whopper Junior w/cheese	1	20.0	8.0	52	364	NA	628
Church's Fried Chicken							
chicken breast fillet sandwich	1	34.0	NA	NA	608	NA	725
fish fillet sandwich	1	18.0	NA	NA	430	NA	675
fried chicken breast	1	17.0	NA	NA	278	NA	560
hush puppies	2	6.0	NA	NA	156	NA	110
Dairy Queen							
banana split	1	15.0	NA	30	540	NA	150
Buster bar	1	22.0	NA	10	390	NA	175

Item	Serving	Total Fat (grams)	Saturated Fat (grams)	Cholesterol (mg)	Calories	Fiber (grams)	Sodium (mg)
Dairy Queen *(cont.)*							
cheese dog	1	19.0	NA	55	330	NA	990
cheese dog, super	1	36.0	NA	100	593	NA	1605
cheeseburger	1	14.0	NA	50	318	NA	790
cheeseburger, big	1	30.0	NA	95	553	NA	980
chili dog	1	20.0	NA	55	330	NA	985
chili dog, super	1	33.0	NA	100	555	NA	1595
choc. sundae							
small	1	4.0	NA	10	170	NA	75
medium	1	7.0	NA	15	290	NA	100
large	1	9.0	NA	30	400	NA	165
Dilly bar	1	15.0	NA	10	240	NA	50
fish sandwich	1	17.0	NA	50	400	NA	875
fish sandwich w/cheese	1	21.0	NA	60	440	NA	1035
float	1	8.0	NA	20	330	NA	85
freeze	1	13.0	NA	30	520	NA	180
french fries							
regular	1 order	10.0	NA	10	200	NA	115
large	1 order	16.0	NA	15	320	NA	185
frozen dessert	1	6.0	NA	15	180	NA	65
hamburger	1	9.0	NA	45	260	NA	630
hamburger, big	1	23.0	NA	85	457	NA	630
hamburger, deluxe	1	24.0	NA	85	470	NA	560
hamburger, super	1	48.0	NA	135	783	NA	690
hot dog	1	15.0	NA	45	273	NA	830
hot dog, super	1	30.0	NA	80	518	NA	1365
hot fudge brownie delight	1	22.0	NA	20	570	NA	225
ice cream cone							
small	1	3.0	NA	10	110	NA	45
medium	1	7.0	NA	15	230	NA	80
large	1	10.0	NA	25	340	NA	110
ice cream dipped in choc.							
small	1	7.0	NA	10	150	NA	55
medium	1	13.0	NA	20	300	NA	100
large	1	20.0	NA	30	450	NA	145
ice cream parfait	1	11.0	NA	30	460	NA	140
ice cream sandwich	1	4.0	NA	5	140	NA	40
onion rings	1 order	17.0	NA	15	300	NA	170
shake							
small	1	11.0	NA	35	340	NA	180
medium	1	20.0	NA	50	600	NA	260
large	1	28.0	NA	70	840	NA	360
Dominos							
cheese pizza 16"	2 slices	10.0	6.0	19	376	NA	483
deluxe pizza 16"	2 slices	20.0	9.0	40	498	NA	954
double cheese/pepperoni							
pizza 16"	2 slices	25.0	13.0	48	545	NA	1042
ham pizza 16"	2 slices	11.0	6.0	26	417	NA	805
pepperoni pizza 16"	2 slices	18.0	9.0	28	460	NA	825
sausage/mushroom pizza 16"	2 slices	16.0	8.0	28	430	NA	552
veggie pizza 16"	2 slices	19.0	10.0	36	498	NA	1035
Godfather's Pizza							
cheese pizza, large	$^{1}/_{10}$	7.0	NA	16	228	NA	464
combo pizza, large	$^{1}/_{10}$	19.0	NA	36	437	NA	1019
Hardee's							
apple turnover	1	12.0	4.0	0	268	NA	245
bacon biscuit	1	24.0	7.0	89	315	NA	983

Item	Serving	Total Fat (grams)	Saturated Fat (grams)	Cholesterol (mg)	Calories	Fiber (grams)	Sodium (mg)
Hardee's *(cont.)*							
bacon cheeseburger	1	39.0	16.0	60	610	NA	973
Big Cookie Treat	1	13.0	4.0	0	250	NA	239
Big Country Breakfast							
w/bacon	1	54.0	9.0	350	754	NA	1661
w/ham	1	47.0	12.0	265	768	NA	2021
w/sausage	1	74.0	16.0	280	1005	NA	1950
Big Deluxe	1	27.0	12.0	58	495	NA	824
Canadian biscuit 'n' gravy	1	22.0	3.0	10	420	NA	1379
chef salad	1	15.0	9.0	114	248	NA	932
cheeseburger	1	13.0	6.0	28	310	NA	681
cheeseburger, ¼ lb.	1	29.0	14.0	60	510	NA	1076
chicken fillet	1	16.0	2.0	61	416	NA	1384
chicken fiesta salad	1	14.0	9.0	128	286	NA	533
chicken stix	6 pieces	9.0	2.0	35	210	NA	678
cinnamon 'n' raisin biscuit	1	17.0	5.0	0	315	NA	515
fisherman's fillet	1	25.0	7.0	40	510	NA	861
french fries, regular	1 order	10.0	2.0	0	226	NA	83
garden salad	1	14.0	8.0	103	208	NA	266
hamburger	1	13.0	6.0	28	310	NA	681
hot dog	1	16.0	7.0	23	306	NA	776
mushroom 'n' swiss burger	1	28.0	13.0	55	516	NA	1031
rise 'n' shine biscuit	1	28.0	6.0	187	478	NA	1550
roast-beef sandwich	1	15.0	6.0	34	338	NA	966
sausage biscuit	1	30.0	9.0	19	448	NA	1053
side salad	1	1.0	0	0	19	NA	14
steak biscuit	1	30.0	6.0	18	521	NA	1425
turkey club sandwich	1	14.0	4.0	45	374	NA	1296
Jack in the Box							
apple turnover	1	24.0	10.8	15	411	1	350
Breakfast Jack sandwich	1	13.0	5.2	203	301	0	871
cheeseburger	1	15.0	7.5	41	310	0	746
cheeseburger, Jumbo Jack	1	35.0	12.0	95	628	1	1000
french fries	1 order	15.0	6.5	11	270	1	200
hamburger	1	11.0	4.9	24	263	0	555
hamburger, Jumbo Jack	1	29.0	10.0	70	551	1	700
Mobey Jack sandwich	1	26.0	8.4	47	455	0	820
onion rings	1 order	23.0	12.0	30	351	0	410
pancakes	1 order	27.0	11.0	83	626	1	1650
scrambled eggs	1 order	44.0	21.1	260	719	1	1110
shake							
choc.	1	7.0	4.3	25	330	0	270
vanilla	1	6.0	3.6	25	320	0	230
taco	1	11.0	5.2	21	189	1	406
taco, super	1	17.0	8.0	37	285	1	765
Kentucky Fried Chicken							
breast	1	18.0	3.6	96	286	0	654
breast, extra crispy	1	21.0	5.3	93	353	0	842
breast fillet sandwich	1	22.5	NA	NA	436	0	NA
chicken nuggets	6 nuggets	17.4	4.2	72	276	0	840
coleslaw	1 order	7.5	1.0	5	121	1	175
corn on the cob	1	2.8	0.5	0	169	1	81
drumstick, extra crispy	1	9.0	2.0	60	155	0	300
drumstick, fried regular	1	6.5	2.0	70	117	0	250
french fries	1 order	6.7	1.6	1	184	1	40
gravy	1	4.0	1.0	2	59	0	398

Item	Serving	Total Fat (grams)	Saturated Fat (grams)	Cholesterol (mg)	Calories	Fiber (grams)	Sodium (mg)
Kentucky Fried Chicken *(cont.)*							
mashed potatoes	1	0.9	0.1	0	64	0	297
thigh	1	17.5	5.0	110	257	0	500
thigh, extra crispy	1	23.4	2.2	105	343	0	740
wing	1	9.0	2.0	50	136	0	300
wing, extra crispy	1	13.5	3.0	55	201	0	400
Long John Silver's							
baked fish dinner	1	19.0	NA	NA	387	NA	1298
catfish fillet dinner	1	58.0	NA	NA	980	NA	1716
Chicken Planks (dinner)	4 pieces	59.0	NA	NA	1037	NA	2433
clam chowder	1	5.0	NA	NA	128	NA	612
clams, breaded	1 order	34.0	NA	NA	617	NA	1170
combo salad w/crackers	1	3.0	NA	NA	377	NA	1051
corn on the cob	1	4.0	NA	NA	176	NA	15
fish dinner	1	70.0	NA	NA	1180	NA	2797
fish & more dinner	1	58.0	NA	NA	366	NA	2124
fish sandwich	1	31.0	NA	NA	560	NA	NA
french fries	1 order	16.0	NA	NA	288	NA	6
hush puppies	3	7.0	NA	NA	153	NA	450
ocean chef salad w/crackers	1	8.0	NA	NA	222	NA	983
ocean scallops dinner	1	45.0	NA	NA	747	NA	1579
oyster dinner	1	45.0	NA	NA	789	NA	763
seafood salad w/crackers	1	30.0	NA	NA	406	NA	1021
shrimp dinner	1	57.0	NA	NA	962	NA	2007
shrimp salad w/crackers	1	3.0	NA	NA	183	NA	658
McDonald's							
apple bran muffin	1	0	0	0	190	NA	230
bacon bits	1 pkg.	1.2	0	0	16	0	95
Big Mac	1	32.4	10.1	103	560	1	950
biscuit w/bacon, egg, & cheese	1	26.4	8.2	253	440	1	1230
biscuit w/sausage	1	29.1	9.3	49	440	1	1080
biscuit w/sausage & egg	1	34.5	11.2	275	520	1	1250
biscuit w/spread	1	12.7	3.4	1	260	1	730
cheeseburger	1	13.8	5.2	53	310	0	750
chef salad w/o dressing	1	13.6	5.9	128	230	1	490
Chicken McNuggets	6 pieces	19.0	4.5	75	314	0	700
chunky chicken salad w/o dressing	1	3.4	1.0	78	140	1	230
cookies							
choc. chip	1	15.6	5.0	4	330	0	280
McDonaldland	1	9.2	1.9	0	290	0	300
croutons	1 pkg.	2.2	0.5	0	50	NA	140
Danish, all varieties	1	18.0	4.5	35	413	0	350
Egg McMuffin	1	11.2	3.8	226	290	0	740
English muffin w/butter	1	4.6	2.4	9	170	1	270
Filet-o-Fish	1	26.1	5.2	50	440	0	1030
french fries							
small	1 order	11.5	5.1	9	220	1	110
medium	1 order	17.1	7.2	12	320	1	150
large	1 order	21.6	9.1	16	400	1	200
frozen yogurt cone	1	0.8	0.4	3	100	0	80
garden salad w/o dressing	1	6.6	2.9	83	110	1	160
hamburger	1	9.5	3.6	37	260	0	500
hash browns	1 order	7.3	3.2	9	130	0	330
hotcakes w/butter & syrup	1	9.2	3.7	21	410	0	640

348

Item	Serving	Total Fat (grams)	Saturated Fat (grams)	Cholesterol (mg)	Calories	Fiber (grams)	Sodium (mg)
McDonald's *(cont.)*							
McChicken	1	28.6	5.4	43	490	0	780
McD.L.T.	1	36.8	11.5	109	580	1	990
McNugget sauce							
barbecue	1	0.4	0.1	0	60	0	309
honey	1	0	0	0	50	0	2
hot mustard	1	2.1	0.5	3	63	0	259
sweet & sour	1	0.3	0	0	64	0	186
pie, apple	1	14.8	4.8	6	260	0	240
Quarter Pounder	1	20.7	8.1	86	410	1	660
Quarter Pounder w/cheese	1	29.2	11.2	118	520	1	1150
sausage, pork	1	16.3	5.9	48	180	0	350
Sausage McMuffin	1	21.9	7.8	64	370	1	830
Sausage McMuffin w/egg	1	26.8	9.5	263	440	1	980
scrambled eggs	1	9.8	3.3	399	140	0	290
shake							
choc.	1	1.7	0.8	10	320	0	240
strawberry	1	1.3	0.6	10	320	0	170
vanilla	1	1.3	0.6	10	290	0	170
side salad w/o dressing	1	3.4	1.5	41	60	1	85
sundae							
caramel	1	2.8	1.5	13	270	0	180
hot fudge	1	3.2	2.4	6	240	0	170
strawberry	1	1.1	0.6	5	210	0	95
Pizza Hut							
thin 'n' crispy pizza							
cheese 10"	3 slices	15.0	NA	NA	450	NA	NA
pepperoni 10"	3 slices	17.0	NA	NA	430	NA	NA
supreme 10"	3 slices	21.0	NA	NA	510	NA	NA
thick 'n' chewy pizza							
cheese 10"	3 slices	14.0	NA	NA	560	NA	NA
pepperoni 10"	3 slices	18.0	NA	NA	560	NA	NA
supreme 10"	3 slices	22.0	NA	NA	640	NA	NA
Shoney's Restaurants							
All American burger	1	32.6	NA	86	501	1	597
baked fish, light	1	1.4	NA	83	170	0	1641
baked potato (10 oz.)	1	0.3	NA	0	264	7	16
charbroiled chicken	1	6.1	NA	85	198	0	491
charbroiled chicken sandwich	1	17.0	NA	90	451	1	1002
charbroiled shrimp	1	3.0	NA	162	138	0	170
chicken fillet sandwich	1	21.2	NA	51	464	1	585
chicken tender	1	20.4	NA	64	388	0	239
country-fried steak	1	27.2	NA	27	449	1	1177
french fries (3 oz.)	1 order	7.5	NA	0	189	3	26
french toast sticks	1	2.9	NA	0	69	0	157
garden salad, typical (9 oz. fresh veg./low-cal. dress.)	1	0.6	NA	0	63	5	601
Grecian bread	1	2.2	NA	0	80	0	94
half-o-pound dinner	1	34.4	NA	123	435	0	280
Hawaiian chicken	1	6.2	NA	85	221	0	492
hot fudge sundae	1	22.0	NA	60	451	0	226
lasagna	1	9.8	NA	26	297	3	870
liver and onions	1	22.9	NA	529	411	1	321

Item	Serving	Total Fat (grams)	Saturated Fat (grams)	Cholesterol (mg)	Calories	Fiber (grams)	Sodium (mg)
Shoney's Restaurants *(cont.)*							
onion rings	each	3.1	NA	2	52	0	43
pancakes	1	0.1	NA	0	41	0	238
rice (3.5 oz.)	1	3.7	NA	1	137	0	765
shrimper's feast	1	22.2	NA	125	383	0	216
sirloin	6 oz.	24.5	NA	64	357	0	160
Slim Jim	1	23.9	NA	57	484	1	1620
soups, Lightside, average	1	1.7	NA	4	73	1	503
spaghetti dinner	1	16.3	NA	55	496	2	387
strawberry pie	1 slice	16.7	NA	0	332	2	247
Taco Bell							
burrito, bean	1	10.8	5.0	13	350	1	922
burrito, beef	1	21.0	8.0	59	466	NA	993
burrito, combination	1	16.0	10.0	59	404	NA	928
burrito, supreme	1	22.0	9.0	35	457	NA	952
enchirito	1	16.9	10.0	56	373	1	1260
frijoles & cheese	1	6.0	5.0	19	232	2	733
taco	1	8.6	4.0	32	162	1	274
tostada	1	6.0	5.0	18	179	NA	670
tostada w/beef	1	15.0	10.0	40	291	NA	764
Wendy's							
baked potato, plain	1	2.0	0	0	270	4	20
baked potato, w/cheese	1	15.0	4.0	10	420	4	310
Big Classic	1	33.0	5.9	90	570	NA	1065
cheeseburger, single	1	34.0	NA	90	580	1	655
cheeseburger, double	1	48.0	NA	165	800	1	760
chef salad (prepared)	1	9.0	NA	120	180	NA	140
chicken sandwich	1	19.0	2.8	60	430	NA	725
chili con carne	1	7.0	2.6	45	230	2	750
crispy chicken nuggets (6)	1	20.0	4.5	50	280	NA	600
fish fillet sandwich	1	25.0	5.0	55	460	NA	780
french fries (small)	1 order	12.0	2.5	0	240	NA	145
Frosty, choc., small	1	14.0	4.8	50	400	0	220
grilled chicken sandwich	1	13.0	2.5	60	340	NA	815
hamburger, single	1	21.0	5.7	70	420	1	890
hamburger, double	1	40.0	NA	160	670	1	500
hamburger, junior	1	9.0	3.3	34	260	NA	570
taco salad (prepared)	1	37.0	NA	35	660	NA	1110
FATS							
bacon fat	1 T	14.0	3.6	9	126	0	126
beef, separable fat	1 oz.	23.3	6.0	24	216	0	5
butter							
solid	1 t	4.1	2.3	11	36	0	26
solid	1 T	12.3	6.9	33	108	0	78
whipped	1 t	3.1	1.9	8	28	0	31
Butter Buds, liquid	2 T	0	NA	0	12	0	170
chicken fat, raw	1 T	12.8	3.8	11	115	0	0
cream							
light	1 T	2.9	1.8	10	29	0	6
medium (25% fat)	1 T	3.8	2.3	13	37	0	6
cream substitute							
liquid/frzn	½ fl. oz.	1.5	0.3	0	20	0	12
powdered	1 T	0.7	0.7	0	11	0	4
half & half	1 T	1.7	1.1	6	20	0	6

Item	Serving	Total Fat (grams)	Saturated Fat (grams)	Cholesterol (mg)	Calories	Fiber (grams)	Sodium (mg)
margarine							
liquid	1 t	4.0	0.6	0	35	0	37
solid (corn)	1 t	4.0	0.6	0	35	0	44
solid, reduced cal	1 t	2.0	0.3	0	18	0	46
mayonnaise							
regular (soybean)	1 T	11.0	1.6	8	99	0	78
reduced calorie	1 T	4.5	0.6	3	44	0	96
no-stick spray (Pam, etc.)	2-sec. spray	0.8	0.1	0	8	0	0
oil							
canola	1 T	14.0	1.3	0	120	0	0
corn	1 T	14.0	1.7	0	120	0	0
olive	1 T	14.0	1.8	0	119	0	0
Puritan	1 T	14.0	1.7	0	124	0	0
safflower	1 T	14.0	1.2	0	120	0	0
soybean	1 T	14.0	2.0	0	120	0	0
pork							
backfat, raw	1 oz.	25.4	6.5	20	192	0	7
separable fat, cooked	1 oz.	23.4	7.8	26	216	0	9
pork fat (lard)	1 T	12.8	5.0	12	116	0	0
salt pork, raw	1 oz.	23.8	8.3	25	219	0	404
sandwich spread (Miracle Whip type)	1 T	7.0	1.1	6	69	0	84
shortening, vegetable (Crisco)	1 T	12.0	3.1	0	106	0	0
sour cream							
cultured	1 T	2.5	1.6	5	26	0	6
half & half, cultured	1 T	1.8	1.1	6	20	0	6
imitation	1 T	2.7	2.3	0	25	0	13
reduced calorie	1 T	1.3	0.6	4	15	0	15
FISH (all baked/broiled w/o added fat unless otherwise noted)							
abalone, canned	3¹/₂ oz.	0.3	0.1	97	80	0	298
anchovy, canned	3 fillets	1.2	0.2	12	21	0	370
anchovy paste	1 t	0.8	NA	NA	14	0	NA
bass							
freshwater	3¹/₂ oz.	2.6	0.7	60	104	0	60
saltwater, baked w/fat	3¹/₂ oz.	19.4	NA	NA	287	0	168
saltwater, black	3¹/₂ oz.	1.2	0.2	50	93	0	68
saltwater, striped	3¹/₂ oz.	2.7	0.7	70	105	0	60
bluefish							
cooked	3¹/₂ oz.	3.3	0.8	50	117	0	51
fried	3¹/₂ oz.	12.8	2.7	59	205	0	78
buffalofish	3¹/₂ oz.	4.2	0.8	72	150	0	34
butterfish							
gulf	3¹/₂ oz.	2.9	0.7	60	95	0	80
northern	3¹/₂ oz.	10.2	1.9	49	184	0	59
northern, fried	3¹/₂ oz.	19.1	2.5	50	275	0	160
carp	3¹/₂ oz.	5.8	1.2	72	138	0	54
catfish	3¹/₂ oz.	3.1	0.7	60	103	0	50
catfish, breaded & fried	3¹/₂ oz.	13.2	2.9	81	226	NA	278
caviar, sturgeon, granular	1 round t	1.5	0.4	47	26	0	150
clams							
canned, solids & liquid	¹/₂ cup	0.7	0.1	25	52	0	45
canned, solids only	3 oz.	2.5	0.2	57	126	0	95
meat only	5 large	0.9	0.1	42	80	0	70
soft, raw	4 large	1.9	0.1	29	63	0	47
cod							
canned	3¹/₂ oz.	0.3	0.1	45	85	0	180

Item	Serving	Total Fat (grams)	Saturated Fat (grams)	Cholesterol (mg)	Calories	Fiber (grams)	Sodium (mg)
cod *(cont.)*							
cooked	3½ oz.	0.3	0.1	40	78	0	60
dried, salted	3½ oz.	1.7	0.4	129	246	0	5973
crab							
canned	½ cup	2.1	0.2	76	86	0	283
deviled	3½ oz.	9.9	3.5	40	188	0	450
fried	3½ oz.	18.0	NA	NA	273	0	NA
crab, Alaska king	3½ oz.	1.5	NA	53	96	0	1062
crab cake	3½ oz.	10.8	1.2	100	178	0	225
crappie, white	3½ oz.	0.8	0.3	60	79	0	104
crayfish, freshwater	3½ oz.	0.5	0.2	115	72	0	45
croaker							
Atlantic	3½ oz.	3.2	1.0	60	133	0	50
white	3½ oz.	0.8	0.3	60	84	0	104
cusk, steamed	3½ oz.	0.7	0.2	NA	106	0	110
dolphinfish	3½ oz.	0.7	0.2	72	85	0	86
eel, American							
cooked	3½ oz.	18.3	4.2	74	260	0	82
smoked	3½ oz.	23.6	4.9	60	281	0	679
eulachon (smelt)	3½ oz.	6.2	1.3	49	118	0	59
fillets, frzn							
batter dipped	2 pieces	31.0	NA	NA	440	0	552
light & crispy	2 pieces	23.0	NA	NA	311	0	345
fish cakes, frzn, fried	3½ oz.	14.0	3.9	102	242	2	567
flatfish	3½ oz.	0.8	0.2	47	79	0	69
flounder/sole	3½ oz.	0.5	0.2	30	68	0	56
gefilte fish	3½ oz.	2.2	0.5	50	815	1	155
grouper	3½ oz.	1.3	0.4	47	87	0	53
haddock							
cooked	3½ oz.	0.6	0.1	50	79	0	58
fried	3½ oz.	10.0	3.0	60	180	0	130
smoked/canned	3½ oz.	0.4	0.1	68	103	0	655
halibut	3½ oz.	1.2	0.5	30	100	0	50
herring							
canned or smoked	3½ oz.	13.6	2.2	66	208	0	734
cooked	3½ oz.	11.3	2.0	70	176	0	90
pickled	3½ oz.	15.1	2.4	70	223	0	786
Jack mackerel	3½ oz.	5.6	1.7	75	143	0	360
kingfish	3½ oz.	3.0	0.8	68	105	0	83
lake trout	3½ oz.	19.9	4.2	74	241	0	82
lobster, northern							
broiled w/fat	12 oz.	24.0	NA	NA	308	0	NA
cooked	3½ oz.	1.9	0.1	65	91	0	325
mackerel							
Atlantic	3½ oz.	12.2	2.9	65	191	0	80
Pacific	3½ oz.	7.3	2.2	50	159	0	80
muskekunge ("muskie," "skie")	3½ oz.	2.5	0.6	70	109	0	75
mussels							
canned	3½ oz.	3.3	NA	NA	114	0	NA
meat only	3½ oz.	2.2	0.7	30	95	0	250
ocean perch							
cooked	3½ oz.	1.2	0.5	40	88	0	70
fried	3½ oz.	13.3	NA	NA	227	0	NA
octopus	3½ oz.	0.8	0.3	48	73	0	NA
oysters							
canned	3½ oz.	2.2	0.8	54	76	0	100
fried	3½ oz.	13.9	3.2	83	239	0	426

Item	Serving	Total Fat (grams)	Saturated Fat (grams)	Cholesterol (mg)	Calories	Fiber (grams)	Sodium (mg)
oysters *(cont.)*							
raw	5–8 medium	1.8	0.6	54	66	0	110
scalloped	6 medium	18.0	NA	NA	356	0	NA
perch, freshwater, yellow	3$^1/_2$ oz.	0.9	0.4	80	91	0	58
pickerel	3$^1/_2$ oz.	0.5	0.1	NA	84	0	NA
pike							
blue	3$^1/_2$ oz.	0.9	0.5	75	90	0	45
northern	3$^1/_2$ oz.	1.1	0.7	40	88	0	40
walleye	3$^1/_2$ oz.	1.2	1.0	80	93	0	50
pollock, Atlantic	3$^1/_2$ oz.	1.0	0.2	70	91	0	85
pompano	3$^1/_2$ oz.	9.5	5.0	55	166	0	65
red snapper	3$^1/_2$ oz.	1.9	0.5	35	93	0	60
rockfish, oven steamed	3$^1/_2$ oz.	2.5	0.8	40	107	0	70
roughy, orange	3$^1/_2$ oz.	7.0	0.1	20	124	0	63
salmon							
Atlantic	3$^1/_2$ oz.	6.3	0.9	55	141	0	43
broiled/baked	3$^1/_2$ oz.	7.4	2.0	50	182	0	60
chinook, canned	3$^1/_2$ oz.	14.0	2.0	60	210	0	800
pink, canned	3$^1/_2$ oz.	5.1	1.3	54	118	0	471
smoked	3$^1/_2$ oz.	9.3	1.0	35	176	0	900
sardines							
Atlantic, in soy oil	2 sardines	2.8	0.4	34	50	0	121
Pacific	3$^1/_2$ oz.	8.6	2.5	50	160	0	310
scallops							
cooked	3$^1/_2$ oz.	1.2	0.2	30	81	0	140
frzn, fried	3$^1/_2$ oz.	10.5	2.3	55	194	0	417
steamed	3$^1/_2$ oz.	1.4	0.2	40	112	0	260
sea bass, white	3$^1/_2$ oz.	1.5	0.6	40	96	0	65
shrimp							
canned, dry pack	3$^1/_2$ oz.	1.6	0.5	155	116	0	150
canned, wet pack	$^1/_2$ cup	0.8	0.3	125	87	0	1956
fried	3$^1/_2$ oz.	10.8	0.9	120	225	0	186
raw or boiled	3$^1/_2$ oz.	1.8	0.7	139	91	0	130
smelt, canned	4–5 medium	13.5	NA	NA	200	0	NA
sole, fillet	3$^1/_2$ oz.	0.5	0.2	30	68	0	160
squid							
fried	3 oz.	6.4	NA	NA	149	0	NA
raw	3 oz.	1.2	0.4	261	110	0	49
surimi	3$^1/_2$ oz.	0.9	0.2	30	98	0	142
sushi or sashimi	3$^1/_2$ oz.	4.9	1.3	38	144	0	38
swordfish	3$^1/_2$ oz.	4.0	1.1	43	118	0	96
trout							
brook	3$^1/_2$ oz.	2.1	0.9	53	101	0	25
rainbow	3$^1/_2$ oz.	11.4	1.2	96	195	0	46
tuna							
albacore, raw	3$^1/_2$ oz.	7.5	0.2	70	177	0	542
bluefin, raw	3$^1/_2$ oz.	4.1	1.3	37	145	0	39
canned, flaked in oil	6$^1/_4$ oz.	29.0	2.1	62	440	0	646
canned, light in oil	6$^1/_2$ oz.	22.1	2.8	35	386	0	650
canned, light in water	6$^1/_2$ oz.	1.7	0.7	70	204	0	950
canned, white in oil	6$^1/_2$ oz.	19.9	2.5	58	381	0	837
canned, white in water	6$^1/_2$ oz.	3.5	1.5	80	237	0	700
yellowfin, raw	3$^1/_2$ oz.	3.0	0.5	57	133	0	41
white perch	3$^1/_2$ oz.	3.9	0.7	65	114	0	45
yellowtail	3$^1/_2$ oz.	5.4	0.9	75	138	0	46

FRUIT

Item	Serving	Total Fat (grams)	Saturated Fat (grams)	Cholesterol (mg)	Calories	Fiber (grams)	Sodium (mg)
apple							
dried	1/2 cup	0.1	0	0	155	5	56
whole w/peel	1 medium	0.4	0.1	0	81	4	1
applesauce, unsweetened	1/2 cup	0.1	0	0	53	2	0
apricots							
dried	5 halves	0.3	0	0	83	6	3
fresh	3 medium	0.4	0	0	51	2	1
avocado							
California	1 (6 oz.)	30.0	4.5	0	306	4	21
Florida	1 (11 oz.)	27.0	5.3	0	339	4	14
banana	1 medium	0.6	0.2	0	105	2	1
blackberries							
fresh	1 cup	0.5	0	0	74	7	0
frzn, unsweetened	1 cup	0.7	0	0	97	7	0
blueberries							
fresh	1 cup	0.6	0	0	82	5	9
frzn, unsweetened	1 cup	0.7	0.2	0	80	4	1
boysenberries, frzn,							
unsweetened	1 cup	0.3	0	0	66	6	2
breadfruit, fresh	1/4 small	0.2	0	0	99	3	2
cantaloupe	1 cup	0.4	0	0	57	3	14
cherries							
maraschino	1/4 cup	0.1	0	0	56	1	2
sour, canned in heavy							
syrup	1/2 cup	0.4	0	0	116	1	9
sweet	1/2 cup	0.7	0.1	0	49	2	0
cranberries, fresh	1 cup	0.2	0	0	46	4	1
cranberry sauce	1/2 cup	0.2	0	0	209	1	40
cranberry-orange							
relish	1/2 cup	0.9	0	0	246	3	44
dates, whole, dried	1/2 cup	0.4	0	0	228	8	2
figs							
canned	3 figs	0.1	0	0	75	9	1
dried, uncooked	10 figs	1.0	0.4	0	477	16	20
fresh	1 medium	0.2	0	0	37	2	1
fruit cocktail, canned							
w/juice	1 cup	0.3	0	0	112	5	8
fruit roll-up	1	0	0	0	50	0	7
grapefruit	1/2 medium	0.1	0	0	39	1	0
grapes, Thompson							
seedless	1/2 cup	0.3	0	0	94	1	7
guava, fresh	1 medium	0.5	0.2	0	45	7	2
honeydew melon, fresh	1/4 small	0.3	0	0	33	1	12
kiwi, fresh	1 medium	0.3	0	0	46	2	4
kumquat, fresh	1 medium	0	0	0	12	1	1
lemon, fresh	1 medium	0.2	0	0	17	1	1
lime, fresh	1 medium	0.1	0	0	20	1	1
mango, fresh	1 medium	0.6	0.1	0	135	4	4
mandarin oranges, canned							
w/juice	1/2 cup	0.1	0	0	46	4	7
melon balls, frzn	1 cup	0.4	0	0	55	2	53
mixed fruit							
dried	1/2 cup	0.5	0	0	243	6	18
frzn, sweetened	1 cup	0.5	0.2	0	245	2	8
mulberries, fresh	1 cup	0.6	0	0	61	3	14
nectarine, fresh	1 medium	0.6	0	0	67	2	0

Item	Serving	Total Fat (grams)	Saturated Fat (grams)	Cholesterol (mg)	Calories	Fiber (grams)	Sodium (mg)
orange							
naval, fresh	1 medium	0.2	0	0	65	4	1
Valencia, fresh	1 medium	0.4	0	0	59	4	0
papaya, fresh	1 medium	0.4	0.1	0	117	3	8
passionfruit, purple, fresh	1 medium	0.1	0	0	18	3	5
peach							
canned in heavy syrup	1 cup	0.3	0	0	190	4	16
canned in light syrup	1 cup	0.2	0	0	136	4	13
canned, water pack	1 cup	0.1	0	0	58	4	8
fresh	1 medium	0.1	0	0	37	1	0
frzn, sweetened	1 cup	0.3	0	0	235	4	16
pear							
canned in heavy syrup	1 cup	0.3	0	0	188	6	13
canned in light syrup	1 cup	0.1	0	0	144	6	13
fresh	1 medium	0.7	0	0	98	5	1
persimmon, fresh	1 medium	0.1	0	0	32	3	0
pineapple pieces							
canned, unsweetened	1 cup	0.2	0	0	150	2	4
fresh	1 cup	0.7	0	0	77	3	1
plantain, cooked, sliced	1 cup	0.3	0	0	179	1	8
plum							
canned in heavy syrup	½ cup	0.1	0	0	119	4	26
fresh	1 medium	0.6	0	0	36	3	0
pomegranate, fresh	1 medium	0.5	0	0	104	2	5
prickly pear, fresh	1 medium	0.5	0	0	42	3	6
prunes, dried, cooked	½ cup	0.2	0	0	113	10	2
raisins							
dark seedless	¼ cup	0.2	0.1	0	112	3	8
golden seedless	¼ cup	0.2	0.1	0	113	3	4
raspberries							
fresh	1 cup	0.2	0	0	61	6	0
frzn, sweetened	1 cup	0.4	0	0	103	12	1
rhubarb, stewed, unsweetened	1 cup	0	0	0	12	6	5
strawberries							
fresh	1 cup	0.2	0	0	45	3	2
frzn, sweetened	1 cup	0.3	0	0	245	3	3
frzn, unsweetened	1 cup	0.2	0	0	52	3	8
sugar apples, fresh	1 medium	0.5	0	0	146	4	15
tangelo, fresh	1 medium	0.1	0	0	39	3	1
tangerine, fresh	1 medium	0.2	0	0	37	3	1
watermelon, fresh	1 cup	0.2	0	0	50	1	3
FRUIT JUICES AND NECTARS							
apple juice	1 cup	0.3	0	0	116	1	7
apricot nectar	1 cup	0.2	0	0	141	1	9
carrot juice	1 cup	0.2	0	0	96	1	65
cranberry juice cocktail							
low cal	1 cup	0	0	0	45	0	3
regular	1 cup	0.1	0	0	147	0	4
cranberry-apple juice	1 cup	0.2	0.2	0	129	1	5
grape juice	1 cup	0.2	0.1	0	155	1	7
grapefruit juice	1 cup	0.3	0	0	96	0	2
lemon juice	2 T	0	0	0	8	0	0
lime juice	2 T	0	0	0	8	0	0
orange juice	1 cup	0.5	0.1	0	111	1	2

Item	Serving	Total Fat (grams)	Saturated Fat (grams)	Cholesterol (mg)	Calories	Fiber (grams)	Sodium (mg)
orange-grapefruit juice	1 cup	0.2	0	0	107	1	8
peach juice or nectar	1 cup	0.1	0	0	134	1	17
pear juice or nectar	1 cup	0	0	0	149	1	9
pineapple juice	1 cup	0.2	0	0	139	1	2
pineapple-orange juice	1 cup	0.1	0	0	125	1	26
prune juice	1 cup	0.1	0	0	181	1	11
tomato juice	1 cup	0.2	0	0	41	2	675
V8 juice	1 cup	0.1	0	0	53	2	600

GRAVIES, SAUCES, AND DIPS

Item	Serving	Total Fat (grams)	Saturated Fat (grams)	Cholesterol (mg)	Calories	Fiber (grams)	Sodium (mg)
au jus, mix	1/2 cup	0.3	0.2	0	24	0	289
barbecue sauce	1 T	0.3	0	0	12	0	127
béarnaise sauce, mix	1/4 pkg.	25.6	15.7	71	263	0	474
beef gravy, canned	1/2 can	3.4	1.7	4	77	0	73
brown gravy							
from mix	1/2 cup	0.1	0	0	4	0	66
hmde	1/4 cup	14.0	NA	NA	164	0	NA
catsup, tomato	1 T	0.1	0	0	16	0	156
chicken gravy							
canned	1/2 can	8.5	2.1	3	118	0	859
from mix	1/2 cup	0.9	0.2	1	41	0	566
giblet from can	1/4 cup	2.0	NA	NA	35	0	320
chili sauce	1 T	0	0	0	16	0	191
dip made with sour cream	2 T	4.8	2.5	8	53	0	300
enchilada dip, Frito's	1 oz.	1.2	NA	1	35	0	NA
guacamole dip	1 oz.	12.0	NA	14	108	0	370
hollandaise sauce	1/4 cup	18.5	5.6	160	180	0	332
home-style gravy, from mix	1/4 cup	0.5	0.1	1	25	0	374
jalapeño dip	1 oz.	1.1	0.4	60	33	0	120
mushroom gravy							
canned	1/2 can	4.0	0.6	0	75	0	849
from mix	1/2 cup	0.4	0.2	0	35	0	701
mushroom sauce, from mix	1/4 pkg.	3.2	1.7	11	71	0	479
mustard							
brown	1 T	0.9	0	0	14	0	200
yellow	1 T	0.7	0	0	11	0	194
onion dip	2 T	4.0	NA	0	60	0	260
onion gravy, from mix	1/2 cup	0.3	0.2	0	40	0	518
pesto sauce, commercial	1 oz.	14.6	NA	NA	155	0	244
picante sauce	6 T	0.6	0	0	48	1	480
pork gravy, from mix	1/2 cup	0.9	0.4	1	38	0	617
sour-cream sauce	1/4 cup	11.9	NA	28	124	0	126
soy sauce	1 T	0	0	0	11	0	1029
soy sauce, reduced sodium	1 T	0	0	0	11	0	600
spaghetti sauce							
canned, w/o meat	1/2 cup	6.0	0.8	0	136	2	615
hmde, w/meat	1/2 cup	18.7	6.9	32	243	1	505
Prego	1/2 cup	5.6	NA	NA	136	NA	670
Prego w/meat flavor	1/2 cup	5.8	NA	NA	142	NA	680
spinach dip (sour cream & mayo)	2 T	7.1	1.8	10	74	1	138
steak sauce							
A-1	1 T	0	0	0	12	0	400
others	1 T	0	0	0	18	0	405
stroganoff sauce, mix	1/4 pkg.	2.9	1.8	10	73	0	493
sweet & sour sauce	1/4 cup	0.2	0	0	131	0	40

Item	Serving	Total Fat (grams)	Saturated Fat (grams)	Cholesterol (mg)	Calories	Fiber (grams)	Sodium (mg)
tabasco sauce	1 t	0	0	0	1	0	NA
taco sauce	1 T	0	0	0	1	0	52
tartar sauce	1 T	7.9	0	0	70	0	75
teriyaki sauce	1 T	0	0	0	15	0	690
turkey gravy							
canned	½ can	3.1	0.9	3	76	0	868
from mix	½ cup	0.9	0.3	1	43	0	749
white sauce							
thin	2 T	2.6	0.9	4	37	0	100
medium	2 T	4.1	1.8	5	54	1	106
thick	2 T	5.2	2.3	7	65	0	111
Worcestershire sauce	1 T	0	0	0	12	0	244

MEATS (all cooked w/o added fat unless otherwise noted)

Item	Serving	Total Fat (grams)	Saturated Fat (grams)	Cholesterol (mg)	Calories	Fiber (grams)	Sodium (mg)
beef, extra lean							
7.5–12.4% fat	3½ oz.	9.3	3.7	75	205	0	67
arm/blade, lean pot							
roast	3½ oz.	9.4	3.5	95	207	0	60
club steak, lean	3½ oz.	12.9	6.1	90	240	0	60
flank steak, fat trimmed	3½ oz.	8.0	2.9	82	193	0	63
hindshank, lean	3½ oz.	9.4	4.0	76	207	0	70
porterhouse steak, lean	3½ oz.	10.4	5.3	90	225	0	60
rib steak, lean	3½ oz.	9.4	5.0	80	207	0	70
round							
bottom, lean	3½ oz.	9.4	3.4	96	207	0	51
eye of round, lean	3½ oz.	4.2	1.5	52	130	0	60
roasted	3½ oz.	7.4	2.7	81	189	0	64
rump, lean, pot-roasted	3½ oz.	7.0	2.5	60	179	0	61
top, lean	3½ oz.	6.4	2.2	89	211	0	60
short plate, sep. lean only	3½ oz.	10.4	5.3	90	225	0	60
sirloin steak, lean	3½ oz.	8.9	3.6	76	201	0	67
sirloin steak, lean & fat	3½ oz.	18.7	7.7	78	278	0	63
sirloin tip, lean, roasted	3½ oz.	9.4	3.9	90	207	0	62
tenderloin, lean, broiled	3½ oz.	11.1	4.2	83	219	0	60
top sirloin, lean, broiled	3½ oz.	7.9	3.1	89	201	0	60
beef, lean							
12.5–17.4% fat	3½ oz.	15.2	3.2	85	264	0	45
chuck, separable lean	3½ oz.	15.2	6.2	105	268	0	70
cubed steak	3½ oz.	15.4	3.3	85	264	0	45
hamburger							
extra lean	3 oz.	13.9	6.3	82	253	0	49
lean	3 oz.	15.7	7.2	78	268	0	56
rib roast, lean	3½ oz.	15.2	5.5	85	264	0	75
sirloin tips, roasted	3½ oz.	15.2	3.2	85	264	0	50
stew meat, round, raw	4 oz.	15.3	3.2	85	294	0	50
T-bone, lean only	3½ oz.	10.3	4.2	80	212	0	66
tenderloin, marbled	3½ oz.	15.2	7.0	86	264	0	61
beef, regular							
17.5–22.4% fat	3½ oz.	19.4	8.1	78	284	0	63
chuck, ground	3½ oz.	23.9	9.6	100	327	0	65
hamburger, regular	3 oz.	19.6	8.2	87	286	0	60
meatballs	1 oz.	5.5	2.0	30	78	0	94
porterhouse steak, lean &							
marbled	3½ oz.	19.6	8.2	80	286	0	60
rib steak	3½ oz.	14.7	6.0	81	286	0	62
rump, pot-roasted	3½ oz.	19.6	8.2	80	286	0	60
short ribs, lean	3½ oz.	19.6	8.2	80	286	0	60
sirloin, broiled	3½ oz.	18.7	7.7	78	278	0	63

Item	Serving	Total Fat (grams)	Saturated Fat (grams)	Cholesterol (mg)	Calories	Fiber (grams)	Sodium (mg)
beef, high fat							
22.5–27.4% fat	3½ oz.	26.5	9.3	84	354	0	50
arm/blade, pot-roasted	3½ oz.	26.5	9.3	84	354	0	50
sirloin, ground	3½ oz.	26.5	9.3	84	354	0	50
T-bone, broiled	3½ oz.	26.5	10.5	90	354	0	65
beef, highest fat							
27.5–32% fat	3½ oz.	30.0	12.0	85	367	0	55
brisket, lean & marbled	3½ oz.	30.0	12.0	85	367	0	55
chuck, stew meat	3 oz.	30.0	12.0	85	367	0	55
corned, medium fat	3½ oz.	30.2	14.9	75	372	0	1726
rib roast	3½ oz.	30.0	12.0	85	367	0	55
ribeye steak, marbled	3½ oz.	38.8	18.2	90	440	0	60
short ribs	3½ oz.	31.7	10.5	90	382	0	55
steak, chicken fried	3½ oz.	30.0	7.0	120	389	0	370
lamb							
blade chop							
lean	1 chop	6.4	2.7	50	128	0	46
lean & marbled	3½ oz.	26.1	14.8	95	380	0	65
leg							
lean	3½ oz.	8.1	3.4	100	180	0	60
lean & marbled	3½ oz.	14.5	9.0	97	242	0	52
loin chop							
lean	3½ oz.	8.1	4.2	80	180	0	68
lean & marbled	3½ oz.	22.5	11.7	58	302	0	38
rib chop							
lean	3½ oz.	8.1	5.0	50	180	0	60
lean & marbled	3½ oz.	21.2	13.0	70	292	0	30
shoulder							
lean	3½ oz.	9.9	5.3	100	248	0	70
lean & marbled	3½ oz.	27.0	14.9	97	430	0	70
miscellaneous meats							
bacon substitute							
(breakfast strip)	2 strips	4.0	0.8	0	50	0	234
beefalo	3½ oz.	6.3	2.7	58	188	0	82
frog legs							
cooked	4 large	0.3	NA	57	73	0	NA
flour coated & fried	6 large	28.6	NA	NA	418	0	NA
rabbit, stewed	3½ oz.	10.1	2.0	60	216	0	35
venison, roasted	3½ oz.	2.5	1.2	111	157	0	54
organ meats							
brains, all kinds, raw	3 oz.	7.4	NA	1701	106	0	106
heart							
beef, lean, braised	3½ oz.	5.7	2.0	195	188	0	65
calf, braised	3½ oz.	9.1	NA	NA	208	0	112
hog, braised	3½ oz.	6.9	1.7	285	195	0	46
kidney, beef, braised	3½ oz.	3.4	1.1	387	144	0	134
liver							
beef, braised	3½ oz.	3.8	1.9	400	140	0	70
beef, pan fried	3½ oz.	10.6	2.8	482	229	0	106
calf, braised	3½ oz.	4.7	2.1	450	140	0	45
calf, pan fried	3½ oz.	13.2	3.4	530	261	0	82
tongue							
beef, etc., pickled	1 oz.	5.7	NA	NA	75	0	NA
beef, etc., potted	1 oz.	6.4	1.5	32	81	0	20
beef, med. fat,							
braised	3½ oz.	16.7	NA	NA	244	0	60
pork							
bacon							

Item	Serving	Total Fat (grams)	Saturated Fat (grams)	Cholesterol (mg)	Calories	Fiber (grams)	Sodium (mg)
pork *(cont.)*							
cured, broiled	1 slice	3.1	1.1	5	35	0	101
cured, raw	1 slice	16.2	4.8	15	156	0	152
bacon bits	1 T	1.0	NA	6	20	0	181
blade							
lean	3 1/2 oz.	9.6	6.1	116	219	0	70
lean, marbled	3 1/2 oz.	18.0	8.4	67	290	0	70
Boston butt							
lean	3 1/2 oz.	14.2	5.3	89	304	0	65
lean & marbled	3 1/2 oz.	28.0	9.6	88	348	0	65
Canadian bacon,							
broiled	1 oz.	1.8	0.6	14	43	0	360
ham							
cured, butt, lean	3 1/2 oz.	4.5	1.5	38	159	0	1255
cured, butt, lean &							
marbled	3 1/2 oz.	13.0	4.0	60	246	0	900
cured, canned	3 oz.	5.0	1.5	38	120	0	1255
cured, shank, lean	3 1/2 oz.	6.3	3.0	59	176	0	1100
cured, shank, lean &							
marbled	2 slices	13.8	5.0	60	255	0	900
fresh, lean	3 1/2 oz.	6.4	1.5	40	222	0	65
fresh, lean, marbled &							
fat	3 1/2 oz.	18.3	6.5	85	306	0	65
ham loaf, glazed	3 1/2 oz.	14.7	6.0	116	247	0	811
smoked	3 1/2 oz.	11.0	4.3	51	175	0	800
smoked, 95% lean	3 1/2 oz.	5.5	1.8	53	144	0	800
loin chop							
lean	1 chop	7.7	3.0	55	170	0	40
lean & fat	1 chop	22.5	8.8	90	314	0	63
picnic							
cured, lean	3 1/2 oz.	9.9	4.4	88	211	0	920
fresh, lean	3 1/2 oz.	7.4	3.2	75	150	0	65
shoulder, lean	2 slices	5.4	3.0	70	162	0	50
shoulder, marbled	2 slices	14.3	6.0	60	234	0	30
pig's feet, pickled	1 oz.	4.1	1.3	30	56	0	261
rib chop, trimmed	3 1/2 oz.	9.9	3.5	81	209	0	67
rib roast, trimmed	3 1/2 oz.	10.0	3.6	83	204	0	65
sausage							
brown and serve	1 oz.	9.4	3.1	24	105	0	366
regular link	1/2 oz.	4.7	1.6	15	52	0	170
patty	1	8.4	2.9	22	100	0	349
sirloin, lean, roasted	3 1/2 oz.	10.2	3.6	85	207	0	70
spareribs, roasted	6 medium	35.0	11.8	121	396	0	93
tenderloin, lean, roast	3 1/2 oz.	4.8	1.6	78	155	0	66
top loin chop, trimmed	3 1/2 oz.	7.7	2.7	79	193	0	65
top loin roast, trimmed	3 1/2 oz.	7.5	2.8	77	187	0	65
processed meats							
bacon substitute (breakfast							
strips)	2 strips	4.0	0.8	0	50	0	234
beef breakfast strips	2 strips	7.2	NA	26	114	0	380
beef jerky	1 oz.	4.0	2.4	30	109	0	280
beef, chipped	2 slices	3.6	1.0	24	114	0	1969
bologna, beef/beef &							
pork	1 oz.	8.0	3.0	15	85	0	200
bratwurst							
pork	2-oz. link	22.0	7.9	51	256	0	473
pork & beef	2-oz. link	19.5	7.0	44	226	0	778

Item	Serving	Total Fat (grams)	Saturated Fat (grams)	Cholesterol (mg)	Calories	Fiber (grams)	Sodium (mg)
processed meats *(cont.)*							
braunshweiger							
(pork liver sausage)	1 oz.	7.8	7.9	28	65	0	473
chicken roll	1 oz.	1.3	0.8	10	30	0	112
corn dog	1	20.0	NA	0	330	0	310
corned beef, jellied	1 oz.	2.9	1.0	3	31	0	150
ham, chopped	1 oz.	2.3	0.8	17	55	0	625
hot dog							
beef	1	13.2	8.8	27	145	0	504
chicken	1	8.8	2.5	45	116	0	616
turkey	1	8.1	2.7	39	102	0	454
kielbasa (Polish sausage)	1 oz.	8.3	2.0	10	80	0	305
knockwurst/knackwurst	2-oz. link	18.9	3.2	36	209	0	560
liver pâté, goose	1 oz.	12.4	3.3	43	131	0	192
pepperoni	1 oz.	13.0	5.4	NA	148	0	600
pork & beef	1 oz.	9.1	3.3	15	100	0	367
salami							
cooked	1 oz.	10.0	6.6	30	116	0	490
dry/hard	1 oz.	10.0	3.0	16	126	0	400
sausage							
Italian	2-oz. link	17.2	6.1	52	216	0	618
Polish	1-oz. link	8.1	2.9	20	92	0	248
smoked	2-oz. link	20.0	9.2	48	229	0	642
Vienna	1 sausage	4.0	1.5	8	45	0	152
Spam	1 oz.	7.4	NA	NA	87	0	432
turkey loaf	1 oz.	2.7	0.8	14	43	0	278
turkey breast	1 oz.	1.5	0.6	12	51	0	21
turkey ham	1 oz.	1.5	0.5	18	36	0	278
turkey pastrami	1 oz.	1.8	0.3	15	40	0	270
turkey roll	1 oz.	4.5	1.1	24	72	0	277
turkey salami	1 oz.	3.7	1.1	23	55	0	266
veal							
arm steak							
lean	3 1/2 oz.	4.8	3.0	78	180	0	70
lean & fat	3 1/2 oz.	19.0	9.0	80	298	0	75
blade							
lean	3 1/2 oz.	8.4	3.5	100	228	0	80
lean & fat	3 1/2 oz.	16.6	7.0	100	276	0	80
breast, stewed	3 1/2 oz.	18.6	8.7	100	256	0	70
chuck, med. fat, braised	3 1/2 oz.	12.8	6.0	101	235	0	80
cutlet							
breaded	3 1/2 oz.	15.0	NA	NA	319	0	NA
round, lean	3 1/2 oz.	12.8	5.2	102	194	0	90
round, lean & fat	3 1/2 oz.	15.0	6.8	101	277	0	90
flank, med. fat, stewed	3 1/2 oz.	32.0	15.8	101	390	0	80
foreshank, med. fat, stewed	3 1/2 oz.	10.4	5.3	101	216	0	80
loin, med. fat, broiled	3 1/2 oz.	13.4	5.4	109	234	0	91
loin chop							
lean	1 chop	4.8	3.0	95	149	0	65
lean & fat	3 1/2 oz.	13.3	7.0	101	250	0	80
plate, med. fat, stewed	3 1/2 oz.	21.2	10.5	101	303	0	80
rib chop							
lean	1 chop	4.6	3.0	100	125	0	65
lean & fat	1 chop	18.4	6.0	100	264	0	65
rump, marbled, roasted	3 1/2 oz.	11.0	6.1	101	225	0	80

Item	Serving	Total Fat (grams)	Saturated Fat (grams)	Cholesterol (mg)	Calories	Fiber (grams)	Sodium (mg)
sirloin							
lean, roasted	3½ oz.	3.4	1.9	90	175	0	80
marbled, roasted	3½ oz.	6.5	2.9	108	181	0	90
sirloin steak							
lean	3½ oz.	6.0	2.3	108	204	0	90
lean & fat	3½ oz.	20.4	9.1	100	305	0	86
MILK AND YOGURT							
buttermilk							
1% fat	1 cup	2.2	1.3	9	99	0	257
dry	1 T	0.4	0.2	5	25	0	103
choc. milk							
2% fat	1 cup	5.0	3.1	17	179	0	150
whole	1 cup	8.5	5.3	30	250	0	149
condensed milk, sweetened	½ cup	14.0	2.1	13	123	0	49
evaporated milk							
skim	½ cup	0.4	0	0	97	0	15
whole	½ cup	10.0	4.5	27	126	0	99
hot cocoa							
w/skim milk	1 cup	2.0	0.9	12	158	0	135
w/whole milk	1 cup	9.1	5.6	33	218	0	123
mix w/water	1 cup	3.0	0.7	5	110	0	149
low cal, mix w/water	1 cup	0.8	0.4	2	50	0	231
low fat milk							
1% fat	1 cup	2.6	1.6	10	102	0	123
2% fat	1 cup	4.7	2.2	18	121	0	122
malt powder	1 T	1.6	0.9	4	86	0	103
malted milk	1 cup	9.9	6.0	37	236	0	223
milkshake							
choc., thick	1 cup	17.2	5.0	32	341	1	333
soft serve	1 cup	7.0	2.3	35	218	1	240
vanilla, thick	1 cup	14.7	5.9	37	274	0	299
Ovaltine, w/1% milk	1 cup	2.8	1.1	33	173	0	201
skim milk							
liquid	1 cup	0.4	0.3	4	86	0	126
nonfat dry powder	¼ cup	0.2	0.2	6	109	0	161
whole milk							
3.5% fat	1 cup	8.0	4.9	34	150	0	122
dry powder	¼ cup	8.6	5.4	31	159	0	119
yogurt							
coffee/vanilla, low fat	1 cup	2.8	1.8	11	194	0	149
frzn, low fat	½ cup	3.0	2.0	10	115	0	55
frzn, nonfat	½ cup	0.2	0	0	81	0	39
fruit flavored, low fat	1 cup	2.6	0.1	10	225	0	121
plain							
low fat	1 cup	3.5	2.3	14	144	0	159
skim (nonfat)	1 cup	0.4	0.3	4	127	0	174
whole milk	1 cup	7.4	4.8	29	139	0	105
MISCELLANEOUS							
Bac o Bits, General Mills	1 T	1.3	NA	0	33	0	130
baking powder	1 t	0	0	0	3	0	426
baking soda	1 t	0	0	0	0	0	821
bouillon cube, beef or chicken	1	0.2	0.1	0	8	0	900
chewing gum	1 stick	0	0	0	10	0	0
choc., baking	1 oz.	15.0	8.9	0	143	1	1
cocoa, dry	⅓ cup	3.6	2.2	0	115	2	2

Item	Serving	Total Fat (grams)	Saturated Fat (grams)	Cholesterol (mg)	Calories	Fiber (grams)	Sodium (mg)
gelatin, dry	1 pkg.	0	0	0	23	0	0
honey	1 T	0	0	0	64	0	1
horseradish, prepared	1 t	0	0	0	2	0	7
icing, decorator	1 t	2.0	0.2	0	70	0	11
jam, all varieties	1 T	0	0	0	54	0	2
jelly, all varieties	1 T	0	0	0	49	0	3
marmalade, citrus	1 T	0	0	0	51	0	3
meat tenderizer	1 t	0	0	0	2	0	1760
molasses	1 T	0	0	0	50	0	3
olives							
black	2 large	4.0	0.6	0	37	1	240
Greek	3 medium	7.1	0.8	0	67	1	631
green	2 medium	1.6	0.2	0	15	0	200
pickle relish							
chow chow	1 oz.	0.4	0	0	8	0	400
sweet	1 T	0.1	0	0	21	0	107
pickles							
bread & butter	4 slices	0.1	0	0	18	0	202
dill or sour	1 large	0.2	0	0	11	1	950
Kosher	1 oz.	0.1	0	0	7	0	350
sweet	1 oz.	0.4	0	0	146	0	268
salt	1 t	0	0	0	0	0	2132
Shake & Bake, Gen. Foods	¼ pkg.	2.6	1.0	0	69	0	600
spices/seasonings	1 t	0.2	0	0	5	0	0
sugar substitutes	1 packet	0	0	0	4	0	0
sugar, all varieties	1 T	0	0	0	46	0	0
syrup, all varieties	1 T	0	0	0	60	0	0
vinegar	1 T	0	0	0	2	0	0
yeast	1 T	0.1	0	0	23	0	10
NUTS AND SEEDS							
almond paste	1 T	4.5	0.5	0	80	1	2
almonds	12–15	9.3	1.0	0	104	1	0
Brazil nuts	4 medium	11.5	2.3	0	114	1	0
cashews, roasted	6–8	7.8	1.3	0	94	2	2
chestnuts, fresh	3 small	0.8	0	0	66	4	1
coconut, dried, shredded	⅓ cup	9.2	10.0	0	135	1	6
hazelnuts (filberts)	10–12	10.6	1.0	0	106	1	0
macadamia nuts, roasted	6 medium	12.3	2.0	0	117	1	0
mixed nuts							
w/peanuts	8–12	10.0	1.5	0	109	2	2
w/o peanuts	2 T	10.1	2.0	0	110	2	2
peanut butter, creamy or chunky	1 T	8.0	1.5	0	94	1	75
peanuts							
chopped	2 T	8.9	1.0	0	104	2	3
honey roasted	2 T	8.9	1.5	0	112	2	150
in shell	1 cup	17.7	2.0	0	209	3	156
pecans	2 T	9.1	0.5	0	90	1	0
pine nuts (pignolia)	2 T	9.1	1.5	0	85	2	0
pistachios	2 T	7.7	0.8	0	92	1	1
poppy seeds	1 T	3.8	0.3	0	44	1	3
pumpkin	2 T	7.9	3.0	0	93	1	4
sesame nut mix	2 T	5.1	1.5	0	65	1	165
sesame seeds	2 T	8.8	1.2	0	94	1	6
sunflower seeds	2 T	8.9	1.0	0	102	1	1

Item	Serving	Total Fat (grams)	Saturated Fat (grams)	Cholesterol (mg)	Calories	Fiber (grams)	Sodium (mg)
trail mix w/seeds, nuts,							
carob	2 T	5.1	0.7	0	87	1	3
walnuts	2 T	7.7	0.3	0	80	1	0

PASTA, NOODLES, AND RICE (all measurements after cooking unless otherwise noted)

Item	Serving	Total Fat (grams)	Saturated Fat (grams)	Cholesterol (mg)	Calories	Fiber (grams)	Sodium (mg)
macaroni							
semolina	1 cup	0.7	0	0	159	1	1
whole wheat	1 cup	0.6	0.1	0	183	5	4
noodles							
Alfredo	1 cup	29.7	9.8	73	462	3	844
almondine, from mix	1/4 pkg.	12.0	NA	NA	240	1	700
cellophane, fried	1 cup	4.2	0.6	0	141	0	6
chow mein, canned	1/2 cup	8.0	1.6	0	153	0	210
egg	1 cup	2.4	0.4	50	200	1	3
manicotti	1 cup	0.4	0.1	0	129	1	1
ramen, all varieties	1 cup	6.5	0.9	0	188	1	978
rice	1 cup	0	0	0	140	1	0
romanoff	1 cup	23.0	11.9	95	372	3	774
rice							
brown	1/2 cup	0.6	0	0	116	2	0
fried	1/2 cup	7.2	0.7	0	181	1	550
long grain & wild	1/2 cup	2.1	0.2	0	120	2	530
pilaf	1/2 cup	7.0	0.6	0	170	1	600
Spanish style	1/2 cup	2.1	0.1	0	106	1	547
white	1/2 cup	1.2	0	0	111	0	0
spaghetti, enriched	1 cup	1.0	0	0	159	1	1

POULTRY

Item	Serving	Total Fat (grams)	Saturated Fat (grams)	Cholesterol (mg)	Calories	Fiber (grams)	Sodium (mg)
chicken							
breast							
w/skin, fried	1/2 breast	10.7	3.0	87	236	0	77
w/o skin, fried	1/2 breast	6.1	1.5	90	179	0	81
w/skin, roasted	1/2 breast	7.6	2.9	70	193	0	72
w/o skin, roasted	1/2 breast	3.1	1.0	80	142	0	70
fryers							
w/skin, batter dipped, fried	3 1/2 oz.	17.4	3.0	95	289	0	85
w/o skin, fried	3 1/2 oz.	11.1	1.0	70	237	0	60
w/skin, roasted	3 1/2 oz.	13.6	3.5	90	239	0	75
w/o skin, roasted	3 1/2 oz.	7.4	1.9	80	190	0	70
giblets, fried	3 1/2 oz.	13.5	3.8	446	277	0	113
gizzard, simmered	3 1/2 oz.	3.7	1.5	393	153	0	58
heart, simmered	3 1/2 oz.	7.9	1.0	194	185	0	67
leg							
w/skin, fried	1 leg	8.7	4.4	99	120	0	92
w/skin, roasted	1 leg	5.8	4.2	105	112	0	99
w/o skin, roasted	1 leg	2.5	0.7	41	76	0	42
liver, simmered	3 1/2 oz.	5.5	1.8	631	157	0	51
roll, light meat	3 1/2 oz.	7.4	1.2	60	159	0	662
stewers							
w/skin	3 1/2 oz.	18.9	5.1	79	285	0	73
w/o skin	3 1/2 oz.	11.9	3.1	83	237	0	78
thigh							
w/skin, fried	1 thigh	11.3	2.5	60	180	0	55
w/skin, roasted	1 thigh	9.6	2.7	58	153	0	52
w/o skin, roasted	1 thigh	5.7	2.4	75	109	0	95
wing							
w/skin, fried	1 wing	9.1	1.9	26	121	0	25
w/skin, roasted	1 wing	6.6	1.9	29	99	0	28

Item	Serving	Total Fat (grams)	Saturated Fat (grams)	Cholesterol (mg)	Calories	Fiber (grams)	Sodium (mg)
duck							
w/skin, roasted	3½ oz.	28.4	9.7	84	337	0	59
w/o skin, roasted	3½ oz.	11.2	4.2	89	201	0	65
pheasant, w or w/o skin,							
cooked	3½ oz.	9.3	3.0	102	211	0	98
quail, w/o skin, cooked	3½ oz.	9.3	3.0	102	213	0	95
turkey							
breast							
barbecued, Louis Rich	3½ oz.	5.0	1.4	56	135	0	860
oven roasted, Louis Rich	3½ oz.	3.0	1.0	35	115	0	786
smoked, Louis Rich	3½ oz.	4.0	0.7	45	120	0	910
dark meat							
w/skin, roasted	3½ oz.	11.5	3.5	89	221	0	76
w/o skin, roasted	3½ oz.	7.2	2.4	85	187	0	79
ground	3½ oz.	14.0	4.0	85	225	0	105
ham, cured	3½ oz.	5.1	1.7	62	128	0	996
light meat							
w/skin, roasted	3½ oz.	8.3	2.3	76	197	0	63
w/o skin, roasted	3½ oz.	3.2	1.0	69	157	0	64
loaf, breast meat	3½ oz.	1.6	0.5	41	110	0	431
patties, breaded/fried	1 patty	16.9	2.0	30	266	0	500
roll, light meat	3½ oz.	7.2	2.0	43	147	0	489
sausage, cooked	1 oz.	3.4	1.5	23	50	0	200
sliced w/gravy, frzn	5 oz.	3.7	1.2	26	95	0	706
wing drumettes, smoked,							
Louis Rich	3½ oz.	7.0	1.8	70	165	0	60
SALAD DRESSINGS							
blue cheese							
low cal	1 T	0.8	0	2	11	0	174
regular	1 T	8.0	1.4	0	77	0	156
buttermilk, from mix	1 T	5.8	1.0	5	58	0	138
Caesar	1 T	7.0	0.9	13	70	0	100
French							
creamy	1 T	6.9	1.0	0	70	0	185
low cal	1 T	0.9	0.1	1	22	0	128
regular	1 T	6.4	0.8	0	67	0	185
garlic, from mix	1 T	9.2	1.4	0	83	0	173
Green Goddess							
low cal	1 T	2.0	0.4	0	27	0	175
regular	1 T	7.0	1.4	0	68	0	173
honey mustard	1 T	6.6	1.0	0	89	0	32
Italian							
creamy	1 T	4.5	1.4	0	52	0	170
low cal	1 T	1.5	0.1	1	16	0	128
regular zesty, from mix	1 T	9.2	1.4	0	85	0	123
Kraft, free	1 T	0	0	0	20	0	120
Kraft, reduced cal	1 T	1.0	0	0	25	0	120
mayonnaise type							
low cal	1 T	1.8	0.3	2	19	0	112
regular	1 T	4.9	0.7	4	57	0	105
oil & vinegar	1 T	7.5	1.5	0	69	0	0
ranch style, prep. w/mayo	1 T	5.7	0.7	4	54	0	105
Russian							
low cal	1 T	0.7	0.1	1	23	0	141
regular	1 T	7.8	1.1	0	76	0	133
sesame seed	1 T	6.9	0.9	0	68	0	153

Item	Serving	Total Fat (grams)	Saturated Fat (grams)	Cholesterol (mg)	Calories	Fiber (grams)	Sodium (mg)
sweet & sour	1 T	0.9	0.3	0	29	0	32
Thousand Island							
low cal	1 T	1.6	0.2	2	24	0	153
regular	1 T	5.6	0.9	0	59	0	109
SNACK FOODS							
bagel chips or crisps	1 oz.	8.8	1.3	0	149	1	140
Bugles	1 oz.	8.0	NA	NA	150	0	150
Cheese Puff balls, Cheetos	1 oz.	10.6	4.8	14	161	0	343
Cheese Puffs, Cheetos	1 oz.	10.0	4.8	14	159	0	348
cheese straws	4 pieces	7.2	6.4	NA	109	0	433
corn chips, Frito's							
light	1 oz.	9.7	0.2	0	144	0	200
regular	1 oz.	9.7	1.0	0	155	0	233
corn nuts, all flavors	1/2 cup	13.9	6.3	0	420	9	651
Cracker Jacks	1 oz.	1.0	0	0	114	1	85
Doo-Dads, Nabisco	1/2 cup	6.0	NA	NA	140	1	393
Funyuns	1 oz.	6.4	0.8	0	140	0	250
party mix (cereal, pretzels,							
nuts)	1 cup	23.0	2.0	4	312	3	722
popcorn							
air popped	1 cup	0.3	0	0	23	1	0
caramel	1 cup	4.2	1.5	5	140	1	208
microwave, plain	1 cup	3.0	0.7	0	47	1	100
microwave, w/butter	1 cup	4.5	1.8	1	61	1	100
popped w/oil	1 cup	2.0	0.5	0	38	1	86
pork rinds, Frito-Lay	1 oz.	9.3	3.7	24	151	0	570
potato chips							
individually	10 chips	8.0	2.6	0	113	0	133
by weight	1 oz.	11.2	2.9	0	159	1	182
barbecue flavor	1 oz.	9.5	2.6	0	149	1	150
light, Pringles	1 oz.	7.8	2.0	0	144	0	152
regular, Pringles	1 oz.	12.9	2.0	0	171	0	215
potato sticks	1 oz.	10.2	2.5	0	152	0	71
pretzels							
hard	1 oz.	1.0	0.5	0	111	0	451
soft	1	0.5	NA	0	175	NA	NA
tortilla chips							
Doritos	1 oz.	6.6	1.1	0	139	0	140
Tostitos	1 oz.	7.8	1.1	0	145	0	140
SOUPS							
asparagus							
cream of, w/milk	1 cup	8.2	2.1	10	161	1	982
cream of, w/water	1 cup	4.1	1.0	5	87	1	981
bean							
w/bacon	1 cup	5.9	6.0	3	173	4	952
w/franks	1 cup	7.0	2.0	12	187	3	1092
w/ham	1 cup	8.5	2.0	3	231	3	1800
w/o meat	1 cup	3.0	1.5	2	142	5	940
beef							
broth	1 cup	0.5	0.2	1	33	0	642
chunky	1 cup	5.1	2.6	14	171	2	867
beef barley	1 cup	1.1	0.5	6	72	1	871
beef noodle	1 cup	3.1	1.2	5	84	1	952
black bean	1 cup	1.5	1.2	0	116	2	1198
broccoli, creamy							
w/water	1 cup	2.7	1.0	5	69	1	981

Item	Serving	Total Fat (grams)	Saturated Fat (grams)	Cholesterol (mg)	Calories	Fiber (grams)	Sodium (mg)
Campbell's Chunky							
w/meat	1 cup	5.1	2.0	30	170	2	887
w/o meat	1 cup	3.7	0.6	0	122	3	1010
canned vegetable type,							
w/o meat	1 cup	2.0	0.7	0	67	1	500
cheese w/milk	1 cup	14.6	9.1	48	230	0	1020
chicken							
chunky	1 cup	6.6	2.0	30	178	2	887
cream of, w/milk	1 cup	11.5	4.6	27	191	0	1046
cream of, w/water	1 cup	7.4	2.1	10	116	0	986
chicken & dumplings	1 cup	5.5	1.3	34	97	0	861
chicken & stars	1 cup	1.8	0.7	5	55	1	875
chicken & wild rice	1 cup	2.3	0.5	7	76	1	815
chicken/beef noodle or veg.	1 cup	3.1	1.2	5	83	1	952
chicken gumbo	1 cup	1.4	0.3	5	56	1	955
chicken mushroom	1 cup	9.2	2.4	10	150	1	900
chicken noodle							
chunky	1 cup	6.0	1.4	18	116	2	900
w/water	1 cup	2.5	0.7	7	75	0	1107
chicken vegetable							
chunky	1 cup	4.8	1.4	17	167	2	1068
w/water	1 cup	2.8	0.9	10	74	1	944
chicken w/noodles,							
chunky	1 cup	5.0	1.4	19	180	2	850
chicken w/rice							
chunky	1 cup	3.2	NA	NA	127	2	1072
w/water	1 cup	1.9	0.5	7	60	1	814
clam chowder							
Manhattan chunky	1 cup	3.4	2.1	14	133	1	1000
New England	1 cup	6.6	3.6	7	163	1	960
consommé w/gelatin	1 cup	0	0	0	29	0	637
crab	1 cup	1.5	0.4	10	76	1	1234
dehydrated							
asparagus, cream of	1 cup	1.7	0.3	0	59	0	801
bean w/bacon	1 cup	3.5	1.0	3	105	2	928
beef broth cube	1 cube	0.3	0.1	1	6	0	1358
beef noodle	1 cup	0.8	0.3	2	41	0	1041
cauliflower	1 cup	1.7	0.3	0	68	0	843
chicken, cream of	1 cup	5.3	3.4	3	107	1	1184
chicken broth cube	1 cube	0.2	0.1	1	9	0	1484
chicken noodle	1 cup	1.2	0.3	3	53	0	1284
chicken rice	1 cup	1.4	0.3	3	60	0	980
clam chowder							
Manhattan	1 cup	1.6	0.3	0	65	1	1336
New England	1 cup	3.7	0.6	1	95	0	745
minestrone	1 cup	1.7	0.8	3	79	0	1026
mushroom	1 cup	4.9	0.8	1	96	0	1019
onion							
dry mix	1 pkg.	2.3	0.5	2	115	1	3045
prepared	1 cup	0.6	0.1	0	28	0	848
tomato	1 cup	2.4	0.4	1	102	0	943
vegetable beef	1 cup	1.1	0.6	1	53	0	1000
gazpacho	1 cup	0.5	0.3	0	40	2	1183
hmde or restaurant style							
beer cheese	1 cup	23.1	11.4	50	308	1	725
cauliflower, cream of,							
w/whole milk	1 cup	9.7	3.0	20	165	1	800

Item	Serving	Total Fat (grams)	Saturated Fat (grams)	Cholesterol (mg)	Calories	Fiber (grams)	Sodium (mg)
hmde or restaurant style *(cont.)*							
celery, cream of, w/whole milk	1 cup	10.6	4.0	32	165	1	1010
chicken broth	1 cup	1.4	0.4	1	38	0	776
clam chowder							
Manhattan	1 cup	2.2	0.4	2	76	2	1808
New England	1 cup	14.0	3.4	5	271	1	914
corn chowder, traditional	1 cup	12.0	4.9	24	251	3	632
fish chowder, w/whole milk	1 cup	13.5	5.3	37	285	1	710
gazpacho, traditional	1 cup	7.0	0.3	0	100	2	1183
hot & sour	1 cup	7.1	1.7	52	134	1	1209
mock turtle	1 cup	15.5	5.3	456	246	2	939
onion, French w/o cheese	1 cup	5.8	0.7	0	93	0	1053
oyster stew, w/whole milk	1 cup	17.7	2.5	14	268	0	980
seafood gumbo	1 cup	3.9	2.7	40	155	3	230
lentil	1 cup	1.0	0.2	0	161	3	1020
minestrone							
chunky	1 cup	2.8	1.5	5	127	2	864
w/water	1 cup	2.5	0.8	3	83	1	1026
mushroom, cream of							
condensed	1 can	23.1	10.1	30	313	1	2000
w/milk	1 cup	13.6	5.1	20	203	1	1076
w/water	1 cup	9.0	2.4	2	129	1	1031
mushroom barley	1 cup	2.3	NA	0	76	1	800
mushroom w/beef stock	1 cup	4.0	1.6	7	85	1	970
onion	1 cup	1.7	0.3	0	57	1	1053
oyster stew, w/water	1 cup	3.8	2.5	14	59	1	980
pea							
green, w/water	1 cup	2.9	1.4	0	164	2	987
split	1 cup	0.6	0.2	1	58	1	600
split w/ham	1 cup	4.4	1.8	8	189	1	1008
potato, cream of, w/milk	1 cup	7.4	1.2	5	157	2	1000
shrimp, cream of, w/milk	1 cup	9.3	3.2	17	165	1	976
tomato							
w/milk	1 cup	6.0	2.9	17	160	1	932
w/water	1 cup	1.9	0.4	0	100	0.5	872
tomato beef w/noodle	1 cup	4.3	1.6	5	140	1	917
tomato bisque w/milk	1 cup	6.6	0.5	4	198	1	1048
tomato rice	1 cup	2.7	0.5	2	120	1	815
turkey, chunky	1 cup	4.4	1.2	9	136	2	923
turkey noodle	1 cup	2.0	0.6	5	69	1	815
turkey vegetable	1 cup	3.0	0.9	2	74	1	905
vegetable, chunky	1 cup	3.7	0.6	0	122	2	1010
vegetable w/beef, chunky	1 cup	3.0	1.3	8	134	2	1340
vegetable w/beef broth	1 cup	1.9	0.4	2	81	1	810
vegetarian vegetable	1 cup	1.9	0.3	0	72	1	823
wonton	1 cup	2.0	NA	NA	92	1	878
VEGETABLES							
alfalfa sprouts, raw	½ cup	0.1	0	0	5	0	0
artichoke, boiled	1 medium	0.2	0	0	53	3	42
artichoke hearts, boiled	½ cup	0.1	0	0	37	3	55
asparagus, cooked	½ cup	0.3	0.1	0	22	2	4
avocado							
California	1 (6 oz.)	30.0	4.5	0	306	4	21
Florida	1 (11 oz.)	27.0	5.3	0	339	4	14

Item	Serving	Total Fat (grams)	Saturated Fat (grams)	Cholesterol (mg)	Calories	Fiber (grams)	Sodium (mg)
bamboo shoots, raw	½ cup	0.2	0.1	0	21	2	3
beans							
all types, cooked w/o fat	½ cup	0.4	0.2	0	124	9	1
baked, brown sugar & molasses	½ cup	1.5	0.2	0	132	4	516
baked w/pork & tomato sauce	½ cup	1.3	0.5	8	123	5	556
baked, vegetarian	½ cup	0.6	0.3	0	235	5	1008
homestyle, canned	½ cup	1.6	0.3	0	132	5	550
beets, pickled	½ cup	0.1	0	0	75	4	301
black-eyed peas (cowpeas), cooked	½ cup	0.5	0.1	0	99	2	3
broccoli							
cooked	½ cup	0.4	0	0	46	7	16
frzn in butter sauce	½ cup	2.3	NA	NA	51	2	296
frzn w/cheese sauce	½ cup	6.2	1.7	5	116	1	417
frzn, chopped, cooked	½ cup	0.3	0.1	0	25	2	18
raw	½ cup	0.2	0	0	12	1	12
brussels sprouts, cooked	½ cup	0.3	0	0	30	2	17
butter beans, canned	½ cup	0.6	0	0	100	4	434
cabbage							
Chinese, raw	1 cup	0.2	0	0	10	2	23
green, cooked	½ cup	0.2	0	0	16	2	14
red, raw, shredded	½ cup	0.1	0	0	10	2	4
carrot							
cooked	½ cup	0.1	0	0	35	2	52
raw	1 large	0.2	0	0	32	2	25
cauliflower							
cooked	1 cup	0.2	0	0	30	3	4
frzn w/cheese sauce	½ cup	6.1	NA	NA	114	2	446
raw	1 cup	0.2	0	0	12	4	7
celery							
cooked	½ cup	0.1	0	0	11	1	48
raw	1 stalk	0.1	0	0	6	1	35
chard, cooked	½ cup	0.1	0	0	18	2	158
chilies, green	¼ cup	0	0	0	14	0	3
Chinese-style vegetables, frzn	½ cup	4.7	0	0	79	3	120
chives, raw, chopped	1 T	0	0	0	1	0	0
collard greens, cooked	½ cup	0.1	0	0	13	2	36
corn							
cream style, canned	½ cup	0.4	0.1	0	93	4	365
frzn, cooked	½ cup	0.2	0	0	67	4	4
frzn w/butter sauce	½ cup	2.6	NA	NA	105	4	275
whole kernel, cooked	½ cup	1.1	0.2	0	89	5	14
corn on the cob	1 medium	0.9	0.1	0	83	4	4
cucumber							
w/skin	½ medium	0.1	0	0	8	1	1
w/o skin, sliced	½ cup	0.1	0	0	7	0	1
dandelion greens, cooked	½ cup	0.3	0	0	17	2	23
eggplant, cooked	½ cup	0.1	0	0	13	2	1
endive lettuce	1 cup	0.1	0	0	8	1	6
garbanzo beans (chick peas), cooked	½ cup	2.1	0.2	0	134	5	6
green beans							
french style, cooked	½ cup	0.1	0	0	18	2	1
snap, cooked	½ cup	0.1	0	0	22	2	2

Item	Serving	Total Fat (grams)	Saturated Fat (grams)	Cholesterol (mg)	Calories	Fiber (grams)	Sodium (mg)
hominy, white or yellow, cooked	1 cup	0.7	0	0	138	3	708
Italian-style vegetables, frzn	½ cup	7.0	0	0	130	2	489
kale, cooked	½ cup	0.3	0	0	21	2	15
kidney beans, red, cooked	½ cup	0.5	0	0	112	8	2
leeks, chopped, raw	¼ cup	0.1	0	0	16	1	5
lentils, cooked	½ cup	0.4	0	0	116	8	2
lettuce, leaf	1 cup	0.2	0	0	10	1	6
lima beans, cooked	½ cup	0.4	0.1	0	108	5	2
miso (soybean product)	½ cup	8.0	1.2	0	284	4	5032
mushrooms							
canned	½ cup	0.2	0	0	19	1	500
fried/sautéed	4 medium	7.4	NA	NA	78	1	NA
raw	½ cup	0.2	0	0	9	1	0
mustard greens, cooked	½ cup	0.4	0	0	13	2	11
okra, cooked	½ cup	0.1	0	0	25	3	4
onions							
canned, french-fried	1 oz.	15.0	6.9	0	175	0	334
chopped, raw	½ cup	0.2	0	0	27	1	2
parsley, chopped, raw	¼ cup	0	0	0	5	0	12
parsnips, cooked	½ cup	0.2	0	0	63	3	8
peas, green, cooked	½ cup	0.2	0	0	67	4	2
pepper, bell, chopped, raw	½ cup	0.2	0	0	12	2	2
pimientos, canned	1 oz.	0	0	0	10	0	5
potato							
baked w/skin	1 medium	0.2	0.1	0	220	4	16
au gratin							
from mix	½ cup	6.0	3.1	6	140	2	538
hmde	½ cup	9.3	5.8	29	160	1	528
boiled w/o skin	½ cup	0.1	0	0	116	2	7
french fries							
frzn	10 pieces	4.4	2.1	0	111	2	15
hmde	10 pieces	8.3	2.5	0	158	1	108
hash browns	½ cup	10.9	3.4	23	163	2	101
knishes	1	3.2	0.8	15	73	1	83
mashed							
from flakes	½ cup	5.9	3.6	15	118	1	349
w/milk & margarine	½ cup	4.4	1.1	2	111	1	309
pan fried, O'Brien	½ cup	12.1	1.5	7	157	3	421
scalloped							
from mix	1 serving	5.9	3.6	10	127	1	467
hmde	½ cup	4.8	2.8	14	105	1	409
w/cheese	½ cup	9.7	NA	NA	177	1	370
potato pancakes	1 cake	12.6	3.4	93	495	1	388
potato puffs, frzn, prep.							
w/oil	½ cup	11.6	3.2	0	183	3	462
twice-baked potato,							
w/cheese	1 medium	9.9	3.3	10	180	1	55
pumpkin, canned	½ cup	0.3	0.2	0	41	4	6
radish, raw	10	0.2	0	0	7	1	9
rhubarb, raw	1 cup	0.2	0	0	29	2	2
sauerkraut, canned	½ cup	0.2	0	0	22	4	780
scallions, raw	5 medium	0.2	0	0	45	4	1
soybeans, mature, cooked	½ cup	7.7	1.1	0	149	4	0
spinach							
cooked	½ cup	0.2	0.1	0	21	3	29
creamed	½ cup	5.7	0.8	1	89	3	312
raw	1 cup	0.2	0	0	12	3	22

Item	Serving	Total Fat (grams)	Saturated Fat (grams)	Cholesterol (mg)	Calories	Fiber (grams)	Sodium (mg)
squash							
acorn							
baked	1/2 cup	0.1	0	0	57	4	4
mashed w/o fat	1/2 cup	0.2	0	0	41	3	3
butternut, cooked	1/2 cup	0.1	0	0	41	4	4
summer							
cooked	1/2 cup	0.3	0	0	18	2	1
raw, slice	1/2 cup	0.1	0	0	13	1	1
winter, cooked	1/2 cup	0.6	0.1	0	39	4	1
succotash, cooked	1/2 cup	0.8	0.1	0	111	3	16
sweet potato							
baked	1 medium	0.1	0	0	118	7	12
candied	1/2 cup	3.8	1.4	8	192	5	73
mashed w/o fat	1/2 cup	0.5	0	0	172	5	107
tempeh (soybean product)	1/2 cup	6.4	0.9	0	165	1	5
tofu (soybean curd), raw, firm	4 oz.	5.4	0.8	0	86	1	8
tomato							
boiled	1/2 cup	0.3	0	0	30	1	13
raw	1 medium	0.3	0	0	24	1	10
stewed	1/2 cup	0.2	0	0	34	1	325
tomato paste, canned	1/2 cup	1.2	0.2	0	110	4	86
turnip greens, cooked	1/2 cup	0.2	0	0	15	2	21
turnips, cooked	1/2 cup	0.1	0	0	14	2	21
water chestnuts, canned, sliced	1/2 cup	0	0	0	35	1	6
watercress, raw	1/2 cup	0	0	0	2	0	7
wax beans, canned	1/2 cup	0.2	0	0	25	2	321
yam, boiled/baked	1/2 cup	0.1	0	0	79	3	6
zucchini, cooked	1/2 cup	0.1	0	0	14	2	1
VEGETABLE SALADS							
Caesar salad w/o anchovies	1 cup	7.2	1.5	19	80	1	145
carrot-raisin salad	1/2 cup	3.7	1.2	49	157	4	762
chef salad w/o dressing	1 cup	4.3	2.0	39	71	1	281
coleslaw							
w/mayo-type dressing	1/2 cup	14.2	0.2	5	147	1	14
w/vinaigrette	1/2 cup	5.5	0	0	77	1	50
gelatin salad w/fruit & cheese	1/2 cup	4.6	0	0	74	0	82
macaroni salad w/mayo	1/2 cup	12.8	2.5	12	200	1	157
pasta primavera salad	1 cup	5.9	0.8	0	149	3	639
potato salad							
German style	1/2 cup	3.5	NA	NA	140	1	NA
w/mayo dressing	1/2 cup	11.5	1.8	85	189	1	662
salad bar items							
alfalfa sprouts	2 T	0	0	0	2	0	0
bacon bits	1 T	1.6	0	6	27	0	181
beets, pickled	2 T	0	0	0	18	0	74
broccoli, raw	2 T	0	0	0	3	0	3
carrots, raw	2 T	0	0	0	6	0	5
cheese, shredded	2 T	4.6	2.5	15	56	0	87
chickpeas	2 T	0.4	0	0	21	1	75
cottage cheese	1/2 cup	5.1	1.5	17	116	0	458
croutons	1/2 oz.	3.0	0.2	0	60	0	189
cucumber	2 T	0	0	0	2	0	0
eggs, cooked, chopped	2 T	1.9	1.0	93	27	0	23
lettuce	1/2 cup	0	0	0	4	0	1

Item	Serving	Total Fat (grams)	Saturated Fat (grams)	Cholesterol (mg)	Calories	Fiber (grams)	Sodium (mg)
salad bar items *(cont.)*							
mushrooms, raw	2 T	0	0	0	2	0	0
onion, raw	2 T	0.1	0	0	7	0	0
pepper, green, raw	2 T	0	0	0	3	0	0
potato salad	½ cup	10.3	1.8	85	179	0	661
tomato, raw	2 slices	0	0	0	2	0	1
seven-layer salad	1 cup	17.8	6.1	105	226	2	336
tabbouli salad	½ cup	9.5	1.4	0	173	3	542
taco salad w/taco sauce	1 cup	14.0	6.4	41	202	2	404
three-bean salad	½ cup	11.2	1.7	0	145	3	307
three-bean salad, w/o oil	½ cup	0.3	0	0	90	3	894
Waldorf salad w/mayo	½ cup	12.7	2.8	11	157	2	123

INDEX